THE CHELSEA PIERS FITNESS SOLUTION

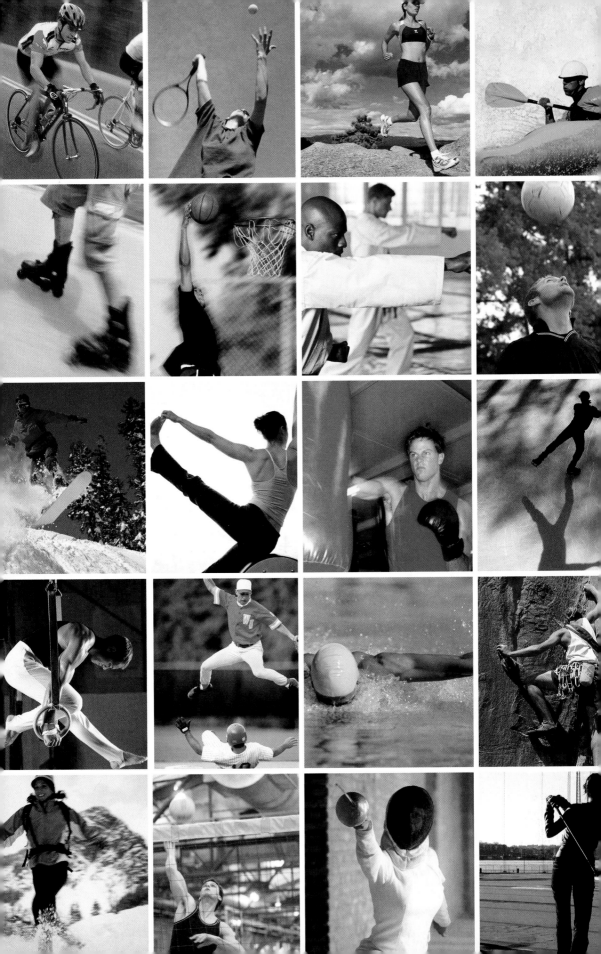

THE CHELSEA PIERS
FITNESS SOLUTION

Achieve a Lifetime of Health and Vitality

ELENA ROVER

BLACK DOG
& LEVENTHAL
PUBLISHERS
NEW YORK

Published by
Black Dog & Leventhal Publishers, Inc.
151 West 19th Street
New York, NY 10011

Distributed by
Workman Publishing Company
225 Varick St.
New York, NY 10014

Manufactured in the United States of America

Design by THINK STUDIO, NYC

ISBN 10: 1-57912-589-1
ISBN 13: 978-157912-589-9

h g f e d c b a

Library of Congress Cataloging-in-Publication Data available on file.

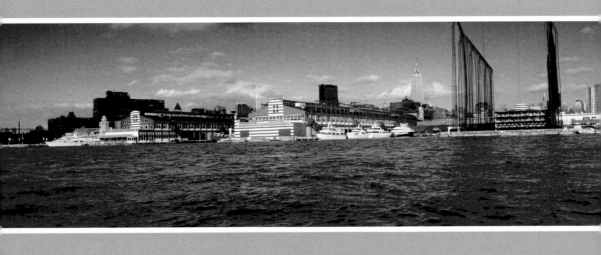

Introduction

THE PROBLEM

Are you having a hard time getting as much exercise as you think you need? Or maybe you're not as fit and trim as you'd like to be. If so, welcome to the club. Only one third of Americans get the recommended minimum thirty minutes of daily activity; and a quarter of us get none at all. Clearly, our current approach isn't working. Witness the escalating rates of obesity, diabetes, heart disease, and other illnesses—all of which could be dramatically reduced if we exercised more. (Eating better wouldn't hurt either.) Indeed, a lack of exercise was linked to 23 percent of deaths from major chronic illnesses, according to the Centers for Disease Control and Prevention.

Some of us have never exercised and don't want—or know how—to start. Others spend mind-numbing hours on cardio and strength machines. Even for die-hard exercise addicts, a busy schedule, illness, family crisis or vacation can force a short break, which can then turn into an extended absence. And the longer you're away, the more insurmountable it seems to get back to your same old fitness routine. For most people, doing the same thing all the time is not attractive or sustainable for the long-term.

THE SOLUTION

The Chelsea Piers Fitness Solution solves these problems by turning exercise into something you want to do, not something you should do. The premise is easy. If exercise is truly fun, you won't need to force yourself to work out: you'll want to get out and play. It's not even required that you know you're exercising. Because *The Chelsea Piers Fitness Solution* is personalized and varied, you get a well-rounded program that delivers all the benefits of exercise while keeping injuries, fatigue, and burnout to a minimum. Better

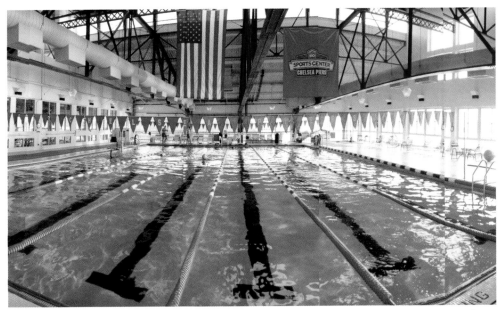

yet, the program incinerates boredom and excuses because you'll want to participate, especially if your teammates or opponents are counting on you. There still may be tough patches when you can't show up, but they won't stretch on for months as you resist the return to working out. Instead, you'll look forward to the day you can get back.

The goal is to develop a sports system that works for you. The method to finding success is to match and mix. First you'll take a short three-part quiz that gets to the heart of your fitness personality and matches you with several activities that suit you well. After the quiz, you'll find information about how exercise works, how to evaluate your current capabilities, and a step-by-step guide to design a routine that's perfect for your body and mind at any age. The workbook pages help you slot your chosen activities into a feasible and fun exercise plan that's customized to your goals, personality, physical abilities, and schedule. That's your mix. Next, you'll learn how to fuel your active lifestyle in the healthiest possible way. There's also a guide that shows you how to combine exercise and eating to produce effective, long-lasting weight loss.

Next come the twenty-seven activities, from boxing to yoga, with each described in detail, from the fundamentals of the sport to what to expect your first time. If you're interested but intimidated, the information should inspire you and help you feel at ease. You'll learn about physical and mental benefits, what gear you need to get started, and how to progress when you want to improve your skills. And you'll meet an athlete just like you, who wasn't sure at the outset if a new sport would be a good fit, but who fell in love with it. You'll also get expert coaching from top trainers.

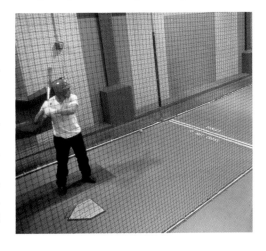

WHY CHELSEA PIERS?

If you need inspiration, ideas, and information for adding sports into your life, Chelsea Piers—the famous 1.2 million square foot sports facility on the Hudson River in Manhattan—can provide it. Step into the Field House or the Sports Center, Sky Rink or the Golf Club, and the energy and enthusiasm are contagious. The facility was built with a mandate to maximize the natural light, fill the space with real sports rather than virtual reality games, and hire the best possible instructors, all in a safe environment open to the public around the clock. In short, it's a playground that provides unparalleled offerings for kids and adults alike.

Anyone can find something fun to do at Chelsea Piers—from playing beach volleyball or ice hockey, to climbing the rock wall, to taking a private fencing lesson—at one of four venues: The Field House covers 80,000 square feet and includes a childcare facility, gymnastics center, courts and fields for soccer and basketball, batting cages, and an indoor rock climbing wall, as well as cardio machines designed specifically for kids. Sky Rink has one rink for recreational skating and lessons as well as a second regulation-sized hockey rink with stadium seating, both of which are open all year. The 150,000-square-foot Sports Center includes the ubiquitous studios for fitness classes, cardio and weight machines, spa and café; but it also boasts a quarter-mile running track, a 200-meter banked track, basketball, volleyball, and sand volleyball courts, a boxing ring, one of the largest indoor rock climbing walls in the Northeast, and a 25-yard, six-lane competition-style pool with three walls of glass that overlook the Hudson. The Golf Club, which has a teaching academy, also offers a driving range with fifty-two hitting stalls in a four-story building that opens over a 200-yard fairway. It's sprinkled with target greens, views of the Statue of Liberty and gorgeous sunsets over the river. And there's also a forty-lane bowling center, a sailing school, and walking promenade and park.

Four million visits a year stand as testament to the variety—and popularity—of Chelsea Piers' activities. Much of the drawing power is due to the top-caliber instruction in twenty-eight sports from more than 250 trainers, among them six Olympians and many career athletes including an NBA pro and boxing trainer. There is an average of sixty-five fitness classes taught each day. And

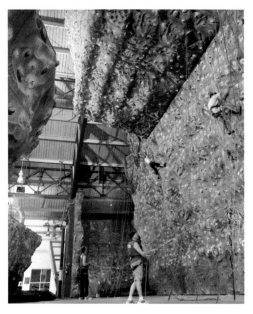

on any given night, almost 600 people play in the leagues at the piers. That's a lot of fit New Yorkers.

Unfortunately, not everyone lives close enough to play at Chelsea Piers. That's why this book is designed to inspire a sports-oriented fitness program in any part of the country. It also includes the expertise—and enthusiasm—of many Chelsea Pier pros (plus a few of the nation's top coaches—such as Lance Armstrong's trainer Chris Carmichael and the top instructor for the U.S. Tennis Association, Bill Mountford) so that you can have a better time taking up a sport or two, wherever you live. They'll inspire you, but also provide trade secrets to help you maximize your potential, even as a beginner. Now, get out and play!

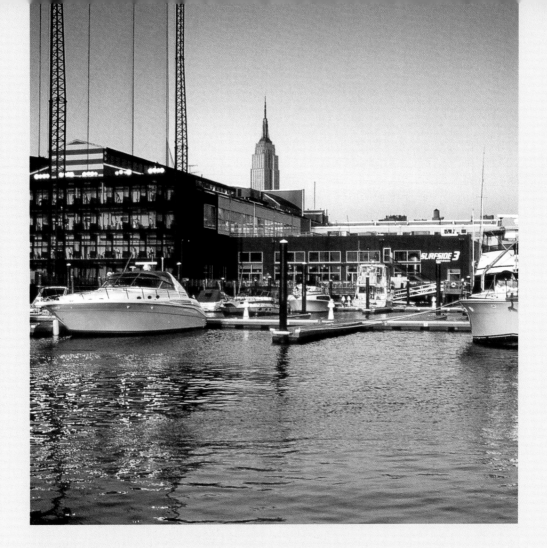

THE CHELSEA PIERS STORY

It's hard to believe, but the bustling, 30-acre complex that is Chelsea Piers was born from one girl's dedication to daily practice. "My daughter Jessie wanted to skate," says Roland W. Betts, a lawyer turned film financier who had played ice hockey in college. "So I took her and a friend to Sky Rink every morning at 5 A.M." The successful businessman became a fixture at the dingy rink, located on the top of a building in midtown Manhattan. And it wasn't long before he was pressed into service to help the flailing nonprofit. Betts teamed up with another ice-hockey player, David A. Tewksbury, and together they turned Sky Rink into a successful venture—only to discover that the lease on Sky Rink's venue was running out and wouldn't be renewed.

Finding a huge space with no columns in the middle of Manhattan proved a daunting task, until a friend recommended a two-story derelict pier on the Hudson, one of several owned by New York State. After a long history as a glamorous passenger terminal (the Titanic was supposed to dock there at the end of her maiden voyage), a military embarkation point and then a shipping dock, the piers were being used to park garbage trucks and had fallen into disrepair. "Upstairs, the roof was falling in, it was full of debris and smelled like dead animals," recalls Tewksbury. But the space was huge and had no columns, and Betts and Tewksbury immediately envisioned two large rinks plus a common area. After much discussion and delay, they discovered that they could not lease the 100,000 square feet they wanted—they had to go to auction and bid on 1.8 million square feet, including three additional piers and the connecting headhouse. Betts' business partner Tom A. Bernstein joined in the planning, and the three men started searching for additional sports to fill the vast space. "If people want to skate, there must be other things people want to do," Betts

thought. Requests started to trickle in, and the idea for a comprehensive sports facility was born. "I set out to build a skating rink for my daughter," recalls Betts. "And it got out of hand."

The next two years were a blur of architects, permits (for twenty-seven different city, state, and federal government agencies), local community boards, and area advocates, and then fundraising and construction crews. "If we knew what we were getting into, we would not have done it," says Bernstein. But in the fall of 1995, Chelsea Piers, an unparalleled collection of sports and fitness offerings in one place, opened to the public. Today, the once run-down section of Manhattan waterfront is revitalized, sprouting a new Frank Gehry building and a number of other high-end developments. But more important, New York residents, old and young, gained access to more sports than any city kid did before the Piers existed. For the rest of us, who don't have this state-of-the-art facility nearby, Chelsea Piers and the experts who share their experience in this book can inspire a return to the youthful urge to run around and play—and to lead healthier lives.

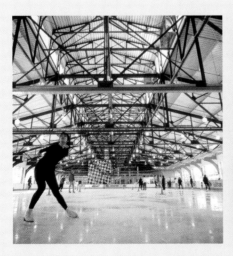
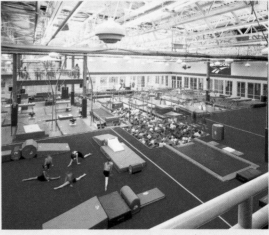

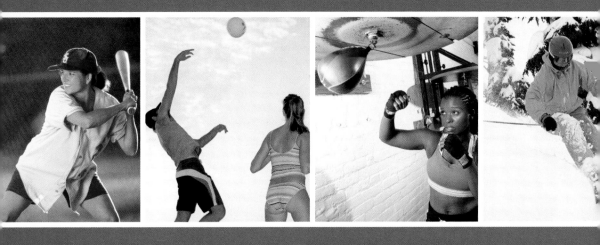

1

Identify Your Fitness Personality

Strolling across my college campus one day, I was stopped by a basketball coach who asked if I wanted to try out for the team. I'm tall and looked athletic, so he figured I might play. When I told him I was trying out for the rowing team, he laughed, saying, "Oh, you're crazy!"

It does take a touch of insanity to row, especially with a 6 A.M. practice schedule, even on Saturdays. But the team was perfect for me—competitive and exciting, but beautiful, too: the water glistens, the boat glides, and there's an elegance to the sport that is infectious. While it's important that an activity suit you physically, the mental match is equally, if not more, essential. I joined the rowing team—and fit right in.

Many people end up trying a sport because a friend or family member is a fan, because they've been tapped by a coach in school, or because the activity is all the rage. Sometimes, the encouragement and excitement is all it takes to find the right choice. But often, an inherited sport is not the best fit. "If you don't enjoy a sport, you're not going to be able to stick with it," says sport psychologist Jeffrey L. Brown, an instructor at Harvard Medical School with a clinical practice at McLean Hospital, the largest psychiatric hospital at Harvard. "People who hate to run or hate to lift weights or hate their aerobics class are motivated by the outcome. They are not seeing themselves as a runner, they see themselves as a size eight," he says. Yet that doesn't inspire the long-term dedication you feel when you have passion for the activity. "Athletes quickly identify with a particular sport," says Brown. "It becomes part of how you perceive your life."

This chapter will guide you in selecting sports you love by first determining your sports personality. Next, the chart provides selections to try first. Finally, the lists help you consider your fitness level, goals, schedule, and logistics. In addition, if you have an injury, consult a doctor, orthopedic specialist, or physical therapist to narrow the field to sports that are well suited to your body.

Once you've compiled your short list, read the later sections about those sports to see which ones sound the most appealing. Then, try a few. Many sports complement each other well in physical and mental requirements as well as skills, making it easy to go back and forth between them. It's good to have options so you can switch from snowshoeing in winter to kayaking in the summer, rock climbing when you can get to the mountains, or yoga when you're stuck at home.

You'll know you've found the right selections when you feel jazzed up enough to play, no matter how busy or stressed your life. Your sport will recharge you physically and mentally, and it won't be a struggle to get suited up and out the door.

THE FITNESS PERSONALITY QUIZ

Because humans are complex beings, you probably won't be able to pick one answer to every question on the quiz. If that's the case, put your choices in order of preference—with the best fit first, followed by the next choice and so on (your second choice can also be a useful tie-breaker, if needed).

PART 1

1. When planning your next vacation, you would love to be able to:
ⓐ head off alone to chill out and/or see some sights

ⓑ go visit a friend or take a romantic vacation with your mate

ⓒ get away with your family to a place that has something for everyone

ⓓ go on a cruise, take a group tour, share a ski cabin, or rent a villa with a bunch of friends

2. When coping with bad news such as a medical diagnosis, you are most likely to:
ⓐ keep it to yourself

ⓑ share your feelings with a trusted confidant

ⓒ tell your close friends and family so they can offer support

ⓓ spread the news so others will understand what you're going through or offer suggestions

3. If you were looking for a new job, you would like to be:
ⓐ an entrepreneur with an innovative product who sinks or floats on your own merit

ⓑ a partner in a top-notch company so you have some support but plenty of autonomy

ⓒ part of a hand-picked team that produces award-winning work

ⓓ the head of a group in a large company with ample resources and prestigious projects

4. For New Year's Eve, if you could have any of these choices, you would love to:
ⓐ pretend it's not a holiday

ⓑ go out on a date with one special person

ⓒ celebrate with a small dinner party attended by your friends

ⓓ go to Times Square or a huge black-tie soirée

PART 2

1. For dinner with friends, you:
ⓐ cook one of your favorite recipes

ⓑ pick up a rotisserie chicken or takeout

ⓒ try a new cuisine

2. For your next vacation, you would love to go:
ⓐ to a spa or beach resort, Disney, or the Grand Canyon

ⓑ gambling in Las Vegas or Monte Carlo

ⓒ rafting in Costa Rica or dogsledding in Alaska

3. When driving, you:
ⓐ tool along in the right lane going the speed limit

ⓑ shift into the left lane and flash your brights at slowpokes

ⓒ bail out on a traffic jam even if you don't know another route

4. Your favorite kind of leisure reading is:
ⓐ the latest literary novel or a romance

ⓑ a mystery or science fiction

ⓒ nonfiction such as travel, history, or a biography

5. Picking out a video for Saturday night, you'd select:
ⓐ *When Harry Met Sally, Shrek, Caddyshack*, or anything starring Tom Hanks or Robin Williams

ⓑ *Speed, Matrix, Thelma and Louise, Miracle on Ice*, or any movie starring Bruce Willis or about James Bond

ⓒ *Mr. & Mrs. Smith, What the Bleep Do We Know?, The Hitchhiker's Guide to the Galaxy*, or any film with *Star Wars* or *Indiana Jones* in the title

PART 3

1. Your dream job would be one in which you were:

ⓐ left alone to get your work done so you can go home at the end of the day

ⓑ the veteran in the group who can show others the ropes

ⓒ promoted into a position that stretches your abilities—you can do it!

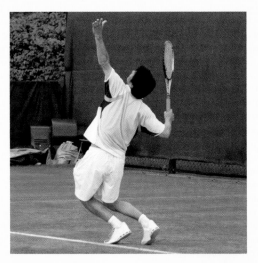

2. In high school, your main goal was to:

ⓐ learn, get decent grades, and graduate

ⓑ get into the college of your choice or land a good job

ⓒ secure a spot on the honor roll or become the valedictorian

3. If you had unlimited time and funds, you would:

ⓐ buy an island getaway

ⓑ visit one place on each continent

ⓒ climb Mount Everest

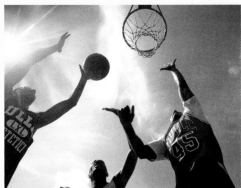

4. In games such as charades, checkers, Pictionary,® Cranium,® or Scrabble,® you most hope to:

ⓐ have fun

ⓑ make a few great moves

ⓒ win

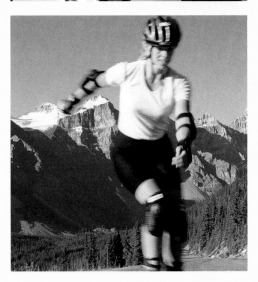

SCORING YOUR QUIZ

PART 1

Which letter answer did you choose two or more times?
ⓐ Solo
ⓑ Partner
ⓒ Group
ⓓ Team

Sports fit into all these categories. You can do an individual activity such as swimming, pick a sport that includes someone else such as tennis, sign up for a small group activity such as golf, or join a team, as in hockey.

Many athletes love to feel like part of a team. They want the camaraderie on the field as well as going out for a beer after practice. A team is a ready-made group of new friends who share at least one interest. For others, the team dynamics are too political and complicated; they'd rather go at their own pace or compete against their own best records. Note, however, that a solo type who is also competitive may be happiest as the star player on a team. Keep this tip in mind when you use the sport selection chart.

Making the choice of solo versus group sports also may be a question of logistics. Are you better at self-motivation, getting into your shorts and shoes when it suits you and heading out on your bike? Or would it help you get going to know that a whole group of people are counting on you to show up to play soccer?

If your answers are spread between the choices, try a sport with options. For example, many individual sports such as cycling can be done alone, with a friend, or in a group.

PART 2

Which letter answer did you choose two or more times?
ⓐ revel in the experience of activities at which you excel
ⓑ go for speed, get out in front and feel exhilaration
ⓒ Love adventure and learning new skills

Your answers to the questions in this section could vary a lot. But if one letter came up two or three times, that's a good start toward discovering the driving force behind how you like to spend your time.

The categories aren't mutually exclusive—you can love both speed and adventure, for example. Perhaps one edges the other out just a bit in importance. Put that category first when picking your sports, but take a look at the other choices that made your list. For example, Lorie Parch, a forty-one-year-old writer in Scottsdale, Arizona, picked (a) three times and (c) twice. Lorie loves yoga, which she is adept at, but she stays engaged because there are always new poses to master, some of which are quite hard for her.

PART 3

Which letter answer did you choose two or more times?
ⓐ not competitive
ⓑ competitive with myself
ⓒ competitive with others

It may seem that all sports are competitive, but some are much more so than others. According to the *Merriam-Webster Dictionary*, a sport is: "physical activity engaged in for pleasure" and the synonym is "fun." If scoring goals (or failing to score) is not your idea of fun, then a competitive sport is not for you. On the other hand, if you need a metric of success, then you can choose between sports that encourage you to beat your own personal best, such as trail running, or the ones in which you either win or lose based on the score, such as tennis.

HOW YOUR SCORE ADDS UP

Use the chart below to find sports that fit your personality. Many sports appear in multiple places on the chart because they can be played in different ways, such as downhill skiing on a pristine powder day with friends versus ski racing at a competition. Keep the variations in mind when heading out. For example, if you want to play noncompetitive volleyball, be sure your teammates aren't cut-throat about winning the game. In the chart below, the solo, partner, and group activities are listed together because you can choose to do most of these sports in all three ways. Each box in the chart does not contain every possible sport that fits in the category but, rather, the best choices for the personality type from among the sports covered in this book.

	Not competitive	Compete w/myself	Compete w/others
Enjoy the Experience	Solo/Partner/Group: cross-country skiing cycling downhill skiing hiking ice skating in-line skating kayaking snowshoeing swimming yoga Team: baseball/softball basketball soccer volleyball	Solo/Partner/Group: cycling golf hiking ice skating in-line skating kayaking rock climbing snowshoeing swimming trail running Team: baseball/softball basketball soccer volleyball	Solo/Partner/Group: cycling fencing golf ice skating in-line skating kayaking rowing snowshoeing tennis trail running Team: baseball/softball basketball rowing soccer swimming tennis volleyball
Need for Speed	Solo/Partner/Group: cycling downhill skiing ice skating in-line skating kayaking rowing snowboarding trail running Team: basketball soccer	Solo/Partner/Group: boxing cycling downhill skiing ice skating in-line skating kayaking rowing snowboarding trail running Team: basketball soccer	Solo/Partner/Group: boxing cycling downhill skiing fencing ice skating in-line skating kayaking rowing snowboarding trail running Team: basketball hockey rowing soccer volleyball
Love Adventure and Learning Skills	Solo/Partner/Group: cross-country skiing downhill skiing gymnastics hiking ice skating kayaking pilates snowboarding snowshoeing trail running yoga Team: basketball tennis	Solo/Partner/Group: boxing cycling downhill skiing fencing gymnastics ice skating kayaking martial arts rock climbing trail running Team: basketball hockey	Solo/Partner/Group: boxing cross-country skiing cycling downhill skiing fencing ice skating kayaking martial arts trail running Team: basketball hockey

NARROWING THE FIELD

Once you have selected a box or a few boxes that seem like a good match, consider next the logistics of each sport, such as access to mountains, whether or not you want to bring the kids along, and the expense of equipment. Also, keep in mind your physical abilities and fitness goals. Some sports are easy to begin, even if you've been completely sedentary, such as hiking and golf—you can proceed at your own pace and tailor the experience to your strengths. Other activities, in particular team sports, are more challenging in terms of stamina and strength requirements, and they are harder to do a little at a time. If you've been getting to the gym or playing a different sport, you'll have more success than the average couch potato. Here are some suggestions to help you choose.

Sports for improving aerobic fitness	Sports for improving strength	Sports for developing calm and inner strength	Sports for an all-around intense workout
baseball/softball	boxing	cross-country skiing	cross-country skiing
basketball	downhill skiing	hiking	gymnastics
cross-country skiing	gymnastics	ice skating	martial arts
downhill skiing	martial arts	kayaking	rock climbing
fencing	pilates	martial arts	rowing
gymnastics	rock climbing	pilates	
hiking	rowing	rock climbing	
ice skating	yoga	rowing	
in-line skating		snowshoeing	
martial arts		yoga	
rowing			
snowboarding			
snowshoeing			
soccer			
swimming			
tennis			
trail running			
volleyball			

Sports that provide mental challenge	Sports to play with kids	Sports that are great for seniors	Sports that require a serious commitment of time
fencing	baseball/softball	cross-country skiing	hockey
golf	basketball	cycling	downhill skiing
hockey	cross-country skiing	fencing	snowboarding
martial arts	cycling	golf	golf
rock climbing	downhill skiing	hiking	fencing
	gymnastics	ice skating	rowing
	hiking	kayaking	rock climbing
	in-line skating	pilates	
	soccer	snowshoeing	
	swimming	swimming	
	volleyball	tennis	
	yoga	yoga	

Sports for those who love gear	Sports you can do if you rarely have free time	Sports that require very little gear/money	Sports to get you started if you've been sedentary
cycling	cycling	basketball	baseball/softball
downhill skiing	hiking	gymnastics	cross-country skiing
fencing	in-line skating	hiking	cycling
golf	tennis	martial arts	golf
hockey	yoga	soccer	hiking
kayaking		swimming	ice skating
rock climbing		trail running	kayaking
rowing			pilates
snowboarding			snowshoeing
			swimming
			tennis
			volleyball
			yoga

Put some advanced thought into how to make your first foray into the sport you've chosen. There are cases in which the sport is a fine choice, but perhaps you're matched up with the wrong teacher or started out on a challenging day. You can see this problem in action at almost any ski slope on any weekend—when a virgin skier or snowboarder is learning from a well-meaning friend who has forgotten what it felt like to get on and off a chairlift for the first time. Teaching someone a sport can be like teaching your own teenager to drive. If a sport is complex, it's generally best to leave the lessons to the professionals. Timing counts, too. If your first snowboarding experience is on an icy hill, you'll likely have less fun than trying the sport after a fresh dumping of two feet of powder that makes for softer landings when you fall.

Don't give up on a new sport until you've given it every chance. If you ultimately decide the activity isn't for you, try to figure out which aspects you didn't like and go back to the chart so you can look for sports that might be a better fit. But remember, there can be a lot of variation within one sport. If a sport you were sure you'd like isn't working out for you, you may simply need to change to another style. For example, if you take up in-line skating, you can go for a roll through the park, take up in-line hockey or speed skating, do obstacle and slalom courses, go to a skateboard park and do tricks on the half-pipe, find a rink and skate around to tunes, go touring on skating vacations, or even try the roller version of figure skating. There's something on that list for every personality. The trick is culling through the possibilities and deciding where to start. The information in the sport chapters will help you make an informed choice and improve your chance of success.

Getting Fit and Having Fun
How and Why It Works

Imagine a week of workouts that goes something like this: You get up on Saturday, pack a picnic lunch, and meet some friends at a park to spend the morning hiking to a pristine lake for a lovely meal al fresco. Don't forget the camera! On Sunday, you and your brother get together for a quick game of tennis first thing before facing the obligations of the day. You beat him handily at the game. Monday at lunchtime there's a great kickboxing class at the gym, so you run over and grab a sandwich on the way back to work. On Tuesday, you can't get away for long, so you squeeze in a few blocks of walking when you go out to get lunch.

The highlight of the week, on Wednesday, is ice hockey. Your team is getting noticed by the league, is really starting to play well together, and you're rising in the rankings. A little tired on Thursday, you look forward to a yoga class in the evening that always leaves you feeling great. On Friday, you want to work on your legs because you think a little more strength will improve your skating ability—so you do a quick session of lunges, squats, and calf raises at the gym. Since you're already sweaty, you toss in some abs and arm moves for good measure. Don't overdo it, though...because the coming weekend's plans include a charity bike ride and a pickup game of soccer.

Yes, you can get fit and have fun at the same time—even if conventional wisdom holds that exercise must include mindless repetitions of weight moves, or session after session sweating it out on the elliptical trainer. There's no rule that says you have to be bored in order to reap the rewards of physical activity. It's not even required that you know you're "exercising." The only key to success is that you work your body harder than usual for a reasonable duration of time. A brisk walk in the park counts, and so does a glorious afternoon of skiing, or a paddle around the lake in a kayak. And the latest research shows that you can even accumulate fitness in short bouts during the day, which reap the same health and fitness benefits as if you did one longer workout.

For proof that a traditional workout isn't essential to fitness, consider your ancestors. In the pre-industrial era, there weren't many people who were flabby. The only people who were overweight were the wealthy or the ill—the ones who had servants, a debilitating injury, or maybe a metabolic disorder. Before we all had desk jobs, people were too active to be unfit (even though they ate bacon and butter by the pound). Now, we live longer, thanks to the miracles of modern medicine, but we don't necessarily thrive in our later years. As aging expert Walter M. Bortz II, M.D., said in the title of his first book: We live too short and die too long.

Not only is it extremely unpleasant to have a debilitating illness, but being unfit and unhealthy ends up costing us billions in medical care as well as in diet and fitness products and services. Using recent data, the Centers for Disease Control and Prevention (CDC) estimates that poor eating habits along with a lack of exercise cause about 300,000 deaths each year. And very few Americans get

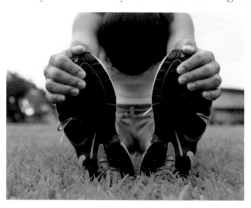

enough exercise—while most of us get none at all. Unfortunately, even the small minority of people who do work out regularly may not be getting the best results, because they tend to stick to a single activity, or maybe just a few favorite workouts. An unchanging routine has a higher risk of injury and burnout as well as fewer benefits than a varied program.

WHAT IS THE EXERCISE PROBLEM?

The problem is that too many people view exercise as work (as in "working out"). And it's almost never an urgent, deadline-driven task. There's always something more pressing than "yet another workout," which you can easily put off until tomorrow. Exercise usually doesn't rise in priority on the to-do list until you've had a serious wake-up call such as a heart attack.

There's a string of excuses for why we don't exercise: We are too tired, have no time, don't have access, have had injuries or illnesses that are difficult to overcome, or think it's too expensive. As we get older, we suffer aches and pains that compel us to skip workouts. We are blocked by these barriers because most of us have far too narrow a definition of what counts as exercise. We think we have to do prescribed workouts such as aerobic classes, cardio machines, and strength training. Unfortunately, very few people succeed in getting to the gym often enough to get sufficient exercise that way. They get bored or busy, and one skipped day turns into a week, then a month, and so on. You need at least thirty minutes a day of moderately intense activity to reap the health benefits of exercise, and it's hard to do that day after day after day—especially when the activity is always exactly the same and never gets more challenging or teaches you new things about your abilities. Even people who enjoy working out tend to stop when they get sick, injured, have a life change, become tired of the routine, or just don't have time. And those who do make it to the gym regularly often have one or two favorite activities instead of a healthy well-rounded program.

WHAT IS THE CHELSEA PIERS FITNESS SOLUTION?

The Chelsea Piers Fitness Solution provides the answer to fitting fitness into a busy life. It's a varied program of fun activities that provides fitness and health benefits without pain or boredom. It's inspired by the everyday people who have become athletes because they have access to Chelsea Piers, a premier fitness and sports facility in New York City. They make their way from near and far every day to play in leagues, swim in the pool, bump the ball on the beach volleyball court, and climb one of the biggest indoor rock walls in the Northeast.

Basically, they come to play.

Even if you've never been to New York, you can look to *The Chelsea Piers Fitness Solution* and create your own version of its basic precept, which is to have fun while you're getting fit. When you find a few sports that you enjoy, you come to look forward to these activities, rather than seeing them as just another chore you need to make room for in your day. You'll show up not just because your program delivers every payoff that being fit has to offer, but also because it's fun and fulfilling. This combination is the only one that stands a chance against the top priorities in your busy life. If you choose well, you will permanently ease your sports selections into your schedule. And if you find you are getting less excited about heading out to play, pick something else or take your sport to another level in order to re-energize your enthusiasm. Fitness should be a pleasant and varied lifelong endeavor, not a single activity, home exercise gadget, or gym membership.

THE COMPONENTS

When you organize your exercise routine around sports, you're likely to get plenty of cardio fitness, but you may not have an optimal mix of strength, flexibility, or other advantages, such as balance. *The Chelsea Piers Fitness Solution* helps you address that imbalance. Here's a look at each of the essential components of exercise, why it's important, and how to be sure that you get enough of each.

PART 1: CARDIO

Your number-one priority in your fitness plan should be to get cardio benefits, because heart disease is the leading killer of Americans, and aerobic exercise trains your heart and circulatory system to be more efficient and effective. Cardio also delivers a high level of calorie burn for the time you spend, which helps with weight control—and thus wards off disease.

Thankfully, you don't need to tromp on machines to get a cardio workout. Any activity that gets you breathing hard will do it. In the body, it works something like this: Your muscles like to have oxygen to burn when they need energy. And while the muscles are working, they produce waste products that need to be carried away (if not, they build to toxic levels, which causes that "burning" feeling you experience when you're working hard). Your heart pumps blood to the muscles, and the blood delivers oxygen and "picks up the garbage." The blood then gets routed to the lungs, where it "dumps the garbage" (which gets exhaled) and picks up more oxygen (which you just inhaled) before heading back to the muscles. The harder you exercise, the more oxygen the muscles need and the more "garbage" they produce. Your blood needs to make the trip faster between the lungs and the muscles, so the heart beats more quickly. You breathe faster so you can swap the garbage deposited in your lungs for oxygen to be sent to the blood.

When you use just your legs, as in cycling, those muscles get the most blood flow. Add your arms as well, as in fencing, and more muscles compete for the blood. Move even more quickly, and the muscles work harder and scream for more blood in order to trade waste products for more oxy-

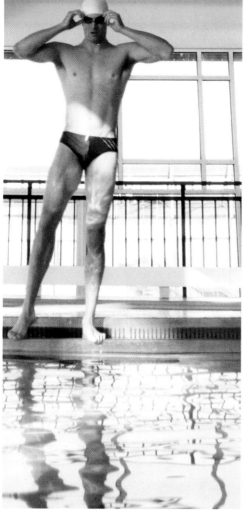

and then quickly recover when the job has been accomplished, which is a key indicator of heart health—called *elasticity*. When you do aerobic exercise, you improve these factors and related heart-health parameters such as blood pressure and cholesterol levels.If you rarely exercise, your heart is like your other muscles—flabby and quick to tire, not efficient and elastic. Toning your heart muscle gives you more energy, cuts your risk of disease, and makes it easier to accomplish your day-to-day tasks without tiring—from running after the dog to jumping over puddles. Perhaps the most compelling benefit is in weight loss: The fitter your heart, the faster you can go. And more speed translates into burning more calories per minute. For example, a 150-pound person who rides a bike at a leisurely ten to twelve miles-per-hour pace for thirty minutes burns a respectable 150 calories. But if the same person picks it up to fourteen to sixteen miles per hour, a vigorous ride, he burns 270 calories in the same half hour. So a fitter heart ramps up your weight loss potential by allowing you to do more.

gen. When there isn't enough oxygen—because your muscles are moving too fast for the heart and lungs to keep up—then the muscles have to switch to a process called anaerobic (or "no oxygen") exercise, which produces less energy and a lot more waste. Eventually, this builds up, your muscles start to burn, and you have to quit, panting for breath to help get that waste out of your system. You can't exercise for long using the anaerobic system.

Like all muscles, the heart gets stronger and fitter every time you challenge it with a workout. A fitter heart actually moves more blood each time it beats, so it doesn't pump as hard to do the same work—just like stronger legs make it feel easier to walk up the stairs. A fitter heart is also healthier because it doesn't have to work as hard to keep up with everyday demands. And a heart that gets a lot of exercise also responds well when faced with a tough task (such as running up stairs). It knows how to rise to the challenge

Better cardio wins

Elite athletes can move a lot faster than the average person before their bodies switch from aerobic to anaerobic exercise (a point called the *lactate threshold*, because lactate is one of the main waste products). A beginner might run one nine-minute mile fairly comfortably before hitting this line and then eking out another thirty seconds before dropping out, whereas a marathon runner might do twenty-four miles at an eight-minute mile in the aerobic zone and then pull off the last two miles at an anaerobic pace before collapsing. That difference can win races.

PART 2: **STRENGTH**

Your next priority is strength training. Any activity that significantly taxes your muscles makes them stronger, which means that a lot of cardio exercises overlap with this category. You build strong muscles from rowing, for example. The key to gaining strength is to push your muscles to the point of fatigue.

Think of your muscles as being a little lazy— they like to rest, and they get flabby if you let them. They'll cheat if they can, getting the work done without breaking a sweat. Like a kid who cheats on a test instead of studying, your muscles will get by on the strength they already have and share the effort with nearby muscles that can help out. If you want to get stronger, you have to push them a bit, compelling them to improve. The best way to build

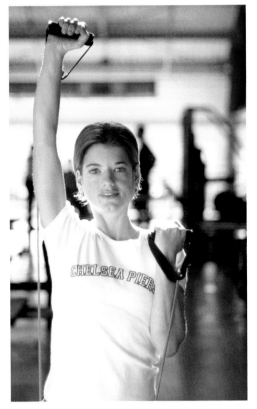

muscle is with intense moves, the ones that make you feel the burn and fatigue in thirty to ninety seconds, says Wayne Westcott, Ph.D., fitness research director for the South Shore YMCA in Quincy, Massachusetts, and author of twenty books on strength training.

Why bother working so hard, especially if you don't want big muscles? The first reason to do so is good health. Strong muscles protect the structures of your body, holding your organs in the proper places and supporting your spine and joints, which prevents injuries. You need muscle tone for good posture, too. And when you work your muscles, they tug on your bones, helping to prevent osteoporosis. Research shows that leg strength is the prime indicator of whether or not you will spend your final years in a nursing home. Weak legs mean you'll become unable to care for yourself.

Toned muscles also look better. Consider your abs: Even if you have fat on top, a firm muscle at the base makes for fewer jiggles and less of a bulge compared to a Jell-O gut. If health and appearance aren't enough to make you improve your muscle tone, there's one more excellent motivator: The more muscle you have, the more calories you burn no matter what you're doing—even sitting still. Muscle is active tissue; it works, it gets broken down, and it gets rebuilt—and all of that requires energy, meaning calories. Fat, on the other hand, is stored energy that's there in case you need it. It requires almost no calories to maintain itself. Whether you strength-train in the gym by lifting weights or with a sport such as rock climbing, you add lean muscle. And the more muscle in your body, the faster your metabolism, meaning the more calories you burn before you even start to exercise.

What is weight-bearing exercise?

You hear a lot about *weight-bearing* exercise to build and maintain your bone mass—and that term is not a synonym for weight lifting. Weight-bearing exercise is any activity in which you carry weight—cycling and swimming don't qualify, but tennis does because you are carrying the weight of your body. Lifting weights does improve your bone health, because every time you move, the muscles pull on the bones where they attach. But activities that involve impact have a more pronounced effect on bones. Even low-impact exercises such as walking fit the bill. The greater the impact, the better the workout for your bones—so jumping jacks do wonders—but keep in mind that these same activities are tough on your joints.

PART 3: **FLEXIBILITY**

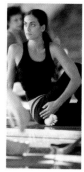

As you get stronger, you must spend some time stretching. Toned muscles are the goal, not tight, painful ones. Many athletes start out thinking they don't have time to stretch. They quickly learn that stretching is essential to avoid painful stiff muscles that cause a shift in body mechanics, which often leads to injuries. If you want to remain active and feel good, make time to stretch the muscles you're working.

It's not inevitable that you'll get stiffer as you get older, either. And you can limber up, even if you feel crotchety now. Plus, some activities such as yoga incorporate a lot of flexibility training along with strength gains, so you can get an efficient session if you want one.

PART 4: **ADDITIONAL BENEFITS**

Cardio, strength, and flexibility are the three main components of your program, but there are other benefits you should pursue. For example, a good sense of balance is particularly important. Unless you work on it, you get a little more wobbly each year, starting at about age fifty. The first sign is having trouble standing on one foot when putting on a sock or shoe. Over time, you'll risk losing your footing in a fall. And the resulting injuries can hamper your future abilities in sports and daily tasks, or could even kill you if you break a hip.

Another secondary benefit of exercise is its effect on your mood. Most people find activities such as gentle yoga or swimming calm and relaxing. On the other end of the spectrum, challenging or competitive activities such as boxing convey a sense of accomplishment and improve self-esteem. One well-documented mood-enhancing effect comes from repetitive exercise such as jogging, the type that can be mindless and boring

if you just slog through the activity. Instead, try turning off the iPod and focusing your attention on your footfalls, your breathing, and your movement. If your mind wanders, let the thoughts dissipate, and bring your focus back to your body. When you're warmed up and the movement is flowing, you'll reach a meditative state that feels calm, clear, and energetic. This experience is often referred to as *flow* or *being in the zone*. Try it next time you're on a cardio machine, out for a walk or run, snowshoeing, or in-line skating. A similar effect happens with repetitive activities done at a higher intensity, such as cross-country skiing or rowing, when a rush of feel-good hormones floods your body, producing a euphoria that is sometimes called the *runner's high*. Being in the zone has strong benefits such as reducing depression, stress, and anxiety, and lowering blood-pressure levels. And it feels great—compelling you to come back to exercise again so you can reach the same euphoria.

PART 5: **REST**

Yes, you read that correctly. Rest is an integral part of your plan. Your body needs to recover from physical challenges in order to get stronger. You definitely can get too much of a good thing, even in exercise, and that leads to burnout and injury. Sometimes our exuberant pursuit of results makes us push too hard, especially at the beginning of a new exercise program. And overdoing it, which is officially called *overtraining*, has some serious downsides: depression, irritability, anxiety, apathy, disturbed sleep, loss of appetite, chronically sore muscles, physical injuries, and susceptibility to colds and other illnesses, to name a few. That's not to say you should never feel sore, catch a cold, or have a bad night's sleep, but when the workouts are nonstop and the symptoms add up, pay attention and cut back on your exercise schedule. Better yet, plan your program to include breaks so you don't overtrain in the first place.

A Guide for the Novice

If you haven't moved your body much in a while, it can be intimidating to think of jumping into a new sport. Happily, it isn't necessary to suffer in order to be active—as *The Chelsea Piers Fitness Solution* illustrates. While it may be hard to take the first steps, moving more will make you look and feel better before long. You'll get some benefits starting from your very first session, such as improved sleep and a mood boost.

In a recent study at the University of Texas, Austin, people with major depression found that a half-hour walk improved their moods and energy levels immediately; and earlier research has shown that over time, a workout routine is as effective as antidepressant medication, and without the side effects. Other payoffs, like gorgeously toned muscles, take longer. The good news: If you've done nothing before, it takes very little effort to get positive results in the areas of health, fitness, and appearance.

Most sports are intense, and a couch potato might not enjoy jumping right into a gymnastics class or an ice hockey game, for example, because the physical demands could prevent you from accomplishing much and leave you very sore. But even as a beginner, you'll find plenty of good options in other sports. Hiking, snowshoeing, and pilates are perfect starting points. Cycling, tennis, and many other sports can be done at a slower pace when you're a beginner and later ramped up as you get more fit. Check the lists at the end of the quiz (see pages 18-19) for guidance on selections that work for most people. Before you head out the door for your first sports outing, here's a checklist of steps to do to get prepared:

STEP 1: GO SHOPPING

Start at the bottom: Your feet take more pounding from sports than during day-to-day tasks, and it's vital to give your body a good base in order to prevent knee and back pain, as well as other problems. Sneakers don't have to be the latest brand or cost a fortune. You can go to a discount sporting goods store or shoe outlet and find something for under $60. Make sure they are fitness sneakers, not a fashion statement. Start with a crosstrainer sneaker, which is designed to

do a decent job in a large selection of activities. When laced up, they should feel comfortably snug so they support your feet. You should notice a bump under your arch that provides support but not too much pressure. If you have a favorite pair, be sure to check the fit for these factors—and if they are a year old or more, replace them with new ones; the materials that cushion and support your feet break down over time, whether worn or not.

STEP 2: THE WALK TEST

If you're starting from scratch, first assess your current fitness level. You don't need fancy equipment or to be an expert to do it. Here's the method: On a day when you can set aside some time (and preferably when you're decently rested), take a walk. Wear comfortable clothes and sneakers that are appropriate for the weather, as well as a watch. Try a variety of different paces and go uphill and down if you can. Make a mental note of any physical problems you encounter so you can correct for them before your next workout. At the end of your walk, write down how long you lasted, what made you stop—for instance, tired legs, shortness of breath—and your *rate of perceived exertion (RPE)* (see *Taking Stock*, page 28).

STEP 3: PICK YOUR ACTIVITIES

The walking test above provides a baseline. You can translate that experience into any fitness activity by using the duration and RPE as a goal toward how much you can do. The main focus of your early workouts is cardio—building up your heart until you can go longer without panting for breath. The goal is to be able to walk for twenty minutes at an RPE of five. To get there, try to do some activity every day, adding up sessions so you get a total of twenty minutes a day. Do five or ten minutes here and there, whenever you can squeeze it in. (Try to keep it to four segments of exercise or less.)

If you spend your day stuck at work, try this plan: Before you leave home, do some moves such as jumping jacks, marching in place, and walking up and down stairs for three minutes. At lunchtime, walk a few laps around the block for five minutes. Dance around for two minutes while you make dinner. Then take a brisk after-dinner walk for ten minutes. Total: twenty minutes.

Does this program sound like other fitness plans so far? Here's where *The Chelsea Piers Fitness Solution* makes it different. Write up a list of fun activities that get you breathing harder, then pick from the list until you get to that twenty minutes of activity a day. Instead of walking on the treadmill, hit tennis balls (against a wall if you don't have a partner). Rather than trying to keep up in a step class, go in-line skating or play tag with the kids. Try some of the unusual offerings at your health club, like belly dancing or kickboxing. Even splashing in the pool counts as a workout as long as you keep moving. Any activity in which you move your body and start to huff and puff a bit counts as cardio. Add ideas to your list for cold, warm, or rainy days—things you can do alone or with others, quick sessions or longer ones. Make sure you'll always have something to choose no matter what the circumstances. The key is to select activities that you like to do so you look forward to the sessions instead of thinking of them as a chore. Your primary goal is to get active every day—and not bore yourself with tedium in the process.

Work toward being able to complete the entire twenty minutes or more in one session. Shorter workouts are fine when you can't manage more, but you should train your heart and your mind to go for twenty minutes straight so you'll have more sports options as you become more fit.

STEP 4: **ROUND OUT THE PLAN**

Once fitness is a part of your everyday life, you can work toward optimizing your program. Ramp up your results by adding some strength and stretching activities. Do a few stretches after your cardio, when your body is warm and you're already in exercise mode. For strength, you can incorporate some moves into the same session, even if you only do a few squats and hold a plank position (like the start of a push-up) for as long as you can, a few times. Those two moves target a lot of muscles. Moves such as squats, push-ups, cartwheels, squat thrusts, handstands, and wall sits are also good examples. But plenty of other enjoyable workouts strengthen your muscles: Spend an afternoon in the garden, lifting, digging, and hoeing. Hiking up hills or skiing down them does wonders for your butt and legs. Kayaking is amazing for the abs, upper back, and shoulders. Boxing tones your arms, abs, and legs. And rock climbing is a terrific head-to-toe strengthener. You can find a fun way to get your toning done without ever setting foot in a weight room or lifting a dumbbell.

Try to stretch every day and do some strength training at least twice a week. Yoga or pilates provides strengthening and stretching in one session. The goal is to strengthen and stretch every major muscle from head to toe each week.

THE ULTIMATE GOAL FOR BETTER HEALTH

A report from the President's Council on Physical Fitness and Sports defines being moderately active as accumulating thirty minutes of activity daily and being able to "walk thirty minutes continuously without pain or discomfort." But they note that this level of fitness would not allow you to jog three miles, walk six miles at a brisk pace, cycle twelve miles, or swim three-quarters of a mile without stopping or suffering serious fatigue. That's the bad news. The good part is that thirty minutes a day is all it takes to get the health benefits of exercise. If you never get beyond this point, you'll still live longer and healthier, cut your medical bills dramatically, and prevent weight gain as you age.

MAKE SURE YOU GET RESULTS

Doing any activity is healthier than doing none, no matter how wimpy the workout. But to reap the benefits of fitness, you must put in a minimum level of consistent participation—whether in the gym or out on the field. Here's how to plan your schedule to get the results you desire. According to research done by John Jakicic, Ph.D., a weight management expert and chairman of the department of health and physical activity at the University of Pittsburgh, in order to get the health benefits of exercise, you need to do about 150 minutes per week of moderate and comfortable activity such as brisk walking. That's only twenty minutes a day, but it's every day. However, if your exercise goal is to lose weight and keep it off, you need to improve your diet and spend 250 to 300 minutes each week working out at a moderate pace, Jakicic says. That sounds like a lot, but it's still only thirty-five to forty-five minutes a day. On the other hand, remember that this amount is a minimum, not the optimal, level. You'll find more details on how to use these guidelines below.

TAKING STOCK

What you'll notice in the recommendations above is that each has a measure of *duration* and *intensity*. Duration is easy: Pick up an inexpensive sports watch with a chronograph (stopwatch) feature, which, for about $15, frees you from constantly checking the clock. Then, for that amount of time, skate, cycle, shoot hoops, or do whatever activities you put in your Chelsea Piers plan.

To track your intensity, you have a few choices. The low-tech method is called *rate of perceived exertion* or *RPE*. To do it you simply make a mental note of how hard you're breathing, how tired your muscles feel, and any other indicators you notice of your workout intensity. Considering these factors, pick a number from one to ten, with one being akin to a gentle stroll and ten being an all-out sprint. Anything below five is comfortable, and above five is a challenge. Studies have

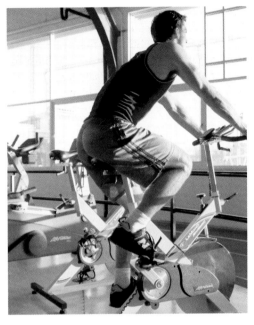

shown that using the RPE scale doesn't require training. With just a little practice, people are remarkably capable of rating their exercise intensity accurately.

Another way to measure intensity is to use a heart-rate monitor, which checks your pulse, to see how hard your heart is pumping while you exercise. Since your heart works harder when you work out harder, your pulse is a logical indicator of intensity. The problem is that your heart rate is also influenced by factors such as your stress level or medications, which could elevate your pulse even when you're not working out very hard. RPE is actually more accurate in such cases, and it's a lot less expensive and doesn't require remembering the gear, strapping it on, or replacing batteries. On the other hand, it's easier to glance down at the monitor instead of thinking through how your body feels. And many people enjoy gadgets or find that numbers are a helpful reminder or can be a tool for motivation. If you fall into that category, by all means use a heart-rate monitor.

If you use heart rate as a guide, you'll need to know your target heart rate or training zone. For most people, 120 to 140 beats per minute (BPM) is a good beginning goal for aerobic workouts. At this intensity, you get the health benefits of exercise, certain fitness benefits, and a decent calorie burn for the effort. But that's not to say that workouts at lower than 120 BPM and higher than 140 BPM are useless. Every type of activity has some benefit, even if it's just a gentle stroll. If that's all you can manage on a particular day, it's still healthier than crashing on the couch with the remote. You'll burn some calories, improve your mood, and might even get an energy boost or actually feel better physically. Your circulation will speed up a little and your breathing might get a little deeper, both of which are good for you. And you should feel less stressed and fatigued when you're done.

On the flipside, if you want to improve your sports performance, you have to increase the intensity in order to push your top exercise capacity higher. But you can't train at your max all the time or you'll burn out, so you need to put together a program that varies the intensity.

Increase the Intensity with Interval Training

One tried-and-true method for making performance gains is called *interval training*. To do it, you alternate between all-out sprints and slower recovery sections within a single workout. Start with a short sprint, maybe thirty seconds, and a longer recovery of one minute. Push as hard as you can on the sprints, then use half the recovery to catch your breath and the other half to prep for the next sprint, hitting the start of the sprint at full tilt. You can use this technique in any sport, and the end result is a higher intensity than if you picked the fastest you could maintain for the entire workout. As you get stronger in your sport, reduce the recovery time until it's the same duration as the sprint (but no less). Another benefit: Interval workouts may be intensely tiring, but they go by quickly because you're mentally engaged the entire time.

BY THE NUMBERS

Now that you know how to exercise by the numbers, it's time to use them to build your personalized program. If you've never worked out before, start with the *A Guide for the Novice* section, on page 26, until you can manage twenty minutes of cardio at an RPE of five. From there, the program plan depends on your goals.

Health Benefits:

The beginner's program is a baseline for basic health and fitness that should allow you to get through your day with ease, whether you are lugging groceries, spending five hours walking around the mall, or doing yard work. That level of fitness is a fine place to stay. If that's your goal, aim for a minimum of twenty minutes of moderate-level cardio (an RPE of about five) and some stretching every day. If you are younger than forty, your weekly workouts should include two fifteen-minute head-to-toe strength sessions. After your fortieth birthday, slowly increase the strength workouts until they are twenty minutes each, and at sixty, bump them up to about a half hour. The longer sessions are designed to counter the natural loss of muscle that comes with aging, which will help maintain your strength and metabolism, making your body seem younger than its years. And starting at age fifty, be sure to get a balance challenge every day, even if it's just standing on one foot while you brush your teeth. At this level, you won't need much time off for rest, but take a break if you have chest congestion or feel burned out.

Weight Loss:

If you want to lose weight, do at least thirty-five minutes of cardio daily and increase the intensity to an RPE of six or seven most days by picking up the pace or the challenge (add hills, switch from doubles tennis to singles, take fewer breaks, etc.). You also need a minimum of ten minutes of daily stretching and fifty minutes weekly of strength work. At age forty, increase the strength work to a total of seventy-five minutes a week, and at age sixty

Sore muscles and rest

When you plan your strength sessions, leave a day of rest between them. You can do cardio on those days, but pick activities that spare the muscles you worked the hardest the day before. Your muscles need the break to get stronger, because you actually do minor damage to muscle fibers with the strength workout (tough cardio sessions can do it too). After the muscles heal, they are stronger than before. If you go at it the next day, the process is destructive and you won't get the healing that adds strength. Your abdominals are the notable exception. This group of muscles is built for endurance, and you can do a moderate abs workout every day as long as the area isn't in pain from the prior day's routine.

The cue that you need rest is a built-in mechanism called *delayed onset muscle soreness* (DOMS) that produces tender, burning muscles a day or two after a tough workout. It's a familiar feeling to any out-of-shape weekend warrior who overdoes it with a favorite activity, such as that touch football game on Thanksgiving. The same thing can happen even if you're in good shape but take on a tough new challenge. For example, if your heart and legs are in great shape from running and you try boxing, your abs and arms are going to protest the next day. Give them a break so they can recover and get stronger.

make it 100 minutes. Do more stretching to be sure to lengthen the muscles you're working. At age fifty, make sure your program includes daily balance exercises.

Performance Goals:

If you want to improve your sports performance, your exercise program has to build. Take your current program and add time, distance, or intensity (not all three) in increments of 10 percent whenever you feel you can. Tailor the schedule to include the three main components plus whichever other factors will help with your sport of choice, from speed to hand-eye coordination. Don't just train in your competitive sport or you'll burn out and suffer injuries; look for other activities that use the same skills or complementary ones, and add those as part of your program.

ROUTINE CHANGES

Once you've made progress toward getting in shape, you must factor in what is called *the law of diminishing returns*. If you keep doing the exact same activities, in short, your routine isn't a challenge to your muscles anymore—they just go through the paces. Your workout is still necessary to stay fit, but you'd get more out of it if you changed it slightly. This training effect happens every eight to twelve weeks.

Change your routine with the seasons. When you put together your list of activities, plan a few to swap in and out with the weather. For example, if you hike a lot in the fall, try cross-country skiing in the winter, in-line skating in the spring, and trail running

When to Expect Results

Be patient while watching for signs of progress. It took you years to get out of shape, and you won't reverse the process in a week or two, although you will quickly stop the downhill slide. The mental benefits can be immediate, but the physical ones take longer. Here's when to expect progress on the three main physical goals.

Strength:
In six to eight weeks—and possibly sooner if you've been completely inactive—you'll be noticeably stronger and more toned.

Aerobics:
In three to four months, you'll notice cardio improvements. Suddenly, it's easier to race up a flight of stairs without huffing and puffing.

Flexibility:
This particular improvement takes the longest. In one study of older exercisers, the participants progressed from barely being able to bend over and touch their knees to reaching their toes in nine months. (They did ten minutes of stretching as part of an hour exercise session five days a week.)

during the summer. Or switch back and forth between hiking and skating every few months. It's not that you shouldn't hike—if you enjoy it and have easy access, by all means do it all year long. But if you want to do the same sport, try to change the challenge to get every ounce of reward for each drop of sweat—such as adding steeper terrain during your hikes or scrambling over boulders.

Professional help

When you're not sure where to start or how to progress to the next level, consider some assistance from a pro. Sign up for a lesson in your sport or a session with a personal trainer. When you're starting out, expert guidance can help you learn the skills properly. Getting it right from the beginning means you won't have to unlearn bad habits, and it helps prevent injuries.

Trainers and coaches are practiced at motivating people, so any time you're in a slump, they can help you get back on track. Describe your goals at the start of the session, and ask for homework tips to use afterward. You don't need to commit to a ten-week program that costs hundreds of dollars, unless you want that level of attention and advancement. Often, a single private session or two can push you ahead to the point where you can continue on your own for a while.

STICKING TO IT

Every fitness routine hits snags. Expect them, plan for them when you can, and accept them when they can't be avoided. If you miss a day, or a week, even a month or two, realize that the gap is a normal part of life, and get back to your sessions as soon as you can. Think of your exercise regimen as if it's a job: You get sick days, vacation time, and the occasional mental-health break. You need to maintain a reasonable level of performance so you don't get fired. If you work hard, you'll get promoted. But a slave-driver of a boss (that's you) will only engender resentment. On the other hand, an unexpected afternoon

off every once in a while builds better morale. And you're making nice payments into the retirement fund. In this job, you don't actually get to retire, but you will enjoy yourself a lot more at sixty-five if you stay fit.

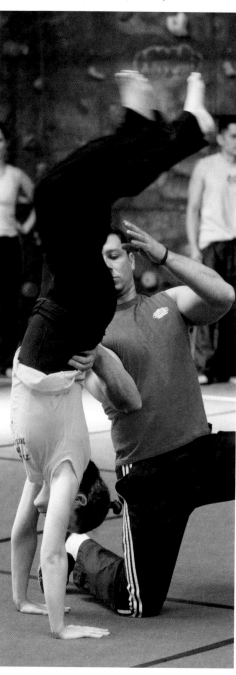

PUTTING THE CHELSEA PIERS FITNESS SOLUTION INTO PLAY

Now that you've finished the equivalent of Exercise Physiology 101, here's the trick to fitting it all in: multipurpose sessions. There's no need to do a separate thirty minutes of cardio and then twenty minutes of strength if you can get both benefits at the same time. The chart to the right provides information on thirty-five activities to help you make selections. Use the *Workbook*, page 34, to design a personalized, well-rounded program.

No matter which activity you choose, there's no free ride. Results are a direct product of how much effort you put in. For example, if you do power yoga with fast moves and sweat flying, you'll get a better cardio workout than that of the average hatha yoga session, which is a great workout but not generally as intense. The chart presents average amounts. Make adjustments based on the intensity of your workouts.

PROOF IN THE POOL

Everyone faces obstacles to regular exercise—from a baby keeping you up all night, to bad arthritis, to too many business trips. But if you find the right sport, you can transform your exercise experience from a struggle into to a joy. One inspiring example is three generations of the swimming Strothenke boys.

Back in Milwaukee, a few years before the U.S. entered World War II, patriarch Robert joined his college swim team. After a few awkward practices in the breaststroke, his coach realized he was a natural backstroker, and Robert enjoyed several years of competition and camaraderie on the team. As a professor, he worked out in the college pool three days a week for almost sixty years, starting with eighty laps and then settling on an even mile for decades. When in his eighties, Robert trimmed back to three-qurters of a mile but kept up the regular schedule even through a diagnosis of advanced cancer, finally quitting when the illness left him bed-bound.

But by that time, Robert's three sons and four grandsons had taken over in the pool. The oldest boys, Bruce and John, spend Friday nights swimming. John, who became quadriplegic after an accident fifteen years prior, swims one-half mile wearing a life preserver and paddling slowly and steadily from end to end. The exercise is a

rare break from the confines of his wheelchair and vital for keeping his muscles strong and his heart healthy. Bruce comes along to help John in and out of the water, then heads to his own lane for a workout. Robert's youngest son, Paul, was a record-setting champ at the same college where his dad taught, and at forty-two continues to swim competitively in the master's program. He won five gold medals in his recent trip to the Empire State Games. And Paul's three sons are all on swim teams: Dan, sixteen, currently holds three team records; Luke, fourteen, qualified for the Junior Olympics; and Mark, twelve, swims backstroke and freestyle. Most recently, Bruce's two-year-old son completed his first swim class at their town pool. Cancer, paralysis, work schedules, teenage shenanigans, and toddlerhood: nothing stopped them from working out because they love it. And if they can do it, so can you—if you find a sport that fits you as well as swimming suits the Strothenkes.

Workout	Cardio	Strength	Flexibility	Balance
Aerobics	Excellent	Some	Some	Good
Baseball	Good	Some	Some	Some
Basketball	Excellent	Some	Good	Good
Boxing	Excellent	Good	Good	Excellent
Calisthenics	Some	Excellent	Some	Good
Cross-country skiing	Excellent	Some	Good	Excellent
Cycling	Excellent	Some	None	Good
Dance	Excellent	Some	Varies	Excellent
Downhill skiing	Excellent	Excellent	Some	Excellent
Elliptical machine	Excellent	Not much	Some	Some
Fencing	Excellent	Excellent	Good	Excellent
Gardening	Some	Good	Some	Good
Golf (no cart)	Good	Some	Good	Good
Gymnastics	Excellent	Excellent	Excellent	Excellent
Hiking	Excellent	Good	Good	Good
Hockey	Excellent	Good	Some	Excellent
Kayaking	Excellent	Good	Not much	Good
Martial Arts	Excellent	Excellent	Excellent	Excellent
Pilates	Not much	Excellent	Excellent	Good
Rock climbing	Some	Excellent	Excellent	Excellent
Rowing	Excellent	Excellent	Not much	Some
Running	Excellent	Some	Not much	Some
Skating	Excellent	Some	Some	Excellent
Snowboarding	Excellent	Good	Not much	Excellent
Snowshoeing	Excellent	Some	Not much	Good
Soccer	Excellent	Some	Some	Good
Softball	Good	Some	Some	Some
Stretching	None	None	Excellent	Good
Swimming	Excellent	Not much	Good	Not much
Tennis (singles)	Excellent	Some	Some	Good
Trail running	Excellent	Some	Some	Excellent
Volleyball	Good	Some	Some	Good
Walking	Good	Some	Some	Some
Weight lifting	Not much	Excellent	Some	Good
Yoga	Not much	Good	Excellent	Excellent

These pages will help you build your own program.

Step 1: **Pick activities**
Fill in the chart below with activities you enjoy, starting with the ones you found as a result of taking the quiz in the previous chapter. Feel free to repeat each one in as many categories as it fits, but don't fill the entire chart with one activity, because you need variety. And don't limit yourself to one choice per box—put in as many as you can—but also don't leave any boxes blank.

	Cardio	Strength	Flexibility	Balance
Indoors:				
Outdoors:				
Easy activity:				
Moderate workout:				
Sweat session:				
Squeeze it in:				
In-depth:				
Alone:				
Together:				
On vacation:				

Step 2: **The short list**
Looking at the chart, which activity repeats in two, three, or four of the columns? That activity is the one with the most benefits, which means you should plan to do it the most often. Continue ranking your activities in order of preference, keeping in mind those you enjoy and those that are easiest to squeeze into your schedule.

My List:

1. _____

2. _____

3. _____

etc.

Step 3: **Goal check**

What do you hope to get out of your program?

_____

_____

_____

_____

_____

_____

Look back to the *By the Numbers* section, page 29, and write down the duration for exercise sessions you need to meet your goals.

Cardio: _____ minutes _____ times per week

Strength: _____ minutes _____ times per week

Flexibility: _____ minutes _____ times per week

Balance: _____ minutes _____ times per week

Step 4: **Plan a week**

Match the results from step 2 and step 3 to outline a plan for one week of workouts, keeping in mind other appointments and activities already in place in your schedule. Be sure to build in flexibility for the weather and your energy level. You can plan a new program every week using the grid below, or repeat the program for the next eight to twelve weeks before scheduling a change.

	Time of Day	Activity	Intensity	Duration
Monday				
Tuesday				
Wednesday				
Thursday				
Friday				
Saturday				
Sunday				

3

Eating Like an Athlete

Taking up a sport could be the motivator that finally gets your diet on track. When you start moving your body more, you need energy and stamina, which are best obtained by eating a steady stream of healthy food (and getting a decent amount of sleep). If you're carrying extra pounds, your exercise sessions will feel harder because the effect is akin to strapping on a backpack with extra weight tucked inside. Think of the liberation you'd feel if you could put that pack down and walk away. Even if you don't diet, you'll probably slim down just by moving more—provided that you're not taking onboard more calories than you're expending on a daily basis.

CALORIES = ENERGY

One of the benefits of a daily fitness program is the effect on your calorie balance. The simple rule is that movement burns calories. The number you see on the scale is predominantly determined by the calories you eat compared to the calories you burn. If you consume more energy than your body uses, you store it away as fat. If you take in fewer calories than your body needs, you use all the calories you've eaten and also burn off some body fat.

There are three main components that add up to the total number of calories your body needs every day:

➡ your metabolism—what you need to keep breathing, pumping blood, and digesting, for example

➡ your regular daily activities such as your work, brushing your teeth, and making dinner

➡ exercise

You can estimate your daily caloric needs by using a variety of Web site calculators. Look for sites that ask how active you are, which can give you an estimate of the second component (calories burned from everyday activities). This number can vary more than you might expect. For example, a 150-pound electrician burns about 1,900 calories a day while the same size office worker burns just 900. If you'd like to see how your job fares, there's a good chance you'll find it (or something similar) in the list at www.calorielab.com on the "calories burned" page. For a customized report based on your food and activity habits, go to www.dietitian.com and complete the two-page Healthy Body Calculator.

To get a quick estimate without logging on, try this technique:

1. Choose your activity level from the chart below.

Activity Level	Description	Multiply by
None	Bed bound	10
Light	You do a little walking in your daily activities plus a lot of sitting	13
Moderate	You do at least thirty minutes of active housework or yard work daily or have a somewhat active job	15
High	You're on your feet all the time, and have a physically demanding job	17

2. Multiply your weight by the number in the last column.

3. If you exercise, add the calorie burn for those activities separately. You'll find a calorie estimate in each sports chapter in this book. If you do a different activity, check the chart below for a rough estimate of the calorie burns per hour.

Pace	Examples	Calories /lb of body weight/ hour	Calories for a 150-lb-person/ hour
Easy	Slow stroll, miniature golf	½	75
Light	Brisk walk, fishing (standing)	1	150
Moderate	Shooting baskets, hopscotch	1½	225
Sweaty	Aerobics class, calisthenics, touch football	2½ to 3	375 to 450
Intense	Run nine-minute mile, competitive racquetball	3½ to 4	525 to 600
All out	Running up stairs, jumping rope fast	4½ to 5½	675 to 825

At the end of this calculation, you have the number of calories you can eat each day without gaining or losing weight. To lose weight, you need to eat less, move more or,

better yet, do both. Studies show that combining exercise with diet improvements is by far the most efficient and effective strategy for successful weight loss and long-term maintenance. Every exercise session burns calories, especially when you compare it to what you'd otherwise be doing. For example, if you weigh 150 pounds, here's what you can accomplish in an hour:

Reading a book	20 calories
Playing the piano	90 calories
Going for a fairly brisk walk	150 calories
Playing singles tennis	420 calories

On the other hand, if you cut out your nightly habit of eating two scoops of ice cream, you've saved about 300 calories a day—or approximately 1½ pounds in a month.

For every extra 500 calories you trim off or burn daily, you lose about a pound of body fat per week (a pound of fat contains about 3,500 calories). The opposite is also true: For every 3,500 calories you consume more than what your body needs, you gain a pound. Unfortunately, one supersized Big Mac meal with a Coca-Cola has about 1,700 calories all by itself. The bad news is that you can consume the meal in about fifteen minutes, but you'd have to jog for almost five hours to burn it off!

Web sites such as www.fitday.com and www.mypyramidtracker.gov can help by providing the calorie counts for different foods and activities, with the exercise measures adjusted for your weight so you don't have to do the math.

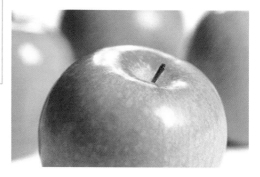

Counting Calories

Trying to count calories every day is too tedious for most of us, but doing it for a brief time is an effective way to jump-start a weight-loss regimen by showing you which foods contribute large chunks of calories and how exercise is helping. This overview will help you find easy changes that can produce results. But don't bother to calculate each meal and workout in detail, because the numbers are not precise. Here are three reasons why:

When you read the calories on a food label, the amount listed could be inaccurate. The FDA allows calorie counts on food labels to be off by as much as 20 percent—which is a lot. That means you can't be sure you're getting the better selection when you choose one brand of chocolate chip cookies because the label says they have 150 calories per serving instead of another, which says 160. Brand A could have 178 calories. If Brand B has 160, they would seem to be lower in calories—but they could have 190 calories. You have no way of determining the actual number. This variance is allowed partly because the methods used to test calorie content aren't perfect. When the calorie difference is small, such as in the cookies, pick the food you prefer. And eat a varied diet so that an error on the label of one food doesn't completely derail your calorie count for the day, week, or month.

Serving size is another issue. While the FDA has attempted to update the amounts listed on labels to match the way Americans actually eat (so you don't see four servings listed for a tiny bag of chips), the given amount might be far less than you really consume. Cereal is a good example: Most boxes show about 1 cup as the serving size, but you probably eat more every morning.

Calculations of the calories burned during exercise are no more precise. The numbers listed on cardio machines are notoriously inaccurate because in most cases they don't ask you to key in your weight—a factor that makes the number shift dramatically. But even if you do the math using your weight (as we do in the sport chapters that follow), the system isn't perfect: Two people who are exactly the same size standing next to each other in the same aerobics class will burn different amounts of calories. The actual burn rate is determined by the amount of muscle being used, so the person who has more muscle or is more energetic will burn more calories. Calorie charts list a variety of intensities for some activities such as running, but others like cross-country skiing will use an average. If you're moving along briskly or climbing hills, expect to burn more than during a slow tour over flatlands. There's no specific formula to adjust your burn rate based on your intensity, but you can estimate whether you think you're doing a harder or easier workout than the average listed.

With all this room for error, it's tempting to give up on calorie counts. But keeping track provides a general idea of what's going in and what's going out. It's enlightening to see approximately how many calories are in a handful of nuts, or a serving of fries, compared to the number burned in an hour-long walk. The numbers are accurate enough to provide guidance on where you can make easy adjustments. If the changes don't work, assume you're consuming more and/or burning less than you need and experiment with other regimens to get the desired outcome.

NUTRIENTS

Food doesn't have to be healthy to provide energy—you can survive on potato chips, if you must. But while the potential exists to eat too many calories of any food, from plums to poultry to pudding, some choices are so filling that you'd have a hard time overdoing it. For example, for a 125-calorie snack, you could binge on twenty stalks of celery or eat two small cubes of cheese. If you eat twenty cubes of cheese you've gotten about half your day's calories in one snack and a hefty dose of fat.

Calorie for calorie, the healthiest foods are the ones that deliver more beneficial nutrients than other choices that bog your body down with junk, including salt and chemicals. Here's a look at some of the major components in your food and how they affect your health and fitness:

daily-protein-gram needs. If you're actively trying to build more muscle, divide your weight by four, then multiply the answer by three (or multiply your weight by 0.75).

To determine how much protein you're getting, check food labels, which list the grams per serving. On average, an ounce of meat, poultry, or fish has 7 grams of protein, and you get 3 ounces in a serving the size of a cassette tape. Milk, cheese, and beans are also good sources of protein.

Despite the popularity of high-protein diets, many major nutrition organizations still recommend that you avoid consuming too much protein because it's taxing for the body. For example, excess protein makes your kidneys work overtime and can cause calcium loss from your bones.

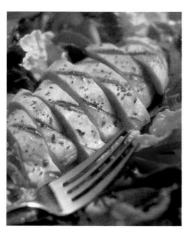 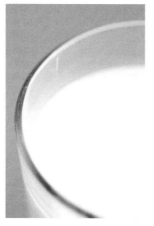 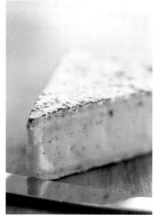

Protein is necessary for almost every function in the body, so we have to eat sufficient amounts in order to stay healthy. Most people should get about 20 percent of the day's calories from protein, which is usually about 45 to 60 grams a day.

To calculate roughly how many grams you need, divide your weight by three. You need more protein if you exercise a lot, because this nutrient supports the maintenance and development of muscle. If you're an endurance athlete, divide your weight by three then double the number (or multiply your weight by 0.6) to get an estimate of

Carbohydrates are a quick source of energy for your muscles and brain, and many types are healthy for you. We tend to equate carbs with starchy foods such as bread and pasta, but fruits and sweets also are a major source of carbs in most American diets. Beans and milk are high in carbs, too. Refined carbohydrates, such as those in white bread and candy, provide calories but few beneficial nutrients. Whole grains are the best choices because they are packed with nutrients such as magnesium and fiber. Recent studies show that three servings of whole grains a day can help prevent metabolic syndrome (the combo

Picking the best carbs

Many of today's popular diets are based on a concept called *Glycemic Index* or *Glycemic Load*, both of which measure the effect of foods on your blood sugar. When you digest carbohydrates, they are converted to sugar, which then is absorbed into the blood. An increase in blood sugar causes the release of insulin so you can use some of the energy immediately and store some sugar for later use, bringing levels down in the blood. (People who have diabetes don't make or use insulin well and have elevated blood sugars that may require medication.) Unfortunately, insulin also damages the body, especially the cardiovascular system, and it causes your body to store energy as fat. The faster and higher a food raises your blood sugar levels, thereby causing it to pump out

insulin in response, the less healthy it is. Although there's no proof that this effect causes weight gain (as many diets claim), there is some logic to it. However, to date, research does not support cutting out carbs completely but rather choosing "good" carbs with a low Glycemic Index rating.

A food's Glycemic Index (GI) is the measure of how much 50 grams of it will raise your blood glucose over the next two hours compared to 50 grams of glucose, a simple sugar. Now popular, the concept of Glycemic Load (GL) takes into consideration a food's GI rating plus the serving size, because eating more of a food can have a bigger impact on your blood sugar—and 50 grams isn't much. The GL has more relevance to the way we actually eat.

Keep in mind as well that what you eat along with carbs has an effect on blood sugar. For example, high-fiber foods such as vegetables are digested slowly, so high GI foods combined with lower GI ones (such as when you put maple syrup on your whole-wheat waffles) have a lower effect on blood sugar, and thus have a lower GI.

For the best health benefits, try to keep your blood sugar even by eating regularly (blood sugar can dip if you go for hours without food) and choosing foods such as whole grains and fruits, which have a low GI (55 or less) or GL (10 or less). These carbs help you stay satiated longer, possibly aiding in weight loss, and they tend to be high in fiber, which is good for your health.

of conditions that lead to a high risk of heart disease and stroke) and boost bone-mineral density.

Most people should get at least half their calories from carbohydrates. You can get an estimate of grams of carbs you need daily by multiplying your weight by two. If

you're athletic, you need more: 3 to 4½ grams per pound of body weight.

Fat has perhaps the worst reputation of the three *macronutrients*. Eat too little, however, and you will have trouble absorbing some vitamins and could get gallstones, constipation, and low HDL ("good") cholesterol

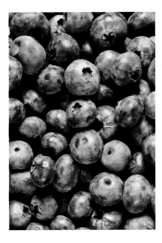
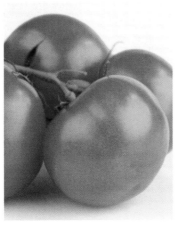
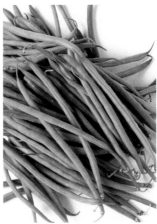

and miss out on nutrients your body needs, such as essential fatty acids. Unfortunately, most of us have the opposite problem and eat too much fat. The key here is balance. The recommendation is to get at least 20 grams of fat a day but no more than 30 percent of your calories from fat (at 9 calories per gram). Like carbs, there are different kinds of fat, some of which are healthier than others.

Within the category of *polyunsaturated fats*, there are two main types to know about: *Omega-6s* are found in vegetable oils and margarines and we tend to eat far too much of these fats. *Omega-3s* are good for your

Health quotient	Fat type	Found in foods such as
Worst	Trans fat	shortening, some margarines/spreads, snack foods made with "hydrogenated" oils
Bad	Saturated fat	Butter, whole milk, cheese, meat, coconut oil, palm oil, cocoa butter
So-so	Polyunsaturated fat	Corn, sunflower, and safflower oils, soybeans and soybean oil, nuts and seeds
Good	Monounsaturated fat	Peanuts, avocado, olive and canola oils

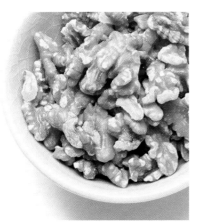
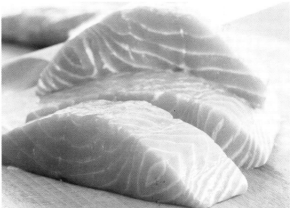

heart and have many other health benefits, especially for preventing diseases resulting from inflammation, which is a hot topic in medicine these days. You'll find high levels of omega-3s in walnuts, flaxseeds, pumpkin seeds, and fatty fish such as salmon and tuna.

Try to consume no *trans fats* (they are now listed on food labels), at most about 20 grams of *saturated fat* (unless you have heart concerns, in which case you should get less), and as much of the rest in *monounsaturates* and omega-3s as you can.

Dietary fat versus body fat

One of the key points of confusion in nutrition is the terminology for fats. Dietary fat is the stuff in your foods. The chunk you pinch on your waist is body fat. Some foods are pure fat, such as butter, oil, and shortening. These foods have about 120 calories per tablespoon or 3,000 to 4,000 calories per pound (that's four sticks of butter or 2 cups of oil). Other foods are a mix of nutrients, with some, such as salad dressing, having more fat than others, such as salad.

But when you eat fat, the calories are not deposited directly onto your belly, thighs, and butt, even if that seems to be the case. Like any other component in food, fat is digested and used for energy if the body needs it. On the other hand, any nutrients—including carbohydrates or protein—will be digested and then stored as body fat if you eat more calories than you need.

Vitamins and minerals are sometimes called *micronutrients* because, while they are vital for health, you need smaller amounts of each. Some are *antioxidants* that help prevent chronic diseases (see more about antioxidants, below). Others work to facilitate key processes in the body, such as the role of calcium and vitamin D in bone building. Your

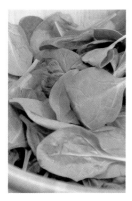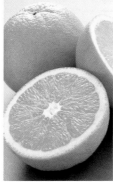

body is adept at storing some of the nutrients it needs, but there are several (such as vitamin C) that you need to consume on a daily basis so your levels don't drop, which often leads to illness.

Many vitamins and minerals are better for you if obtained from foods rather than supplements, because the pills may not deliver everything listed on the label in a way the body can use. Fruits and vegetables are good sources of many important ones, with each type and color of produce containing a different variety. For example, citrus fruits are high in vitamin C, while spinach is a good source of vitamin A and magnesium. Therefore, eating a rainbow of these nutrient-packed low-calorie foods is an important part of a healthy diet.

Since few Americans get the recommended five servings a day, however, many doctors and dietitians suggest that most people take a multivitamin daily. While you need to get enough vitamins and minerals, it's also important not to overdose on some nutrients because they can cause damage—especially

the ones that can be stored by the body and may accumulate at toxic levels. Overdoses rarely happen from foods; it's usually megadoses of supplements that cause problems. Pick a multivitamin from a reputable brand, with doses of vitamins and minerals that generally don't exceed 100 percent of the *Percent Daily Value* (%DV), which is the amount scientists have determined is necessary and safe. Although there is always debate and new information that leads to changes in these recommendations, they are a good place to start.

Some essential micronutrients are not abundant in fruits and vegetables but are found in meats, fish, nuts and beans, whole grains, and dairy products. As long as you eat a varied diet, you probably consume enough of these nutrients. But if your menu is limited to a few favorite selections, the daily multivitamin will help prevent deficiencies. Don't, however, think that taking a multivitamin gives you license to eat poorly.

Antioxidants are beneficial chemicals in foods that help prevent damage to your cells. Researchers continue to discover new antioxidants and the ailments they help prevent. For example, lycopene in tomatoes and some other red foods, such as watermelon, has been shown to help stave off prostate cancer and heart disease. There's sulforafane in crucifers such as broccoli, cauliflower, and cabbage. The health benefits of dark chocolate, red wine, and green tea are also thought to result from their antioxidant content. For example, quercetin in red wine (and apples, leafy greens, and other foods) works to help lung function and may be beneficial for people who have allergies and respiratory diseases. This antioxidant may also be beneficial in preventing heart disease and some cancers. Red wine also contains resveratrol, another antioxidant.

The best way to be sure you're getting plenty of antioxidants is to eat a variety of fruits and vegetables of all colors, if possible, even more than the recommended five servings a day—although most of us have trouble just getting that much.

FUEL FOR ACTIVITY

To some extent, your muscles don't care what fuels them over the course of the day. But when it comes to providing energy for your muscles, carbs are king. As a matter of fact, people who adhere strictly to a no-carb diet may find they feel tired because they lack carbohydrates—although that's no license to munch French fries before every workout. Actually, when carbs are coupled with a high fat content, they are digested slowly and are less effective in providing quick energy; they may even cause indigestion and discomfort. Plus, eating too many calories (and fats are calorie-dense), leads to weight gain, which hampers your ability to exercise. Sugar-laden foods do provide quick energy, but again they are high in calories and low in necessary nutrients. The nutrient content explains why 100 percent juice is generally a better choice than soda, juice drinks, or sports drinks, even if the calories and sugar content are equal.

When you have a strenuous game coming up or a long event, such as an all-day cross-country ski trip, you can prepare your body with a light version of a technique called *carbo loading*. Several studies have shown that athletic performance in prolonged events is enhanced if you take in 200 to 300 grams of carbs three to four hours before a tough workout. Since there are only 40 grams of carbohydrate in a cup of cooked spaghetti, you'll be eating quite a lot to get the full dose. And if you're not competing in a marathon or the Tour de France, you don't need to down an entire box of pasta the night before. Instead, choose your favorite healthy carb-based dishes such as spaghetti with marinara sauce or a rice-and-bean burrito (go light on the cheese, sour cream, and guacamole).

Shortly before exercise, you can get the energy your body needs by having a snack that's low in fat and fiber so you'll digest it quickly and not suffer discomfort during the workout. Foods packed with carbs and fairly light on protein are the best choices for providing energy. Try a banana, a bagel with peanut butter, or a low-fat yogurt. And if you are going to be intensely active for more than two hours, try to eat snacks while you're working out or follow the session with a carb-rich meal that has a good dose of protein.

It's not unusual to be hungrier when you first start exercising. But be careful not to eat more than you burn off—unless you want to gain weight. If you go out with the team after the game, keep in mind that two beers contain as many calories as you burned by playing about an hour of baseball. And it's not just beer—a Gatorade and a Powerbar add up to just as much.

CHEAT SHEET

To turn all of this information into an easy meal plan, consider stopping at the Web site for the USDA food pyramid: www.mypyramid.gov. Click on "My Pyramid Plan" and enter your age, gender, and activity level to receive a personalized recommendation for the number of servings to eat in each food group per day so that you'll get the nutrients you need in the right proportions. For example, a forty-year-old woman who works out for less than thirty minutes a day will get the following diet:

- ➡ 6 ounces of grains (at least half whole grains)
- ➡ 2 cups of vegetables
- ➡ 1 cup of fruit
- ➡ 3 cups of milk
- ➡ 5 ounces of meat and beans
- ➡ 5 teaspoons of oil
- ➡ limit solid fats and sugars to 195 calories

These proportions are based on a 1,800 calorie weight-maintenance diet, so you must further adjust the amounts to reflect how many calories you should eat.

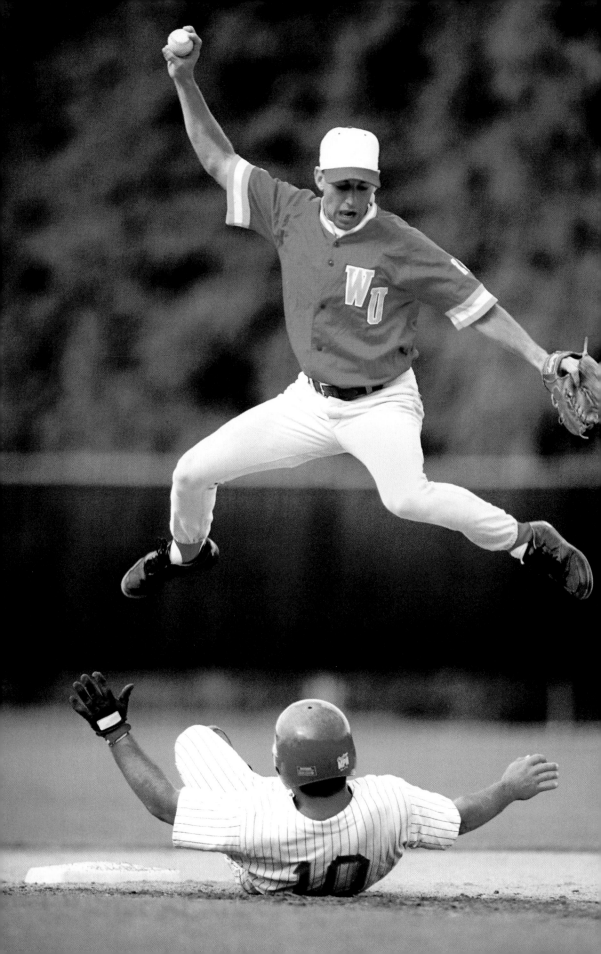

4

BASEBALL/SOFTBALL

YOU'LL LOVE THIS SPORT IF YOU:
- want to improve your strength, reaction time, and sprint speed
- love strategy—like a mental challenge in addition to a physical one
- prefer a sport that's easy to start, but one in which you can improve for years
- want to be so engaged that you don't know you're exercising
- dream of competing
- enjoy team sports, camaraderie, and social activities
- like to have a set role because you play a specific position on the team (although you don't have to if you prefer to float amongst positions as needed)
- prefer a sport where it's easy to get together a pick-up game

YOU MIGHT NOT LOVE THIS SPORT IF YOU:
- are completely lacking in coordination and aim
- are afraid of getting hit by a ball
- don't like to share the glory or suffer losses because of others
- prefer to set your own schedule rather than rely on teammates

In the 1988 classic baseball film "Bull Durham," Tim Robbins as a rookie pitcher with great promise explains the game: "A good friend of mine used to say, 'This is a very simple game. You throw the ball, you catch the ball, you hit the ball. Sometimes you win, sometimes you lose, sometimes it rains.'" Of course, almost every American, and quite a few people from other countries, know there is quite a bit more to the sport than that description.

Baseball began as a children's pastime with stick-and-ball games going back centuries to ancient Egypt and Greece. Thousands of years later, the sports of cricket and roundball were popular with British kids and imported to the U.S. when the colonies were first settled. In roundball, a batter ran around the bases and fielders caught outs. But there were notable differences: A fielder could throw the ball at the runner to "plug" him out.

Legend had it that modern American baseball was invented in 1839 in Cooperstown, New York, by Abner Doubleday (a misconception that led to the building of the Baseball Hall of Fame there). In reality, the game evolved from roundball a few years earlier. In the summer of 1845, a group of New Yorkers formed the Knickerbocker Base Ball Club and codified the rules, replacing plugging with tagging out the runner, and adding foul lines to mark the field. The Knickerbockers were trounced in the first organized game against another New York team the following summer, marking the official start of baseball as an adult sport, similar to the version played today. "The New York Game," as it was then called, benefited by spectators being able to line the newly created foul lines to watch without getting in the way, and thousands of fans did so during the 1850s. Fields sprang up in the northeast, with admission charged to cover the fees and maintenance, but the players were not paid. Then, during the Civil War, Yankee soldiers introduced Southerners to the game. And the north and the south agreed on one thing: baseball was a hit. What followed were decades of growth, with the start of professional teams, bigger and better ball fields being built, strikes, scandals, home-run heroes, and more.

Softball—which can be a less strenuous form of the same game—was derived from baseball in 1887, first as an indoor game and then as an outdoor version. Like baseball, the game was spread by soldiers, but this time it was World War II fighters who introduced it

SCORE

A 150-pound person playing an hour of baseball or softball will burn an average of 240 calories (or 1.6 times your weight in pounds). When playing a relaxed game of catch, the same person will burn about 90 calories an hour (or 0.6 times your weight in pounds).

around the globe. Today, both games are played internationally, although they only reach American-level devotion in a few countries such as Japan, the Dominican Republic, and Cuba. Baseball was a demonstration sport in six Olympics, before it became a medal sport in 1992, but was voted out of the London games in 2012. Women's softball entered the Olympics in 1996 and has been the sole women-only sport in the games, but will also be dropped for 2012. The sports have not been replaced on the roster, so there's a chance that they will return in 2016, and representatives from South Africa, Spain, Australia, and Brazil are taking up the cause, along with those from other countries where the game is well-loved.

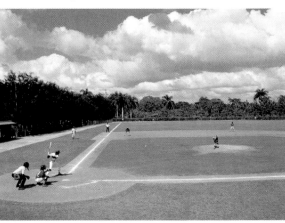

One of the reasons for baseball's and softball's ongoing popularity as pickup sports is that you can actually get a great workout and have a lot of fun with just a bat, ball and glove, and a handful of people. It's easy to designate a few bases or find a field, and you can readily locate a game or a league to play in. The individual skills are fun to practice, from playing catch to getting into a batting cage to hit. And many players develop decent skills in a short amount of time.

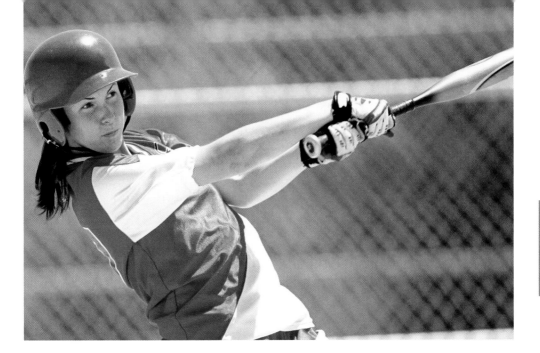

Other than the size of the ball, there are a few distinct differences between baseball and softball. Baseball games have nine innings while softball games have seven. Softball fields are smaller than baseball fields, with the pitcher closer to the hitter and smaller distances between the bases. There are three distinct types of softball, defined by the pitching style. In *slow-pitch*, the ball is thrown underhand in a high arc. In *fast-pitch*, the pitcher swings his arm back and forth prior to an underhand release or windmills the arm in a full backward circle before snapping an underhand pitch with great speed. For *modified fast-pitch*, the pitcher's arm is not allowed to make a full circle. Slow-pitch softball is the dominant variety for corporate leagues and recreational play because it's easier to hit the ball. Also, while baseball and fast-pitch teams field nine players, slow-pitch teams have ten players on the field, making for slightly less running around. And in slow-pitch games, players are not allowed to bunt the ball or steal bases.

As in most sports, once you've mastered the basics of throwing, hitting, and catching, there is plenty more to learn if you want to excel. Strategies for where to hit, when to run, how to field, and more can keep you challenged for many years. But most of all, you can get outdoors on sunny days with a bunch of like-minded athletes and have fun.

GEARING UP

To play ball, you'll probably want to start out owning a glove. You can head to any sporting goods store and buy a decent glove. You don't need anything fancy, just a regular utility or outfielder's glove—not a catcher's glove or a first-baseman's mitt, both of which are distinct. Softball gloves tend to be a little larger than baseball gloves because you'll be catching a larger ball. Try on a variety of gloves to get a sense of how they fit and pick one that feels comfortable. Gloves come in a variety of materials, from kangaroo to cow leather. As a beginner, don't spend a lot on fancy materials—select the best fit at a reasonable price.

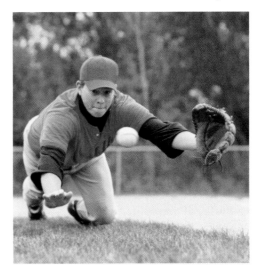

If you need to break in your glove, ask for instructions at the store. You'll need to rub a small amount of petroleum jelly or a softening cream into the palm, bend it in a few places to loosen it up, and then put the ball in the glove and lace it firmly shut with rope. After the overnight treatment (which you can repeat as needed), use the glove to catch lots of balls and you'll complete the process of breaking it in over time. Gloves can be purchased already broken in, which feel better

you. Today, many players prefer aluminum bats for the combination of their light weight, strength, and good drive on the ball—and the fact that the metal ones don't break. Leagues may have rules limiting the weight-to-length ratio of bats (lighter and longer bats are more powerful), so be sure to check before buying if you'll play in an organized group.

You can play recreational ballgames in sneakers, but when you start playing more often

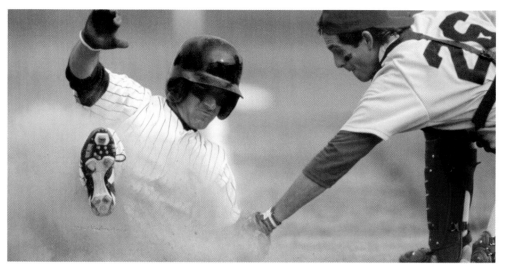

off the shelf but may not last as long. Also consider buying a batting glove so your sweaty palms won't slip on the bat, and purchase your fielding glove to fit over the batting glove, which will protect it from sweat.

Entry-level bats can be inexpensive, so if you want to pick one up to hit some balls at home, just swing them at the store until you find one that feels right. But put off the purchase if you can borrow a bat so you'll have the incentive to try a variety of styles, from wood to metal and different weights. Here's a test to find the right weight: Hold the bat in one hand and raise it to your side. If you can't hold it straight out at shoulder height, it's too heavy. Test bats at the field and go to batting cages where you can try different materials and weights. Hit hundreds of balls before you decide which one works best for

you'll probably want cleats for added traction. Start with cleats that have molded plastic spikes on the bottom rather than metal, because metal cleats are dangerous to other players. Many leagues ban metal cleats for this reason.

Any athletic clothes will work for the average baseball or softball game, but league players have uniforms—a jersey that's typically worn over a T-shirt, pants and athletic socks, plus the ubiquitous baseball cap. Recreational leagues may have printed T-shirts instead of jerseys.

Catchers also wear protective pieces that vary from baseball to the different forms of softball. If you play catcher, check with the league to determine what you need, what you must purchase (such as an athletic cup) and what you can borrow (possibly a face mask or chest pads, for example).

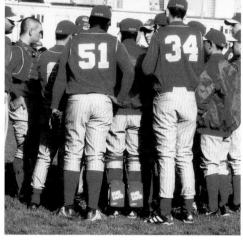

YOUR FIRST TIME

Your teammates may assume you know the basic rules, so it's good to familiarize yourself with the game and positions before trying to play. Start by watching some games, especially amateur-level contests that you can attend in person, because it's easier to learn that way. And consider some time with a coach or a friend who knows the sport in order to get some pointers on hitting and catching as well as fielding and where to throw the ball. Even if you've been practicing in the backyard, try visiting a batting cage a few times to experience what it's like to hit some solid pitches. The cages will have a variety of pitching speeds for baseball plus softball options.

When you arrive for your first organized game, the coach will have a batting order, or will develop one after talking to the players and will also assign you a position to play in the field. The home team takes the field first while the visiting team bats.

Before play begins, the pitcher and catcher are generally allowed a few practice throws. The batters will then hit and run until there are three outs. Then the teams switch for the bottom of the inning. Play continues until the losing team completes the ninth inning or, in the case of a tie score after nine innings, when an inning ends with one team ahead.

ATHLETE IN ACTION

Robert Applegate, 61

Growing up in San Diego, Robert Applegate was a busy young man—he ran track and wrestled in high school, but also started working at 14, was married at 18, and became a dad at 19, which didn't leave much time for ballgames. But when he was about 47 years old, he developed asthma from smoke exposure and was close to a health-forced retirement from the local fire department, so he decided he needed another way to stay in shape. "I had never played at all and had no idea what to even do," he recalls. "But I had an old mitt my dad had given me." So he took his mitt, went down to a casual Sunday softball game, and started to play. "I was in good shape as a fireman, but I was still hurting pretty bad that first season," he says.

When he retired and moved about an hour away, the husband of his real-estate agent invited him to join a slow-pitch game in his new neighborhood. Over the next few years, some teams sprouted up nearby and then fizzled, and Applegate learned the game as he played. A shoulder injury sidelined him for a year, and when he was ready to return to the field, there were no spots open on the local teams.

"Someone suggested the senior league," says Applegate. It was an hour from his new home, but he eventually decided to do it in order to get back into the game. "They first put me on a B-league team and wanted to have someone run for me," he recalls, noting that older players who first get into the game often pull a hamstring, a painful injury. "But I ended up hitting the ball over the fence, and they moved me to the A team." For three of the last four seasons, Applegate has been the top-draft pick when the teams are selected.

He says his talent comes from keeping the game simple but working extra hard. "I see the ball, hit the ball, catch the ball, and throw it to somebody," he says. "I still don't have all the finesse and strategy, but you don't need to know a lot. I pitch most of the time now, so I try to run into the right spot so that if the ball is overthrown, I'm backing up if the person misses it." Now, he plays four days a week, sometimes substituting for an absent player in a second game, and is physically up to the challenge. "I stand in as a pinch runner for others, but I'm not tired when I get home after two games." And while he's competitive, doing everything except cheating to win, he still has a sense of humor and humility about the game. "They'd say 'You're playing second base,' and I'd say 'Is that the one over there?'" he jokes.

SECRETS TO SUCCESS

As a beginning ball player, the fear is that you'll make a mistake and play poorly. And, of course, the catch-22 is that being jittery won't help your performance. "It's impossible not to be nervous," says Joe Wagner, a baseball coach at Chelsea Piers who played two years in the minor leagues. "The best you can do is to try to concentrate on the ball. Try to know what you are going to do with it before it comes to you." It can take years to learn every nuance of the game, so don't feel embarrassed to ask for pointers. Getting a few tips on how to play your position can make all the difference. "If you aren't sure what to do, you'll make a mistake if you are mentally unprepared, even if you're physically capable," says Wagner.

On the days between your games, be a spectator. "Watch with intent," says Wagner. Pick a player in a certain position and try to anticipate what he'll do. Learn from how he plays, how he reacts, when he runs, and when he stays put. If you try to watch the entire game, you won't learn as much about the individual strategy you'll need on the field. Amateur games that you can attend in person are the best ones for observation because the action is often slower than it is in pro ball. The players are closer to your ability level and you have your choice of viewing angle.

In addition to the strategy, you'll need to learn how your own psyche works. Some ballplayers hit best when they are

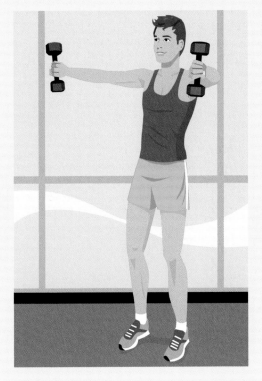

v raises

Hold something heavy in each hand, such as 5-pound dumbbells or cans of soup. Stand in a stable position, legs hip-distance apart, knees slightly bent, abs firm, head up. Start with your arms hanging comfortably by your sides, shoulders down and back. Rotate both hands in until your thumbs face back, palms face out and pinkies face forward. Lift both arms straight up to form a V, stopping when your hands are at shoulder height. Lower to your sides in a slow and controlled motion to complete 1 repetition. Take care not to hunch your shoulders as you lift and lower 12 times. Start with 1 set. Work up to 3 sets of 15 reps.

calm and happy, while others play at their peak ability when their team is down to their last out or they need to make the catch to win the game. Pay attention to the feelings that motivate your best play, stay alert on the field, and try to get into the zone that suits you.

And then there are the physical skills. Like any sport, you'll play better if your hitting, catching, and throwing are ingrained, with no need to think in order to perform—this is called *muscle memory*. That level of skill takes plenty of practice. In addition to playing catch and getting in the batting cage, Wagner says, "Work on hitting and throwing in front of a mirror, because you get immediate visual feedback." As often as your coach might tell you what

to correct, it's different when you can see it for yourself.

While it's tempting to spend most of your time practicing your batting, remember that you'll spend more time in the field than at the plate. Fielding skills can make you the team hero more often than hitting a few home runs will. And, poor fielding can lose the game.

Wagner advises improving your throwing abilities and protecting yourself from injury by strengthening your shoulder muscles, which you can accomplish by doing the exercising below. To prep your legs or improve your speed around the bases, work on footwork.

Try the exercises below:

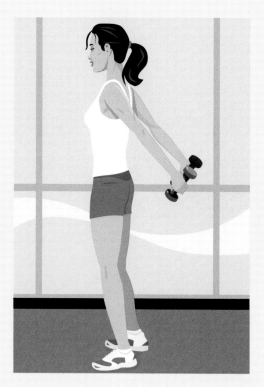

kickbacks

Hold something heavy in each hand, such as 5-pound dumbbells or cans of soup. Stand in a stable position, legs hip-distance apart, knees slightly bent, abs firm, head up. Start with your arms hanging comfortably by your sides, shoulders down and back. Without moving your torso, press both arms back, keeping the hands as close together as possible. Press your arms as high as you can comfortably go, then slowly lower back to the start in a slow and controlled motion to complete 1 repetition. Take care not to hunch your shoulders as you lift and lower 12 times. Start with 1 set. Work up to 3 sets of 15 reps.

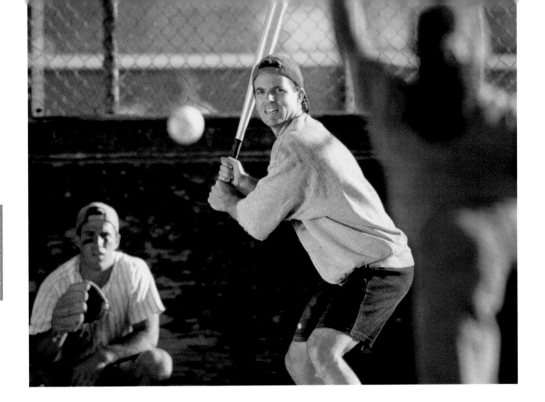

TACKLE THE TRUTH

I'm the only person who didn't learn to play ball as a kid	Adult beginner sessions at fields all over the country get plenty of players learning the game for the first time. While many Americans come up through the ranks of Little League, there are plenty more who were too busy, or played other sports as kids and never took up baseball or softball. The basics of the game are easy, so if you're interested, try it.
You have to be a great hitter to play the game	Hitting looks like the most important skill in baseball and softball, and it's not optional, but every team must have a variety of talent to succeed—and some players are prized for their pitching or fielding abilities while they work on improving their batting average. A team that only has star hitters will often lose to a well-rounded group of opponents.
Baseball and softball are about sitting and standing around, and you won't get fit	In the field, the best players are moving all the time, adjusting to the action that might come their way, backing up other fielders, and staying primed for quick movement. The same goes for runners on base, who must be prepped to sprint at any chance. And the distance between the bases is further than it looks on television— 90 feet in a baseball game. Pro players make it look easy because they're in great shape. After all that exercise, a little time in the dugout is a welcome break—and three outs can go by fast, putting you back out on the field in short order. If you want more physical challenge, be the catcher. You'll squat, stand, and throw with every pitch.

GET MORE FROM YOUR SPORT

Baseball and softball players frequently take up running and cycling to crosstrain while building endurance in the leg muscles. Soccer and basketball are even better for crosstraining because these activities incorporate footwork along with teamwork. And basketball jump shots will improve your throwing technique.

If you enjoy the camaraderie of recreational games, consider taking up volleyball and tennis as well, or martial arts or boxing if you're fast on your feet and love strategy.

Most softball and baseball camps in the U.S. are oriented toward children or advanced adults. If you want to take your game to a higher level, contact a local college team and ask the staff if they moonlight-teach private lessons. If not, get their suggestions for local coaches or players who might be interested. Also contact the league coaches for the local parks department and the YMCA to find out if they have suggestions for finding an instructor. They might also be able to direct you to leagues at your level that have good coaching.

When you've advanced to being a solid player, you can treat yourself to a baseball fantasy camp, where you get to play alongside former Major League players.

RESOURCES

➡ **www.baseball-articles.com** is aimed mainly at coaches of kids' teams. But browse its article archive to find tips on fielding a pop fly, drills to improve sliding, and the proper grip for throwing a curve ball.

➡ **www.pitchsoftball.com** is devoted to pitching instruction, with sections for beginners as well as more advanced players, analyses of the different types of pitches, and a warm-up guide.

➡ **www.asmi.org/SportsMed/throwing/thrower10.html** has a video demonstration of ten shoulder-strengthening exercises designed to keep you injury-free while improving your power.

➡ *Play Better Baseball: Winning Techniques and Strategies for Coaches and Players* by Bob Cluck includes information on throwing with greater accuracy, effective sliding techniques, and conditioning.

➡ *The Rules of Baseball* by David Nemec not only tells you the rules but explains their origins and some of the controversies that led to them.

➡ *Softball Skills & Drills* by Judi Garman covers the execution of the basic skills of the game along with drills to improve them.

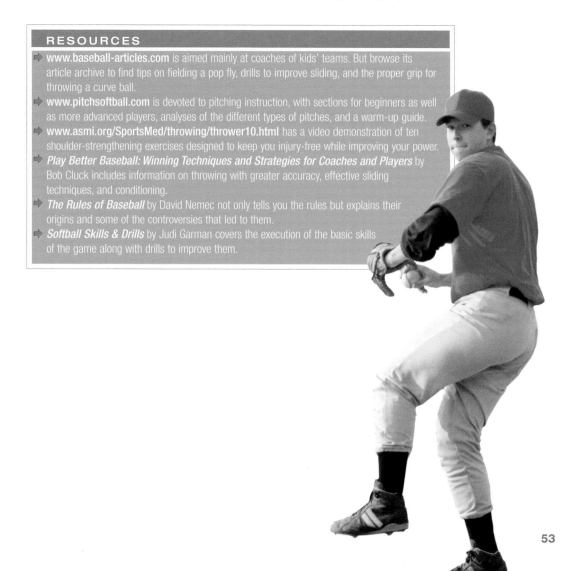

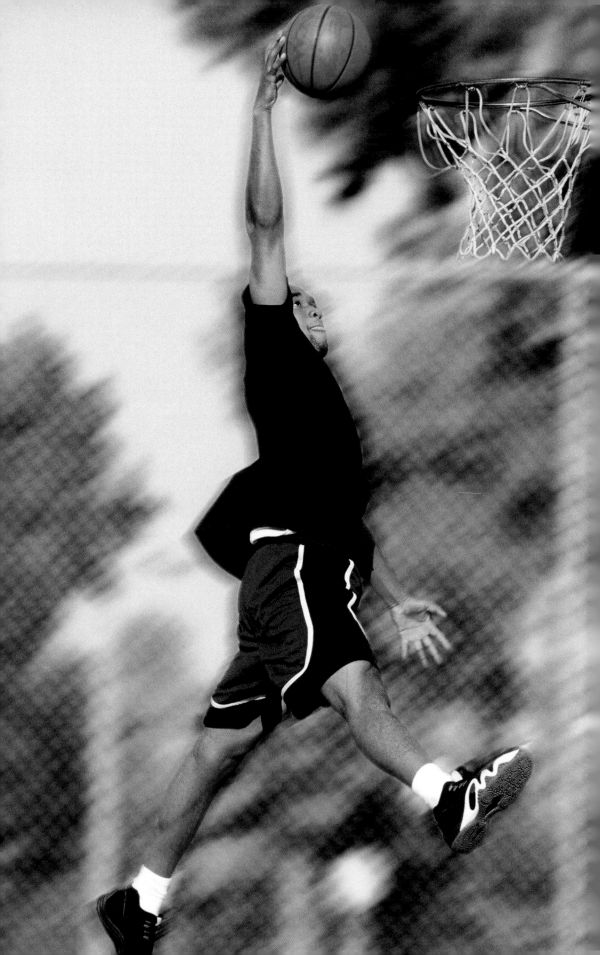

5

BASKETBALL

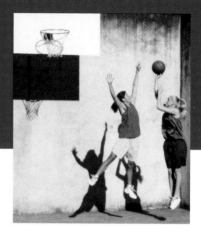

YOU'LL LOVE THIS SPORT IF YOU:
• want to improve your cardiovascular fitness, balance, and agility
• love strategy—want a mental challenge in addition to a physical one
• prefer a sport that's easy to learn, but one in which you can improve for years
• are quick on your feet
• want to be so engaged that you don't know you're exercising
• dream of competing
• enjoy team sports, camaraderie, and social activities
• prefer a sport where it's easy to get together a pick-up game

YOU MIGHT NOT LOVE THIS SPORT IF YOU:
• are completely lacking in coordination and aim
• have chronic knee pain
• prefer to set your own schedule rather than rely on teammates

The best thing about basketball is the variety of ways the game can be played. You can shoot hoops alone to practice your aim and ball-handling skills, play one-on-one for a sweaty challenge, get into a pick-up game that's three-on-three for some fast action, or join a league and play organized games with five players on a side plus a referee. There are basketball hoops almost everywhere—in parks, driveways, schoolyards, and gyms across the country. And portable hoops can be easily installed, making this sport one of the simplest to access, whether you live downtown in a concrete jungle or on a farm. There are even hoops for kids and some that change heights to accommodate players of all sizes.

To an older player just learning the ropes, the game may look too intense, especially if you're judging by the professional play you see on television, but you can play at your own level. As your stamina improves, so does your heart health and general fitness. Running up and down the court, even on half-court games, will burn calories at a rapid pace and tone your legs all around. You'll slim down (unless you eat more) and get a firm butt and core from quick changes in direction you must make in order to keep up with the action. And if you get serious about the game, you'll improve your speed and agility as well as your aim, hand/eye coordination, and jumping ability.

Like other court sports, basketball is all about strategy and instinct. You must know when to dribble the ball, when to pass, and when to shoot. You'll stay mentally engaged and won't often find your mind wandering to other matters while you're on the court, making this a terrific game for relieving stress.

Basketball, now one of the most popular sports in the world, was invented in 1891 by gym teacher James Naismith who was tasked with finding indoor-recreation opportunities during the winter at a college in Massachusetts. He mounted peach baskets on the balconies of the gym to act as hoops, and the players used a soccer ball, which had to be retrieved from the peach basket after each goal by someone climbing a ladder. The first games did not allow dribbling, and the players could not move with the ball but instead had to pass it. The women's game, which was started a year later, was even more unusual because women were not supposed to get as much physical activity, and therefore the sport had rules to limit movement, such as dribbling only three times and players not being allowed out of one of three zones. (These rules didn't change until the 1960s.)

SCORE

A 150-pound person shooting baskets burns about 210 calories in an hour (or 1.4 times your weight). The same person practicing basketball for an hour burns about 300 calories (your weight times two). And an hour of competitive basketball burns about 420 calories (or 2.8 times your weight).

The popularity of basketball quickly spread, spurred by the fact that it required little equipment. It was played in YMCAs, on military bases, and in colleges. By 1914, there were 360 colleges fielding teams, although it was quite a few years before rules were standardized and official tournaments were formed. Basketball remains predominantly a winter sport, with games running roughly from November to April for college players as well as men's professional teams. The professional women's teams play in the summer.

The official Olympic history discusses basketball as a question of "who would finish second," as the U.S. men's team has won three-quarters of the gold medals. Professional players from the National Basketball Association (NBA) were allowed to play in the Olympics starting in 1992, when the best American players formed the Dream Team. The women's competition has been less predictable, with serious contenders from several countries, although the U.S. women's team has taken home the last three gold medals.

No matter where it is played—indoors or out, with a couple of players or teams of five—the rules are roughly the same. The object, of course, is to get the ball through the hoop, but how and where you do that determines how many points your team is awarded. Lines on the court indicate how many points you score—a basket made from close to the hoop generally counts for two points; if you sink one from further away, you can earn three points. Fouls such as pushing or holding can result in one, two, or less often, three *foul shots*, also called *free throws*, which are taken from the foul line directly in front of the basket by the fouled player. Each successful shot counts for a point. Outdoor games may be played on a half-court using one basket for both teams, but the traditional

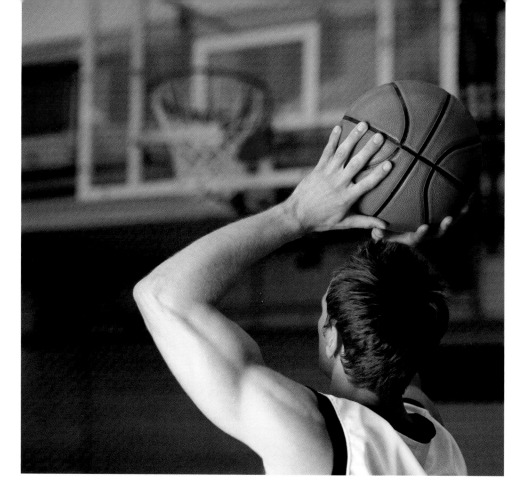

game is played on a full court, with a basket at each end, one per team. After that, depending on who is playing, there are differences in the length of games, number of periods, and height of the basket, among other things.

GEARING UP

A basketball and rim are essential for the game, but easy to find if you don't own one. You can buy a regulation-sized ball in any sporting goods store. In international competition, basketballs must be leather, but molded balls are common elsewhere because they are less expensive and more durable.

Indoors, basketball is generally played in shorts (some players wear compression shorts underneath) and a top—any T-shirt will do. These days, basketball shorts tend to be quite long, with NBA and college players wearing styles that reach to their knees. Recreational players wear anything that doesn't constrict, and since the activity level is intense,

dress lightly. If you need help keeping your hair and sweat off your face, consider wearing a sweatband.

Basketball sneakers are essential. With its quick starts, stops, and pivots, the game is tough on the feet. In the wrong shoes, you are likely to suffer a rolled ankle, blisters, and painful jammed toenails. Most serious players wear high-top sneakers to help support the ankles to prevent strains and sprains. Basketball shoes have excellent traction and stability for lateral movement and sudden stopping. While full-leather styles look sleek, mesh inserts allow more air circulation to keep feet cooler, which also helps avoid blisters. Each player's needs are slightly different, with some combination of cushioning and support plus light weight for speed. Try on a variety of styles until you feel you have an appropriate balance for your feet and playing style. Be sure to jump around when trying on sneakers to check for any spots that rub or shift. And select well-fitting socks that wick moisture away from your feet to help prevent blisters.

YOUR FIRST TIME

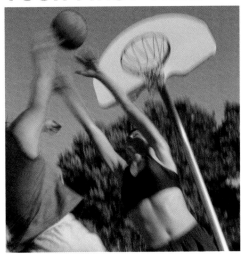

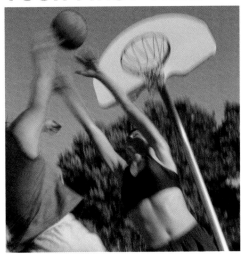

Basketball is a game that you can learn mostly on the court, although it helps to read up on the basic rules and strategies first in a book or online (see Resources). To find a game, inquire at your gym, local YMCA, or YMHA, or town recreation department. You can get into a pick-up game almost anywhere, but be sure the play is somewhere close to your level or you'll be left standing watching the action. Better yet, recruit a few friends to help get some experience on the court.

In a formal recreational league, such as those at the Y, the game will be broken into four eight-minute quarters. The game begins with a *jump ball*: The referee (or, if there's no ref, a player) tosses the ball up in the air and one player from each team tries to gain control of it. Whichever side gets the ball becomes the offense and the other team plays defense. The offensive team then has a set amount of time, typically twenty-four to thirty-five seconds, to attempt a shot on the basket. The time is counted on a *shot clock*, and if a shot hasn't been taken by the time the clock runs out, the ball is given to the other team. Pick-up games may be more informal, without time limits on periods of play or shot clocks, but the basics of play are generally the same. One caveat: Fouls are rarely called in these games because there isn't a referee.

Defense can be played *man-on-man*, when each player guards a specific person on the other team, or *zone*, when the players each defend an area of the court from any offensive players who try to enter it. Zone defense is a necessity in informal play when your team has fewer players than your opposition, but it is also used in regular games because it can be effective for preventing the offensive team from passing well. The team playing defense will try to intercept passes or steal a ball that's being dribbled to gain possession. And when a shot on the basket misses, both teams will scramble to get the rebound and the shot clock is restarted. After a basket is made, the team that had been playing defense gets control of the ball.

The player who has the ball may only run or walk when dribbling it or he gets a violation called *traveling*. When he stops dribbling, he can pivot on one foot to maneuver into a better position to pass or shoot, but can't lift the pivot foot with the ball in his hands. On offense, the team is divided into three positions: Two *guards* generally bring the ball up the court. Two *forwards* play closer to the basket, generally one on each side. The *center*, the tallest person on the team, positions him or herself somewhere between the foul line and the basket.

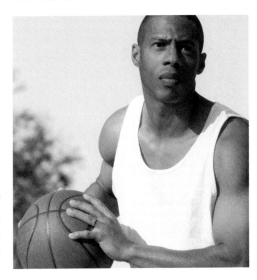

Lynnea Seidlinger, 66

Until she was 55, Lynnea Seidlinger stuck strictly to the sidelines of any sport as a spectator or scorekeeper during her children's games. But when she read a local article about the San Diego Senior Women's Basketball Association, a league for women 50 and older, she liked the idea, figured that it would be good exercise and that she knew plenty about the game from watching, so she went down to the YMCA to try out.

Now it's her children and grandchildren who come to watch her play.

She's won two gold medals and a silver at the national Senior Olympics, and says "I'm a really good player." But unlike her teammates, Seidlinger isn't competitive. "A week later, I can't remember if we've won or lost," she says. "I'm just there for fun and exercise." She also loves meeting the people, making friends, sharing advice about life, but steadfastly ignoring basketball pointers. She just likes to play her own way.

The games aren't what you'd picture from a group of grandmas.

"We play three-on-three, half-court," Seidlinger says. "And it's pretty intense." It took her about three months to build up the stamina to play for ten minutes; now she can play for two hours. Tall and slim, she hadn't felt the need to exercise but, she says, "I always thought that if I could find something that didn't feel like work, I'd do it." Swimming and golf didn't pass the test, but basketball did. She's now been playing three times a week for the last eleven years.

BASKETBALL

TACKLE THE TRUTH

Everyone who plays decently learned as a kid	Childhood experience is not a prerequisite for recreational play. Often, adults who played as kids have bad habits that interfere with their abilities. Learning from scratch means you won't have to unlearn poor technique in order to pick up the proper way to play. Also, adults generally play smarter, by not trying to overpower their opponents but instead by out-thinking them.
You have to be a good shooter to play basketball	Scoring is an essential part of basketball, but not everyone on the team has to do it in every game. Some players excel at defense, assisting and rebounding, which can be just as important as adding to the score directly. A team must include a variety of talents— everyone can't be the star shooter.
You have to be fast to play basketball well	Speed certainly can be an asset on the court, but a lack of it shouldn't deter you from playing. Many players find they get quicker as they learn the game, and others appear to be faster as they become better able to anticipate the movements on the court and maneuver into an advantageous position in time to make a great play.

SECRETS TO SUCCESS

The main trick in basketball is suppressing your ego, says Sean Green, a trainer at the Sports Center at Chelsea Piers who spent four years in the NBA and six years playing professionally overseas. In many ways, it's the ego that stands in the way of becoming a good player on the team—and he doesn't just mean because athletes would rather shoot than pass the ball. He's also talking about improving your skills. "You have to practice the thing you stink at," says Green. "We all want to focus on what we're good at, but if you're a good shooter, don't work only on your shot." By putting the training time toward the areas that need improvement, you gain the most. Unfortunately, adults especially

don't like to look bad, but in fact, it's a necessary aspect of development.

"Don't keep repeating a skill the wrong way and hope it will improve," says Green. "Ask for help; expose your weakness to someone good, and get better by learning to do it correctly." Then practice the new technique over and over again. The process, he says, is humbling, but it's the best way to turn into an exceptional player.

In addition to specific skills in shooting, strategy, and ball-handling, you can improve your game by working on your balance and agility. Most of the time, you won't have the ball, which means you need to be prepared for the next move.

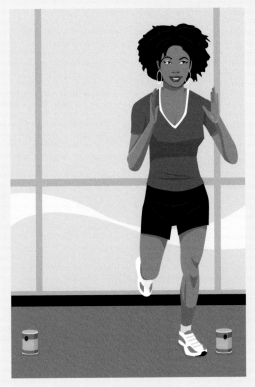

jump and stick

Place two marks on the ground (coins, chalk marks, soup cans) about 3 feet apart, or further if you're tall. Stand between the marks, your left foot up against the left mark. Bend your knees into a slight crouch, torso leaning forward a bit, hands in front of your chest as if holding a basketball, head up. Explode into the air to the right, landing on your right foot just inside the right mark, your left leg hovering in the air, your body in the same crouch position. Immediately jump with your left leg to the left marker, letting your right leg hover. You've completed 1 repetition. Start with 3 sets of 10 reps, concentrating on form over speed so your knees and hips absorb the impact of the landings, and your butt and thighs do the work. Build to 3 sets of 30 reps.

Any time you're standing tall, you're not ready to move rapidly. Instead, keep your knees slightly bent. In the same way, don't put your hands on your hips during a game because they're not ready to play in that position. Keep your legs primed for quick movement by setting them shoulder-width apart with one foot in front of the other. Work on this stance and repeat moves you'll need such as pivoting, passing and receiving the ball, and shooting starting from the proper body position and returning to it after you make a move. This type of practice will improve your agility and quickness on the court, contributing to your success.

Another factor that can elevate your game to the next level is jumping ability. You'll jump for rebounds, to block shots your opponents are trying to make, and to make your own shots. While the average recreational player need not levitate to stuff the ball through the rim like a pro, working on the spring in your step can improve your abilities and also make you faster on your feet. Try jumping rope, footwork drills, and increasing the height on your jumping jacks.

Try these exercises to build explosive leg strength for running and jumping plus core strength for quick stops and starts.

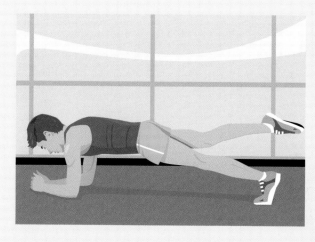

super plank

Start in plank position: From your hands and knees, lower to your elbows so they are directly under your shoulders; extend your legs to rest on your toes, forming a straight line from head to heels. Once you are solidly in position, raise your right foot off the floor slightly, keeping your hips even. If you're able to, also lift your left arm, extending it straight out in the opposite direction from your feet at shoulder height. Hold for as long as you can, up to 30 seconds. Then lower your limbs and repeat on the opposite side. Build up to 3 sets of 1 repetition, resting in between.

GET MORE FROM YOUR SPORT

Basketball players often do jumping and running sports to improve their leg strength, balance, and jumping ability. Try trail running to improve ankle stability, balance, body awareness, and speed. Other court sports are great for crosstraining, especially volleyball, which has a lot of overlap in technique and teamwork.

In addition to joining adult leagues, you can attend camps to get intensive coaching and opportunities to play day after day. One group, Never Too Late (www.nevertoolate.com), runs weekend camps during the off-season (April through October) with plenty of coaching, lots of games, and a videotaped review of your skills. To improve your shooting skills, take a day or two of lessons from coach Hal Wissel, who also helps NBA players; his Shoot It Better Mini Camps are run around the country and can be arranged for your group (www.basketballworld.com).

RESOURCES

➡ **www.guidetocoachingbasketball.com** is geared towards coaches, but this site provides excellent advice for players on topics such as stance and dribbling.

➡ **www.hoopsvibe.com** is top-heavy with information about the NBA, but click on the "coaching" section to find explanations of referees' hand signals, passing tips, and a program for improving your vertical jump.

➡ **www.usabasketball.com** has a chart comparing some of the main rules variations for international, professional, and college games.

➡ *Basketball Steps for Success* by Hal Wissel offers instruction on the basics of basketball as well as tips for correcting common errors.

➡ *Basketball Fundamentals* by Jon Oliver covers the skills you need to play and includes drills, strategies, and rules.

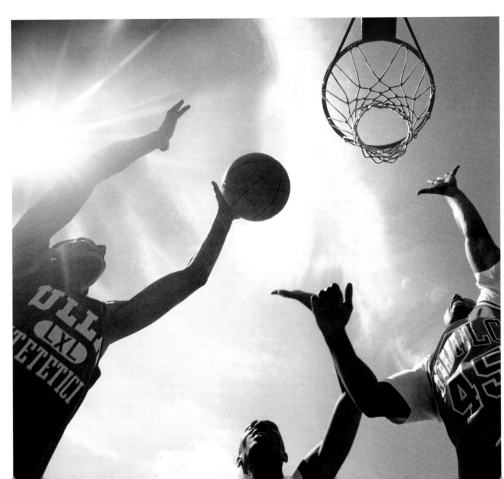

Fitness for Your Feet

About two-thirds of Americans think it's normal for their feet to hurt. Perhaps that explains why few of us ever see a podiatrist even though 75 percent of us have experienced foot pain at some point in our lives. The irony is that while we lace up to protect our feet, shoes actually cause damage, from blisters to bunions and more serious conditions such as nerve pain called a *neuroma*.

Even a small foot injury can sideline your sports ambitions and fitness goals. And, a small problem with your foot can often create bigger problems elsewhere in the body. As you imperceptibly adjust your body mechanics to avoid aggravating the sore spot, you can trigger aches in your back, hips, and other areas.

The simple solution is to wear shoes that fit—and while you may think your shoes do fit, chances are good that they don't. Adult feet spread, changing size and shape as we age. When shopping for shoes, you need to get the width and length of both feet measured. Also, always try on the left and right shoe because it's normal to have one foot that's larger than the other. Buy to fit the larger foot. If the smaller one feels like it's moving around too much, get an insole for a snug fit.

Try on many brands until you find the most comfortable shape and size for your foot. The heel should be snug and your toes should have room to wiggle. Most athletic shoes should fit comfortably right out of the box, not need to be broken in. The exceptions are rock climbing shoes, thick leather hiking boots and figure skates. Use moleskin or gel-filled padding to protect points of friction (called *hot spots*).

Your shoes should have sufficient arch support. There shouldn't be a large gap or uncomfortable pressure under your arch. If you find a shoe that fits well in all aspects except the arch, try replacing the insoles.

You don't need a specific pair of sneakers for every sport. For a variety of sports you play every once in a while, an all-around shoe called a crosstrainer will serve you well. But if you start putting in more time or distance, focusing on a particular sport, look for shoes designed for that activity. If you play several sports often, consider a closet of three pairs: one designed for forward motion (such as a running shoe), one court shoe for side-to-side motion (for basketball, tennis, soccer, etc.) and a crosstrainer that can handle varied activities such as a cardio class.

The next priority is socks. Cushioning often gets top billing, but thinner is generally better—even for cold-weather sports. Thick socks tend to bunch up and cause your feet to sweat. The result is a damp lump of material under your foot that can cause a blister. And, with ski boots, for example, extra material may feel warmer at first, but it may reduce circulation, leaving your feet colder and at risk for frostbite. Also, if your feet sweat while you ski and then cool during the ride on the lift, the damp, sweaty socks will cause a chill. For moisture management, look for synthetic socks that wick sweat away from your feet and dry quickly. Cotton athletic socks are a poor choice for any sport.

With the right socks and shoes, you should be spared many foot problems. But if you do succumb, don't just live with it. For blisters, corns, calluses, and warts, clean and cover the area with a Band Aid. Do not pop blisters or you risk infection. Any condition that doesn't improve within a few days should be evaluated by a doctor.

More tips for pain-free feet:

* Always wear flip-flops in the locker room to avoid athlete's foot and warts, which thrive on the damp floor.

* Wash and dry feet daily, especially between the toes. Never put lotion between toes.

* Alternate shoes to give your feet variety and let your footwear air out and dry.

* If you find a style of shoe that is comfortable, stick with it even if it's expensive. Owning the right shoes will always be cheaper than a lot of doctor's bills.

* Don't buy shoes online unless you've worn the same exact pair and know it fits well.

* Replace shoes at least once a year, even if you don't wear them often. The materials break down over time.

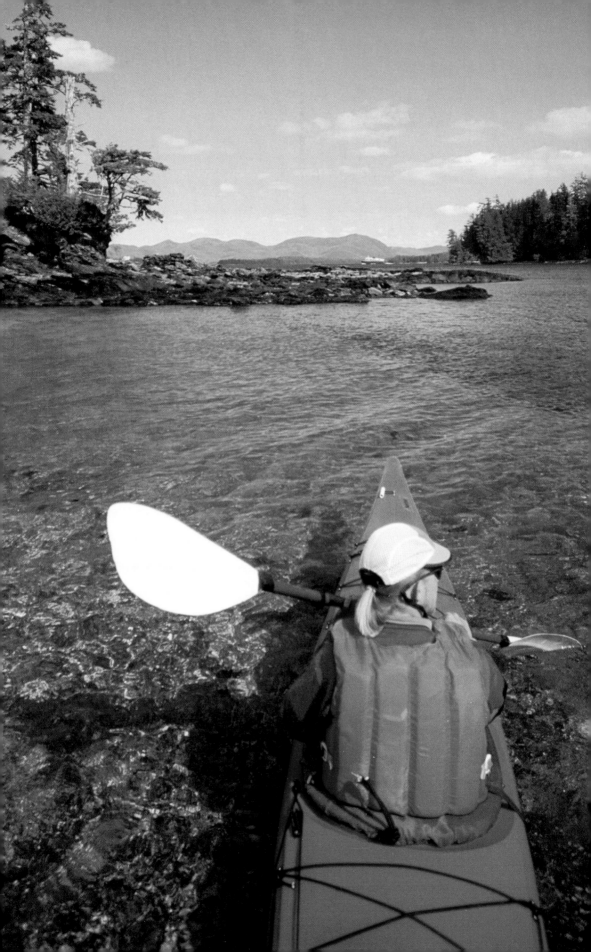

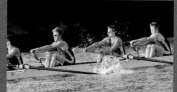

6

BOATING:
ROWING AND KAYAKING

YOU'LL LOVE THESE SPORTS IF YOU:
- want to improve your stamina, strength, and balance
- prefer to work every muscle in your body with one activity
- want an intense calorie-burn without high impact
- enjoy being out on the water in a boat
- want to have so much fun you won't know you're exercising
- enjoy having the option for camaraderie or going out alone
- love activities that are graceful and yet intense
- enjoy competition

YOU MIGHT NOT LOVE THESE SPORTS IF YOU:
- don't have access to water
- can't swim—you need to be able to stay afloat in case you capsize
- don't like to navigate
- can't carry the boat to the water

There's something serene about being on the water, even if you're pulling so hard your arms ache and your heart is pounding. That's part of the beauty of boating in a rowing shell or kayak. But those who truly love these sports wax poetic about the glide. These boats are very different, but they share one main feature: You sit low, with a thin hull between you and the water, feeling the swells underneath your seat. And when the oars or paddles slice through, grab, and propel you, the boat lifts up slightly and flies. With proper form, every ounce of your energy is translated into motion, and the feeling is exhilarating. This glide is one of the main differences between these sports and a row in a rowboat, canoeing, or sailing.

Intense effort means major rewards in calories burned and cardiovascular fitness. These sports deliver tremendous payoff because they use a lot of muscle. And both sports are low impact, which means your joints are protected from abuse.

Another characteristic the two sports have in common is balance. It's easy to capsize in a slim, long boat that's low to the water. If you prefer to stay in the boat, you quickly learn that although balance starts in your hips, every other part of your body plays a role as well. Even moving your head too far in the wrong direction can send you swimming. While some boats such as sea kayaks and racing shells with four or more rowers, are designed to be more stable, you need to work harder to keep the boat balanced in thinner models and smaller boats that hold one or two people. And although you can kayak and row alone— and plenty of people do—many boating enthusiasts enjoy having camaraderie. Being out on the river or lake with fellow rowers or paddlers means sharing the highlights of the scenery around you and having others to help shoulder the burden, including carrying the boat to and from the shore or dock. Also, boats can be expensive, which is why it's helpful to join a group that already owns them. Rowing or paddling together, you can cover for one another when fatigued and coax one another to go faster or longer distances. And the chances are good you'll get a better workout because of your companions.

SCORE

Rowing tends to be done at a fairly intense pace, which is why an hour burns about 660 calories for a 150-pound person (or 4.4 times your body weight). If the same person takes a more leisurely row, he will burn about 360 calories in an hour (or 2.4 times your body weight). The average recreational kayaker who weighs 150 will burn 240 calories in an hour (1.6 times your weight). By comparison, rowing in a rowboat burns about 150 calories per hour for a 150 pound person (or one time your weight).

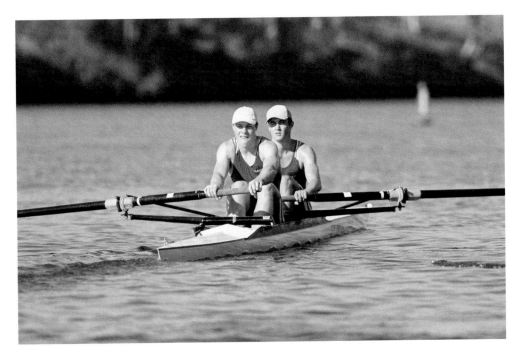

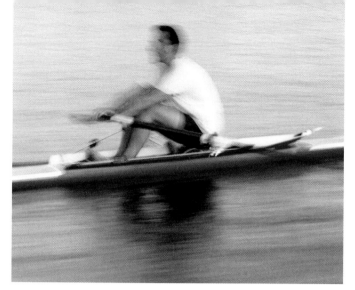
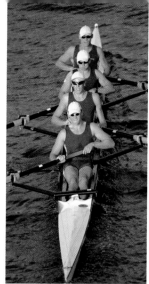

ROWING

You can row in any rowboat with oarlocks and oars, but the type of exercise you get in a dinghy is as unrelated to rowing in a shell as hamburger is to filet mignon. Unlike the average rowboat, a racing shell is typically not much wider than your hips, with a *foot stretcher* attached to the bottom of the hull, in which you secure your feet, and a seat on runners called a *slide*.

Although rowers are sometimes said to be part of a *crew*, one never goes *crewing*. In a shift in jargon, you now belong to a *rowing team* and not a *crew team*. There are two distinct types of rowing: sculling and sweeps. In sculling, each rower has two oars, one on either side of the boat. In sweeps, each rower has one longer oar that is held with both hands, and with few exceptions, the oar sides alternate from one seat to the next. As in rowboats, the rowers sit with their backs facing the direction of travel. (Port oars are on your right, starboard on your left—the reverse of what you'd expect because you are traveling backward.)

Sculling shells are singles, doubles, and quadruples (quads), or—rarely—an octuple. Sweeps shells are typically pairs, fours, and eights. Eights will have a *coxswain* (pronounced cox-en, but usually shortened to *cox*) who steers the boat and provides motivation and feedback. Singles and doubles don't have a cox but pairs, fours and quads may be *straight* (uncoxed) or *coxed*. In most boats, the cox sits in the stern facing the rowers, but

some shells have an almost-hidden dugout for the cox in the bow. Coxed boats don't row against noncoxed boats, as the weight differential would make the competition uneven. And although the coxswain doesn't row, she typically trains with the team when doing land workouts as a sign of solidarity. In boats that don't have a cox, one rower must steer, usually the bowman, by turning around to watch the course and controlling the rudder with a wire that runs to one foot.

Rowing started out as a necessary method of transportation for shore dwellers in ancient civilizations such as Egypt, Greece, and Rome, and later developed into a competition. The earliest known races date back to the 13th century in Venice, but the British brought the sport to its full potential starting in the early 18th century. The famous collegiate rivalry between Oxford and Cambridge began in 1829, followed by that of Harvard and Yale in 1852. Rowing was on the roster for the first modern Olympics in 1896 but had to be cancelled because of rough seas. The first medals were awarded in 1900. Women's events were added in 1976.

In the U.S., all large multiteam rowing races are referred to as *regattas*. *Head races*, such as the famous Head of the Charles in Cambridge, Massachusetts, use a staggered start and boats are timed, so the winner is not obvious. These races are held in the fall and winter and consist of a minimum distance of 2,000 meters (slightly less than a mile) but most are about three miles and can be far longer. To begin the race, the boats power up to the starting line at full speed. Spring and summer races are run in a head-to-head format, where all the boats line up together and begin racing from a dead stop; truncated strokes are used to increase speed quickly. These races

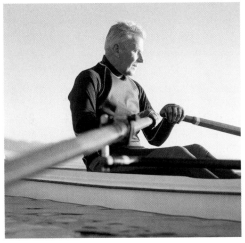

typically last 2,000 meters, but may be as short as half that distance. It's unusual to see more than six boats in one race at a time, but there may have to be a number of rounds to eliminate crews along the way to finals.

The pace of races is taxing. The motions remain controlled but strong and fast; precision is necessary to reduce drag and maximize power. The rowers are at a full-tilt sprint for the entire race, which is why rowing is one of the most intense sports. Training is oriented toward increasing aerobic capacity as well as the ability to sprint for the long haul, making rowers some of the fittest athletes—with a reputation for dedication that borders on obsession.

Races may be divided into some combination of categories by experience, age, gender, and weight (lightweights, who must all be under a certain weight—generally no more than 160 pounds for men and 130 pounds for women—and heavyweights). For example, you might have an LW8+, a light-

weight women's eight with cox. Some races now feature fun events as well, such as parent-child categories. As in other sports with weight categories, some rowers engage in unhealthy weight-loss techniques to stay in the lightweight categories.

GEARING UP

Crew shells are expensive, which is why it's good news that you don't need to buy a single one. To get access to shells, look for a community rowing club in your area (check the yellow pages or wander around the shore to scope out the scene) or ask at the closest college for information about area groups.

When you sign up for a rowing program, you don't need much gear. You won't even be wearing shoes in the boat, so wear a pair you can kick off easily and won't mind leaving on the dock. However, it's advisable to wear socks to avoid blisters. Clothing typically includes skin-tight shorts called *trou* (bike shorts work fine) and a tank top or T-shirt. Elite rowers wear a sleek *unisuit*. If the weather is cool, add a pair of close-fitting sweatpants and a jacket. For rain, you can wear a lightweight waterproof shell, but you'll likely be more comfortable just getting wet (as a novice, you'll probably get splashed anyway). Your top needs to stay clear of the seat's slide, so the best ones can be tucked in or fall at your waist or higher. Baggy bottoms will also get fouled in the wheels, so keep the profile slim. If your group uses older boats, your calves will make contact with the slide with each stroke, which can cause tears or dark marks on the backs of your pant legs. Newer boats have virtually eliminated this problem. Although rowers are prone to blisters on their hands from turning the oar(s) with every stroke, they almost never wear gloves because the material compromises the grip. When you're starting out, or if you don't row often enough to form calluses, you may want protection for your hands. Consider making a wrap using a long piece of thin medical tape between each finger and then secure the strips by wrapping the tape around your hand just below the knuckles. Make the wrap tight enough that it won't shift without restricting your ability to grip. Leave finger rings home, if possible.

As a general rule, you shouldn't bring gear into the boat. That being said, do tote along a small water bottle. And on sunny days, consider adding a cap (unless it's windy) or sunglasses to protect against the glare on the water.

YOUR FIRST TIME

First-timers typically sign up for a learn-to-row program at a boathouse. While you probably want to get right out in a boat, the stroke mechanics are complex and it's easier to learn elsewhere, if another option is available. There are three good choices: a rowing machine, which rowers call an *erg* (short for ergometer); a tank, which is a shallow pool with a fixed faux boat and skeleton oars; or a barge, a double eight with a platform in the middle for the coach. When you first actually row in a shell, the experience will go like this: As the rowers gather at the boathouse, spend some time stretching. When everyone is present, the coach will assign seats starting with number one in the bow and up to eight (the stern pair and bow pair are often coveted spots). Next, you'll carry the oars down to the dock. Then the rowers will gather at the boat and the cox (or bow in a coxless boat) will call commands to lift the boat, carry it, and place it in the water. Boats are heavy and expensive, and there is no chatting allowed from the time you first lay hands on the boat— serious crews don't talk again until the boat is back in the boathouse.

Once the boat is in the water, one person holds it close to the dock while the others

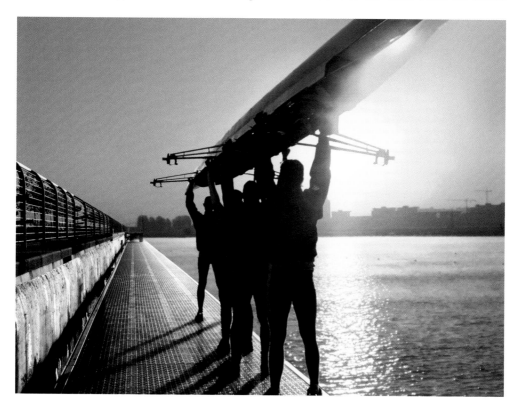

secure the oars in place. The cox or bowman will then supervise everyone getting in, the push-off, and the maneuvers to get the boat a safe distance from the dock (a tad tricky, but they'll explain how). After that, with your oar(s) tucked under your arms, you'll slide up and adjust your foot stretchers to the proper position, securing your feet and doing any other checks or adjustments you need; then indicate you're ready. In the interim, you may need to take an occasional stroke if the boat is drifting to an undesirable location (if your boat is coxed, only do this when asked). If a coach will be on the water with you, he usually rides in a small motorboat called a *launch*.

The first rows are done in small groups, with some oarsmen sitting still with their oars resting on the water to keep the boat set. The rowing motion is far from intuitive. You start at the *finish*, the end of the stroke, with your legs flat, torso leaning back slightly, hands near your chest, elbows tight, and oar blade(s) parallel to the water. First you push your arms straight out and follow with your back without moving the slide at all. When your hands are over your shins, your knees start to come up as you turn the oar(s) to *square* (you'll probably row *on the square* at first without turning the oar, called *feathering*). When you are in a fully compressed position at the front of the slide, you lift your hands slightly to bury the blade(s) in the water, which is called the *catch*, and immediately start to reverse the stroke, driving the legs down without changing position in the upper body, then opening the back, and last, drawing in the arms as your legs come flat. At the finish, you slightly lower your hands to lift the oar(s) from the water, turning them so the blade(s) feather to the flat position for reduced wind resistance.

The pattern of the stroke conveys your energy into the oar(s) efficiently because your legs hold the most power. By keeping your back and arms in position as the legs drive, you hang on the oar, putting every ounce of leg strength into the stroke. Keeping

your arms extended as you open your back serves the same purpose. And finally, your relatively weak arms complete the stroke, letting the boat run as you return up the slide, which is called the *recovery*.

When you row, you follow the person in front of you, doing each part of the stroke exactly when she does. If you move up the slide more quickly, the boat will wobble. If you catch first, the boat will dip. The rowers in a boat should move as one, with the oars making a single splash. The rower in the stern, called the *stroke*, sets the pace and everyone else must match it.

Listening to directions and working together is vital in rowing. The cox, or bowman, and coach must direct the boat safely around obstacles such as rocks, the shoreline, and water traffic. In addition to the rudder, the boat is controlled by commands to the rowers to pull harder on one side, which you must hear and heed. To rotate the boat, you may need to hold the oars steady on one side, square in the water, and row on the other side or row backward (pushing the oar forward in the water instead of pulling it) on one side and forward on the other. Commands will be called by seat number or the side of the boat, as in "ports to row, starboards back."

Even with some rowers sitting still to set the boat, early rows will include the boat flopping from side to side because of a lousy set, making the oars slap the surface rather than moving smoothly through the air. This causes a sensation of instability as you try to stroke and recover. Don't let this deter you from the sport, even if it lasts for weeks. As you and your teammates learn to balance your bodies and hold your hand heights steady, the boat will settle and you'll feel the rush as it slices through the water. The cox (or bowman) and coach will help by suggesting who needs to move their hands in which direction, so be sure to pay close attention to this seemingly minute detail of instruction. It makes all the difference.

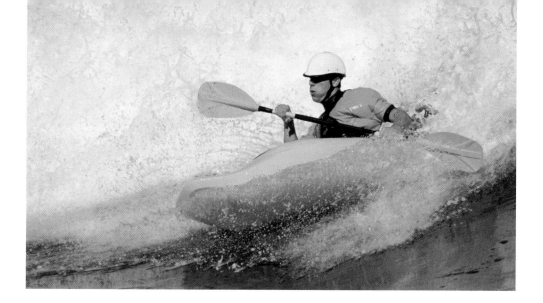

KAYAKING

From a placid paddle on the smooth waters of a pond to whipping down a white-water river, kayaking is a sport that can match any mood or personality. It takes just a few minutes to master the basic stroke. And while it takes longer to become comfortable with the more exhilarating and energetic style of whitewater kayaking, an athletic person with good swimming skills can learn the introductory techniques quickly.

Kayaking is an excellent workout because you tend to stay out for hours, getting far more exercise than you do in the average gym session. With proper technique, you'll work every muscle from the hips up, firming your core intensely and developing strong shoulder and arm muscles. Depending on your route, you may also portage your kayak over obstacles, which adds to the physical demands. And while kayaking is generally thought not to involve the leg and butt muscles, some of the advanced tricks such as flips can be full-body maneuvers. No matter which style of kayaking you do, your body awareness will improve as you use small adjustments to balance the boat. The back-to-nature aspect of the sport also provides an opportunity for soothing the psyche.

Kayaks were originally used by Eskimos in the Arctic areas of Greenland and North America for hunting, fishing, and transportation. The first boats were made from the skins of sea lions, which were stretched over frames made of bone and wood and then rubbed with whale blubber to form a waterproof coating. Inuits would sew their coats to the kayaks to create a water-proof seal for protection from frigid waters.

Kayaks, which have a closed top called a deck, are considered a cold-water variation of a canoe. But there are also other differences. Canoe paddlers operate in a kneeling position, using a single-blade paddle, while kayakers sit with their legs extended forward and use a paddle that has a blade at either end. Canoeing became somewhat popular as a sport during the mid-1800s, with the founding of the Royal Canoe Club of London by a barrister-turned-travel-writer named John MacGregor, and shortly thereafter the New York Canoe Club was founded.

Canoeing—including kayaking races—became a full Olympic sport in 1936. Today, male Olympians race in either canoe or kayak events, while women race only in kayaks (yet the women's sport is still called the Olympic canoe event). Kayak racers compete in singles, doubles, and quads. Olympic kayak flatwater races, which are conducted in lanes, are as much as 10,000 meters long (that's a 10K or about 6.2 miles), but modern competitions (including the Olympics) involve much shorter races, from 200 to 1,000 meters. These racers line up together at the start and paddle all-out in a straight line to the finish.

Whitewater racing is a considerably newer sport and only started in 1933, not making it into the Olympics until 1972—and then not again until 1992. The slalom races require competitors to maneuver around gates in whitewater, with some marked to be negotiated against the current, so that competitors must be able to turn, stop, and maneuver in a circuitous path while getting bounced about by rapids. The kayaker's score is based on the time it takes to complete the run, as well as penalties for missing or hitting the gates. In the U.S., whitewater is divided into ratings, with the calmest at Class 1 and the most treacherous at Class 6. Whitewater paddlers wear helmets and life jackets.

Outside the Olympics, some kayakers compete in events such as *paddlecross* and *kayak rodeo*. For example, at the Teva Mountain Games in Vail, Colorado, there are two rodeo events in which paddlers perform tricks such as flips and cartwheels in short, highly maneuverable boats. Rodeo is also called *playboating* and does not involve much of a course but instead has specific spots where tricks are performed. In paddlecross, a small group of kayakers bombs down a narrow run in a flurry of crashing paddles. Another event at the Teva games, the *Eight-ball sprint*, pits paddlers against guards in boats who attempt to knock them out of the course.

Aside from competitions, many people enjoy kayak excursions. Touring around lakes, wetlands, and rivers is a fun way to spend a day exploring. Sea kayaks are designed for slightly rougher waters off the coast, allowing you to travel to nearby islands, cliffs, and caves or secluded beaches. Some kayak tourists also go bird-watching, fishing, camping, or hiking in conjunction with their paddling trips.

GEARING UP

Kayaks can be a reasonable purchase, with introductory plastic models sold for a few hundred dollars at sporting goods stores and even wholesale clubs. But that's no reason to rush right out and purchase one. Renting a boat for a few outings will help you make some good decisions when you're ready to buy. Kayaks come in a number of different styles—touring, open-water, whitewater, sit-on, playboating, even folding and inflatable styles, and more—as well as various materials, proportions, and configurations, such as tandems and singles. And while there aren't quite as many styles and materials for paddles, there are enough to suggest delaying your decision until you've settled on a style of boating and have tested some gear.

You can rent everything you need, from life jackets (called *personal floatation devices* or *PFDs*) to wetsuits for cold water runs. A kayaking jacket, worn under the PFD, has closures at the neck and wrists to snug down and help keep water out. And for many types of kayaking, you'll wear a *spray skirt*—a stretchy device that you secure around your waist to create a closed seal when attached around the cockpit after you're seated in the kayak, keeping water out of the boat. You may also wear a helmet.

Rental shops may not provide kayaking gloves for rental, so if you'd like a little extra protection against blisters, pick up a pair. For your first time out, you can wear bike gloves. Wear quick-dry clothes such as a bathing suit and water shoes, so you can wade into the water to get going. Leave on shore anything that reach forward slightly from the hips, extending both arms. Tip both arms to the right, digging the right blade into the water and pulling back using your arm, shoulder, and upper back muscles while bending your right elbow and pressing your left hand forward to the right to push the paddle away. Now draw the left hand

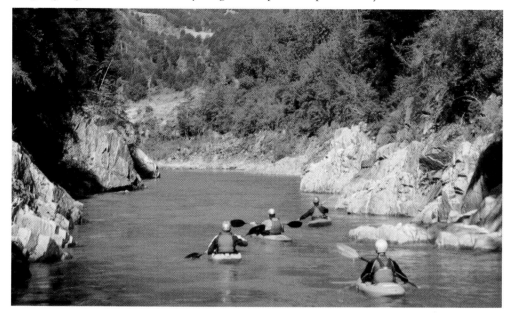

can't get wet or shouldn't get lost. Wear sunscreen and consider bringing a water bottle and sunglasses or a cap that you won't mind losing. A waterproof disposable camera is a nice idea, too, for recording the event. Get one with a rubber-band strap so you can secure it around your upper arm, out of the way.

YOUR FIRST TIME

Your first kayaking experience depends on the style you choose: flatwater or whitewater. For a calm excursion, you probably won't wear a spray skirt. You'll simply grab your paddle and get into the boat (stay low and centered). You can do it in shallow water and simply paddle off, or try getting in with the boat partly on the shore and then push in with your hands or hop on your butt. Next, practice stroking with the paddle. Grasp the paddle with a wide grip and

across and down to the left while pressing up and forward with the right hand to repeat the motion on your left side. Your torso will flex, side to side, as you move, using your abdominals to keep the boat from rocking too much so you won't capsize.

For whitewater kayaking, you'll want an instructor or an experienced friend to show you the techniques and accompany you for safety. The excursion starts much the same way, except that you'll wear a spray skirt and need to learn the *wet exit* in case you turn over. To do the exit, which happens when you are upside down in the water, you reach around to find the front loop of the skirt, tug forward and up to free it, then place both hands on the sides of the cockpit and push out. After that, grab the boat and find your paddle. You can then try to get to a shallow spot to get back into the boat. You can also try to learn an *Eskimo roll*, which is a complex maneuver to right yourself without unhooking the skirt and exiting the boat. This skill is best learned in a lesson in a pool because it is tricky, and the learning process leaves you at risk from fatigue while underwater—also, submerged rocks are not helpful.

Whichever style of kayak excursion you choose, first, rock your hips, move your legs, reach in all directions, and get a feel for how the boat balances while you're still in calm, shallow water. You may need this training later to intuitively correct your set and avoid flipping the boat.

One advantage to making your first foray with an outfitter is that he will map the route to make a loop or arrange transportation from the destination back to your car.

ATHLETE IN ACTION

**Jane Carmody, 48
Michael Carmody, 49**

Jane and Michael Carmody started rowing in 2003 as an almost accidental goodwill gesture. Their son, Sean, had recently joined his high-school team. Then Jane went to a meeting of the local Pelham Community Rowing Association (PCRA) in Pelham, NY. She heard that the fledgling club needed to fill its adult classes. To share the sport with Sean, Michael reluctantly followed Jane's suggestion to sign up. "I knew it was hard, and the first six-week course lived up to every bad expectation I had," says Michael. "Practice was held at 6:30 A.M. on Saturdays and Sundays and nobody in the boat knew how to row, so it flopped side to side."

Jane had a better time. "I thought it was a great thing almost at once," she says. "The women bonded immediately." The couple did the indoor workouts all winter, returned to the water in the spring, and encouraged their daughter Megan to take up rowing over the summer. "So now I couldn't beg off," says Michael. "And we were more confident." The parents switched to sculling in the second season, which they found to be an easy transition.

Then, in mid-June, the coach asked Michael if he and Sean would row in a parent/child race in the Independence Day Regatta in Philadelphia. "For the two weeks before the race, I'd leave work a little early and meet Sean as he came off the water with his school team to go out on the lagoon with me," says Michael, a lawyer with his own firm in New York. Jane was proud. "Michael was the first adult in our program to race, and it was a turning point for all of us to realize that we could be training to race," she says. The Carmody men didn't set any speed records, but the family and their teammates had a great time, because, like all regattas, there were plenty of fans, picnics, and an air of festivity that is infectious.

Jane entered her first race in the fall. Again with little notice, she put together a quad that hastily scheduled extra practices and had a decent race. "We didn't win any medals, but we didn't come in last either—and to go from not knowing what a port oar was to doing OK, it was a nice accomplishment," says Jane. "If we weren't hooked before then, we were after it."

A year later, Jane and Michael competed together in a mixed double. "We teased that we'd get on the water at noon, race at twelve-thirty and meet the divorce attorney at two," says Jane. And while they finished ahead of a few other boats, "the next event was already coming down the river," recalls Jane. But they enjoyed the day—and the Carmody clan has gained much more than race standings from the season. Michael lost twenty-five pounds, Jane is in spectacular shape (her nontraditional lawyer's hours allow her to row in the afternoons), and, more important, they share a great family experience. The adults are on the parents' committees for Sean's school and PCRA, and Jane is on the PCRA board. When Michael can't get home in time for practice, Megan often takes her dad out for a late row. And when Megan entered the indoor rowing ergometer race called the Crash-Bs, Michael was able to coach her through the grueling event. Megan is now being scouted by college crew teams, with the potential for a scholarship.

As for future regattas, "we could get the Carmody quad into a race," says Michael. "Megan and Sean are really good, and I want to get better, which happens sitting behind them. I know what it means to row well, because I've been in the boat with my family."

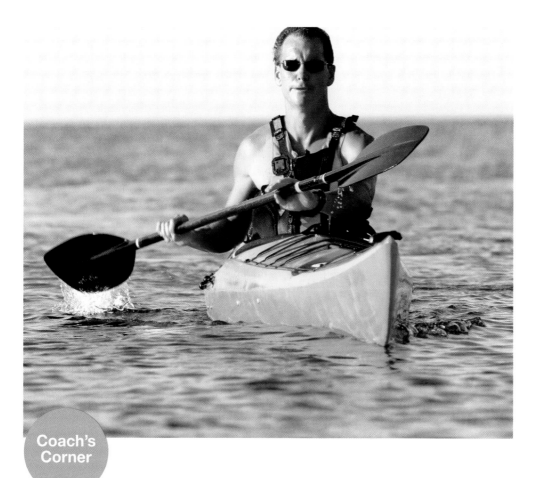

SECRETS TO SUCCESS

One reason that rowers and kayakers are often in prime physical condition is that these sports inspire passion, which brings commitment and intense training. When you're starting out, keep in mind that these sports can be addictive, because the strenuous activity paired with rhythmic repetitive motion delivers a strong meditative euphoria, like an intense runner's high. While you don't have to be competitive to row or kayak, the focus for rowing, in particular, tends to center on the events—perhaps to keep you going through tough practices, or because the feeling of the boat flying through the water is such a mental rush. But you can have a relaxing experience on the water if you pick your group carefully, or go solo.

Rowers pride themselves on being tough, and part of the culture is a predawn practice schedule. Many learn-to-row programs maintain the early hours, in part because it takes time to row and 6 A.M. is the best way to fit it in before work and school obligations. But there are also programs with afternoon and evening hours for rowers at every level. And watch for the U.S. Rowing annual Learn to Row Day, which takes place at schools and clubs across the country every June (www.usrowing.org).

A leisurely kayak outing takes less preparation and not as many participants as the typical row, making it easier to slip one in at any time. Kayaking is also easier to learn for those who just want to paddle around and have fun. "Most people can jump in and get from point to point in one session," says Melanie M. Onufrieff, head coach for the women's team at Columbia

University and a recreational kayaker. "And after that, you can spend years honing your paddling technique to take on white-water or competition."

In contrast, rowing is more challenging to learn and then demands intense physical training if you want to excel. "In a stable boat, you can get the basics in a single lesson," says Onufrieff, "but it will take a number of sessions before you're ready to add power to your stroke." And the longer the duration between lessons, the more you forget, so it helps to practice on a rowing machine in between. "If you go once a week, you could be ready to race by the end of the season," she says. But like the Carmody family, you should go to your first regattas for the fun of it, not with the expectation of winning a medal, because you'll be pitted against rowers

with years of experience and daily training routines.

For the best experience as a novice, look for a program that offers instruction using boats designed for the purpose. You need a stable boat to understand the stroke mechanics and not be panicked about falling in. If you are learning solo, a single scull or kayak with a wide hull is the least likely to flip. When it comes to capsizing, kids have an advantage, because they generally don't mind going for a swim.

Try to relax and be patient on your first few outings. If you push for speed and power, you're more likely to flail or flip. To learn the stroke properly and avoid aches later, be very careful to follow instructions. Both of these sports have subtle techniques that protect you from

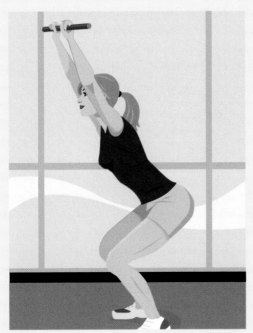

stick squat

Hold a stick such as a broom handle with an overhand grip, hands shoulder-width apart. Lift your arms overhead, drawing your shoulderblades together and pressing the stick as far back as you can. Stand with your legs hip distance apart, weight balanced on both feet. Holding the stick in position, keep your head up and abs firm as you bend your knees as far as you comfortably can, as if you were about to sit in a chair. Press down through your heels and squeeze your glutes as you return to standing. Start with 12 reps. Build up to 3 sets of 15 reps.

injury and maximize your staying power—and they aren't intuitive.

To do land training that improves your performance in the boat, try any exercise that involves sitting on a ball to hone balance, as well as cardio routines that emphasize duration and shifting intensity. The rowing machine is great training for both sports, as long as you get good coaching so you can do it properly. Work on 2,000-meter sessions, which will take about fifteen minutes for most beginners; competitors do it in less than ten. For both sports, tone your core, back, shoulders, and arms. For rowing, work on explosive leg strength with jumping exercises.

Try these two exercises to improve your stability and strength in the boat:

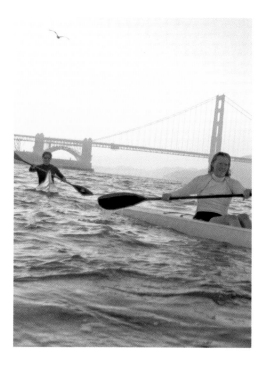

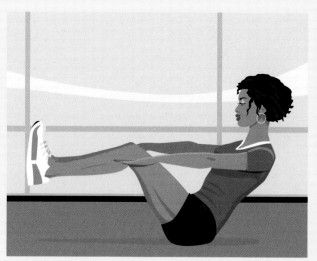

v seat

Sit on the ground with your knees bent, feet flat on the floor. Lean back slightly, keeping your back erect and head up. Press your legs together, then lift your feet until your shins are parallel to the floor. Reach your arms towards your feet. Press your feet out and simultaneously lower your torso back down as far as you can without touching the floor. Contract your abs to return to the start position. Do 10 to 20 repetitions. Build up to 3 sets of 30 reps.

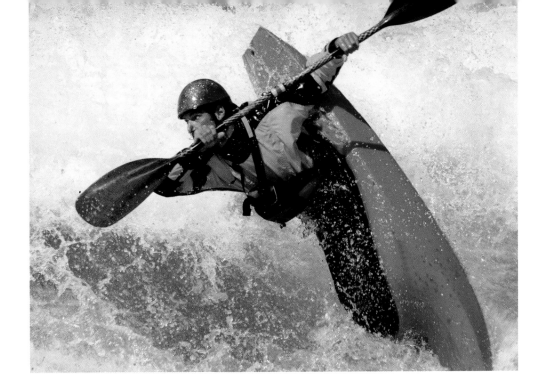

TACKLE THE TRUTH

I'll definitely capsize if I take up rowing or kayaking

Depending on the style you choose, you can stay dry. Sure, big water or bad technique can cause anyone to flip; and because the fear of capsizing can limit your ability to relax and enjoy the experience, some instructors suggest taking an intentional dunk just to get it over with and prove that it's no big deal. But if you row in larger boats, you may never go over. And with good balance, you can stay upright in smaller shells and kayaks, so long as you stay out of whitewater and away from rocks. You can row or kayak for years and suffer no more than a splash.

Rowing and kayaking will only strengthen my arms

One of the main misconceptions about boating is what muscles you use. In kayaking, you work every muscle from the hips up, including a lot of abdominals and back and shoulder muscles. Your arms are not exerting most of the power if you're doing it right. In rowing, you use even more muscle. The main propulsion comes from the legs, butt, and back, the largest muscles in the body, which can generate tremendous force. Rowing is one of the most intense full-body sports, along with gymnastics and cross-country skiing.

Paddling and rowing are bad for your back

If you use proper body mechanics, rowing and kayaking are both safe motions, using natural movements to generate power. Of course, if you twist and pull while overextending your reach, you can wrench your back. But rowing on the ergometer is also commonly used in rehabilitation of back injuries, because the motion strengthens the back and abdominal muscles. If you are concerned about your back, stick to the two-oar motion of sculling, which is more centered.

GET MORE FROM YOUR SPORT

Because the rowing season is limited in much of the country, many rowers and kayakers crosstrain as well as do indoor training. Aerobic sports such as running and cycling tend to top the list, but you'll often find that these athletes gravitate to rock climbing, hiking, trail running, mountain biking, and other outdoor sports.

Along with the competitions, one of the great joys of boating is finding beautiful places to ply the waters. You can kayak all over the world, with adventure-travel companies offering any type of trip, from paddling among the sea otters in Monterey to whitewater in Costa Rica or slipping between icebergs off the coast of Greenland. Rowing getaways often involve trips to regattas. And both sports provide opportunities to travel to a camp for daily instruction. For a paddling lesson merged with a getaway, head to the Nantahala Outdoor Center in North Carolina, a renowned multisport camp and resort with a variety of kayaking courses (including playboating) that was cofounded by a paddler who is in the International Whitewater Hall of Fame (www.noc.com). The premier rowing center is Craftsbury in Vermont, which offers sculling programs during the summer as well as a sculling and yoga retreat (www.craftsbury.com).

RESOURCES

➡ **www.row2K.com** is a rowing portal with news and tips, plus links to various sites about rowing, and classifieds where you can find other rowers. The site was started by Ed Hewitt, former women's coach for Columbia University and a veteran competitor.

➡ **www.paddling.net** should be the first online stop for novice paddlers. Article topics run the gamut from how to get in the kayak to how to "answer Mother Nature's call" once you're in. Best of all is the Places2Paddle section, with directions to scenic paddling sites throughout the country.

➡ *Essential Sculling: An Introduction to Basic Strokes, Equipment, Boat Handling, Technique and Power* by Daniel J. Boyne is as close as you can get to a coach in a book. The manual covers beginner technique as well as more advanced drills and skills.

➡ *Skillful Rowing* by Ed McNeely and Marlene Royle is a training guide for technique and drills aimed at intermediate and advanced rowers.

➡ *Kayaking Made Easy: A Manual for Beginners with Tips for the Experienced* by Dennis Stuhaug explains the basics of maneuvering a kayak and includes information on navigation and safety.

➡ *Kayaking (Paddling Basics)* by Cecil Kuhne is an illustrated guide to kayaking fundamentals, including separate sections on water hazards and navigating river currents.

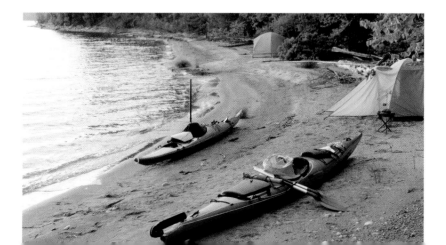

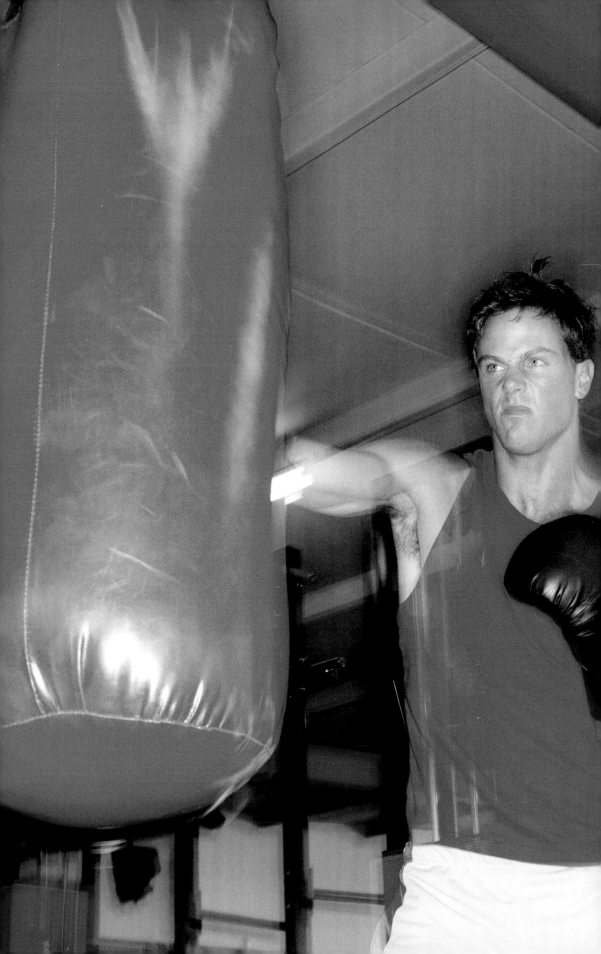

7

BOXING

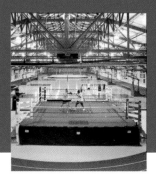

YOU'LL LOVE THIS SPORT IF YOU:
- prefer a full-body workout in one activity that pushes your personal limits
- want to improve your stamina, cardiovascular fitness, strength, speed, and balance
- need a mental challenge in addition to a physical one; love strategy
- want to be so engaged that you don't know you're exercising
- dream of competing
- like to work with a coach
- enjoy sports that have a code of conduct
- want to feel that you can defend yourself

YOU MIGHT NOT LOVE THIS SPORT IF YOU:
- never want to risk an injury—even punching the bag can cause a hand injury
- don't like to work hard; boxing is intense
- already have a chronic injury such as knee or lower-back pain
- don't like to take direction or follow rules

BOXING

If you think you're in decent shape, wait until you try boxing. The physical and mental intensity of the sport are sure to *whup* you. Try it out: The next time you're on the treadmill or out for a walk or run, spend three minutes throwing quick, snapping punches at chin height in time with your feet. Your heart rate is guaranteed to spike.

In boxing, fast footwork and defensive maneuvers will have you sweating in no time, which translates into unparalleled physical benefits. The sport will improve your aerobic endurance and stamina, speed and agility; it will tone your core, legs, butt, and arms; and it will improve your sense of body awareness. Mentally, the sport will build focus, because wandering thoughts will leave you vulnerable to your opponent or unable to maintain your rhythm when shadowboxing.

Boxing is also a release for pent-up tensions and can give you confidence as you feel more capable of self-defense. The training improves your flexibility, because you need to move the body fluidly to segue from a punch to a defensive move and back again. Stiff people are less able to bob away from an incoming punch and more likely to take a blow if it's heading their way.

There are two types of people who take up boxing: Those who want to get in the ring and punch an opponent and those who don't. Many people learn the skills and drills for fitness reasons, with no intention of ever getting hit. One main attraction is the sleek physique boxers develop. Of course, some boxing students discover a hidden talent for throwing a right hook, and the desire to go a few rounds inside the ropes is suddenly born.

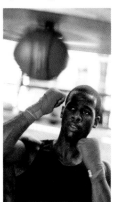

People have always pummeled each other for play and dominance. The history of boxing as a sport traces back to 3,000 years ago in Egypt. Boxing was part of the Olympics in ancient Greece. Competitors wore soft leather wraps over their hands and wrists for protection. Ironically, the most famous boxer from ancient Greece, Melankomas of Karia, did not strike his opponents or allow them to land a blow, thanks to his fast and light footwork; he won by outlasting the other fighter.

In contrast, the Romans made boxing a contest to the death, which they sped along by switching to hand wraps loaded with metal—basically brass knuckles. After the Romans, boxing history is blank for centuries. Amateur boxing became an organized sport

SCORE

If you weigh 150 pounds, you'll burn an average of 660 calories an hour inside the boxing ring. (To calculate your hourly burn rate, multiply 4.4 by your weight in pounds.) Punching a bag will burn 300 calories an hour (that's two times your weight) and sparring burns 480 calories an hour (or 3.2 times your weight).

during the 1880s in Britain and returned to the Olympics in 1904 in St. Louis (the U. S. won because it entered the only team). In Olympic competition today, boxers are required to wear head protection, electronic scoring is used, and both semifinalists are awarded bronze medals.

Women's boxing bouts have been recorded as early as the 1700s and a women's boxing exhibition was held in the 1904 Olympics. Later, the sport was banned in many states until the 1970s, when several women who wanted to box petitioned to hold sanctioned fights. In 1999, the professional debut of famous fighter Muhammad Ali's daughter Laila brought a round of attention. The first world championships for women's boxing were held in 2001, but the International Olympic Committee rejected a bid to include female fighters in the 2008 games in Beijing. Of all the competitions of the summer Olympics, boxing is the only sport other than baseball that excludes women (and baseball has been voted completely off the roster after Beijing).

A boxing bout is held in a ring that's 24 feet square. Modern competitions are based on a set of guidelines drafted in 1867 called the Queensbury rules, which include the restriction not to hit below the belt, the wearing of boxing gloves, and rounds lasting three minutes each (two minutes for novices) with a minute of rest in between. Three-minute rounds may seem like an easy schedule, but boxing is intensely physical. Boxers rarely stand still, generally bouncing and bounding on their feet, because it's better to be a moving target than a sitting duck. Every punch is a full-body experience, coming from a strong stance through a solid core and through the arm. The whole body twists in order to put power into each blow. When you take up boxing, you will be amazed at how long three

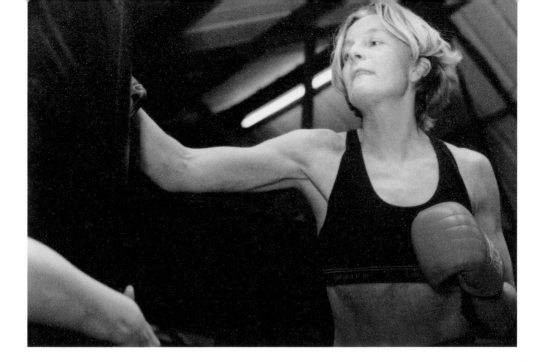

minutes can feel and how much you sweat while you wait for the bell that marks the end of the round.

In amateur boxing, including the Olympics, the object is to land clean punches and score points. Amateur boxing is scored electronically by judges pressing a button when a punch is landed. The top event for amateur boxers in the U.S. is the Golden Gloves. In professional boxing, the bout lasts twelve rounds (reduced from fifteen in the late '80s after a fight in which a boxer died during the fourteenth round). In the Olympics, there are only four rounds. Professional fighters compete in title bouts and win a belt. There are several governing bodies, including the World Boxing Council, World Boxing Association, World Boxing Organization, International Boxing Federation and others. A boxer will have to hold several titles by winning "unification" bouts against other title-holders to be considered the undisputed champion. Some of the organizations have been tainted by corruption and scandals. Further fodder for the sport's seedy reputation is the colorful characters who are professional boxing promoters. But unless you plan to turn pro, you won't be introduced to this side of the sport.

A boxer wins a bout in one of three ways: by knocking out the opponent for a count of ten (a *knockout* or *KO*), by rendering the other fighter too injured to continue (a *technical knockout* or *TKO*) or, if both fighters are still standing at the end of the last round, by scoring more points. There are eleven divisions in boxing, separated by weight class, from *light flyweight* for fighters less than 48 kg (105.6 pounds) to *super heavyweight* for those more than 91 kg (200.2 pounds). Competitive boxers often diet in extreme ways to remain in a certain weight class, because there's an advantage to being the biggest fighter in your weight class and not the smallest guy in the next larger group.

Safety is a serious concern in boxing, of course, since the sport is all about intentionally hitting your opponent. Blows to the head are an effective fighting technique, but they can cause a variety of injuries including serious eye problems. Some professional boxers suffer brain damage—most famously Ali, who was diagnosed with pugilistic Parkinson's in 1984. The headgear worn by amateur fighters helps protect against some injuries but does not prevent concussions or serious injury to exposed areas. However, in amateur fights the referee will be quicker to stop the bout if a boxer is in danger than he would in a professional match. A total mismatch that might put the weaker boxer at risk is avoided because if one boxer is ahead twenty points, the match is ended. For boxing enthusiasts who don't take to the ring, the concerns are more mundane, from the potential twist of an ankle to hand injuries from hitting the bag too hard.

GEARING UP

When you're going to your first class or lesson, bring a water bottle (or two!) and a towel. You are going to sweat. Regular sneakers and gym clothes will work well for boxing; but don't wear anything too warm, unless it's a layer you can peel off. And call ahead to find out if you need to purchase hand wraps or gloves.

There are twenty-seven bones in each hand—eight near the wrist, five in the palm, two in the thumb, and three in each of the four fingers. The muscles and ligaments hold the bones in place, but the structure is fairly delicate and easily damaged, broken, or misaligned compared to, say, a thigh bone that is surrounded by strong muscles. Throwing hard punches at a fairly solid object—whether a heavy bag or someone's chin—is a quick path to injury if your hands are not properly protected. A boxer's hands are wrapped in cotton bandages (there are companies that make hand wraps specifically for boxers) held in place with surgical tape. There are rules about how much padding and how much tape can be used, which vary depending on the organization overseeing the fight. Tape cannot be used across the knuckles, because it can add power to the punch. When preparing for a bout, the taping of the hands is watched by an official to ensure it's done to the proper standards. On top of the hand wraps go the gloves. They lace on and provide further protection for the hands so you can throw hard punches.

For amateur fighters, headgear is required, as is a mouth guard to protect the teeth and gums. All competitive boxers wear a groin protector and women also wear a plastic chest protector. Boxing shorts are long, covering a large portion of the thighs but not falling below the knees. The waistband sits high at the top of the hips to mark the technical boundary, since boxers are not allowed to hit "below the belt." In the Olympics and some other competitions, boxers wear a singlet—a one-piece uniform that incorporates a sleeveless top and shorts with a clearly marked belt line. Professional male boxers typically do not wear shirts in the ring. Boxing footwear is supportive to help prevent twisted ankles yet light because the boxer will be moving a lot.

A boxer also needs gloves, of which there are several styles. Gloves for competition meet either amateur or professional regulations for weight, padding, and appearance. Boxers may use slightly smaller, more maneuverable gloves for practice sessions, such as when hitting the bag or punching at mitts worn by a trainer. There are also weighted gloves for building arm muscle endurance. Cardio boxing gloves have much less padding and slip on and off easily for use in fitness classes. Ask if the gym has gloves and hand wraps you can use during class or for suggestions on where to purchase them.

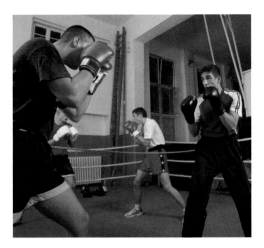

YOUR FIRST TIME

Unless you are lucky enough to know a boxer who can show you the ropes in a private setting, there are two places to get started in boxing: a fitness center or a boxing gym. At a health club, there are two main styles of cardio boxing classes—those that use punching bags and those that don't hit targets but instead use shadowboxing techniques (throwing punches at the air) without gloves. If you sign up to hit bags, you'll need to wrap your hands and put on gloves for protection. The trainer should show you how to do this properly. The most common punching bags used in classes are the *heavy bag*, a huge barrel that hangs from a chain to simulate the large body of an opponent, and a *speed bag*, the small teardrop-shaped target that simulates hitting someone in the face. In either style of class, your heart rate will be high for the whole time thanks to quick moves such as throwing punches, ducking, bobbing, and defensive footwork plus jumping rope, running on a mini-trampoline, and skipping. Some sessions use other gear, such as a medicine ball, and may include a section of targeted abdominal training. Often, the class is broken up into three-minute intervals of intense activity to mimic the pacing of a boxing bout, with one minute of rest or light aerobics between intervals. Gym classes generally don't prepare you for a bout in the ring, although there are exceptions. In most clubs, you train like a fighter to get the body and a bit of the mindset without getting hit.

A boxing gym is a completely different environment in which competitive boxers get coached to take their place in the ring. Amenities such as the locker room usually offer just the basics—you're not going to find high-end fluffy towels. The attitude is gruff, too: The goal is to produce tough fighters, and part of the process includes verbal abuse and nothing that comes close to coddling. Some boxing gyms are crossing over and offering workouts to a larger variety of customers, including cardio boxing fans. These studios may have a more congenial vibe.

Walk into the classic boxing gym and chances are good there will be no front desk at which to inquire about coaching or classes. Everyone in the place will be busy—nobody will greet you or even look up from what he is doing. It's intimidating, and the clients and owners like it that way. Boxing takes determination, and this is your first test. Remember, nobody is going to hit you, and your job is easy: Wander around and take a look. If you're going

to sign up for lessons, you'll want to observe what you're getting into. Watch the trainers to learn their styles. If it's a busy gym, you'll probably notice some trainers who you'd get along with well and others who might not be a good

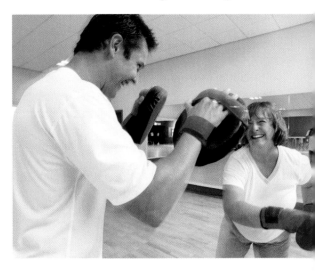

fit. You'll want to choose carefully because it can be hard to switch to a new trainer later.

If nobody approaches to ask what your business there is after a few minutes of scoping out the scene, wait ringside for a break in the action and you should get a chance to ask a few questions—such as who manages the gym (a good person to talk with first) and which trainers work with beginners. Ironically, once you get past the first awkward visit, you'll find that boxers are often laid-back people—perhaps because they channel any negative emotions into punches.

Learning to box is a multidimensional process. You will build strength and stamina through drills, calisthenics, and intense cardio sprints. You'll learn the classic boxer's stance: light on your feet, ready to move, arms poised for defense, and ready to strike. And you'll learn the classic punches and defensive maneuvers, from the jab to the uppercut, how to block, deflect, and evade blows. When you know the basic moves, you'll string them together in a sequence. Now, you're ready to burn some serious calories.

SECRETS TO SUCCESS

Boxing looks deceptively easy—until you try it. "When you're good at boxing, you engage in an extreme form of cardiovascular exercise that combines stamina and speed to push your body to its limits," says Jason Lee, director of boxing at the Sports Center at Chelsea Piers. But it's the mental challenge that often comes as the bigger surprise. You mustn't hesitate, but still you need to be purposeful in your moves yet quick to retract and change tactics if a blow didn't deliver. While you concentrate on the punch you're throwing, you're also planning your defense and your next offensive strike. At the end of a session, you will be completely exhausted and drained, in a good way.

Because of the sport's intensity, be patient with your progress, says Lee.

During lessons, you'll spend a lot of time working on basic punches, but you'll also spend plenty of time on conditioning, coordination, and wrist strength with exercises such as jumping rope. If you aren't adept or aerobically ready to do three minutes jumping rope, skip instead, pumping your arms and bringing your knees high in front. Skipping uses the same cross-the-body angles you'll need for throwing a punch. Boxers tend to do a lot of jumps in their training, which helps improve leg strength and stamina.

To box, you need to constantly evaluate how close you are to your opponent and how to get out of the way of punches coming in your direction. You need to move quickly, shifting and ducking, without losing your balance. Fast footwork is

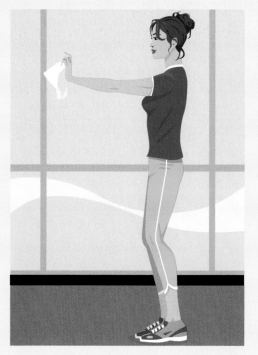

wrist repair drill

Standing or sitting comfortably, hold your left arm out directly in front of you at shoulder height. Bend your wrist so that the palm faces forward, fingertips up. Place a piece of paper in your palm and—without moving your wrist or arm—crumple the paper in your fingers. Repeat 10 times on each side.

an advantage, which you can build by doing obstacle-course training using small, rapid steps to move along a grid on the ground as in a hopscotch pattern or ladder. Running up stairs is also a classic boxer's training technique.

Once you're able to go three minutes without calling for oxygen and have learned how to toss a left hook, upper cut, right cross, and a jab, you may feel ready to get in the ring. Your trainer may not agree—and you have to wait for permission because it's a right you earn.

When you do get into the ring, it's tempting to square off against another novice. A better plan is to spar with someone experienced so you don't get hurt by an accidental move. A seasoned fighter has tremendous control and awareness, which will keep you safer (so long as you're respectful and don't beg to get popped).

Your wrists will absorb a lot of impact, whether you're hitting a bag, pads, or a person. In addition to wrapping them in padding and covering them in gloves, you'll want to develop the muscles that keep the bones stabilized. Many of us have minor wrist problems prior to boxing, thanks to activities such as driving and typing.

Here are some moves to get you started on conditioning so you can spend more time in your boxing lesson learning how to box:

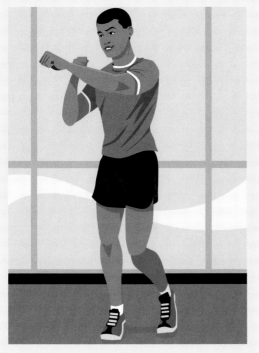

dip and swing

Stand with your feet hip-distance apart, knees soft, and both hands in fists near your chin. Bend your knees to a slight squat and center your weight on your heels. Step to the right with your right foot, straighten, stepping your left foot closer and punching with your right hand toward the head of an imaginary opponent. Repeat to the left. Continue as fast as you can, using good form, for 3 minutes.

ATHLETE IN ACTION

Anne Yih, 43

"I always thought I was in good shape—I played team sports, worked out, did the treadmill, weights, the predictable stuff," says Anne Yih, a former television producer who discovered boxing at Chelsea Piers. "Using your arms and bouncing up and down takes a lot of energy," she says. "The three-minute bout seems like an eternity—it's harder than running six miles—and the one minute of rest feels like the quickest New York minute in the world."

Yih's trainer, Steve Small, was a fighter who introduced her to a few punches about four years ago. She was nervous. "You're up in the ring, it's so foreign. I thought I was going to suck—and everyone is looking at you." Instead, she discovered she had a natural left hook. "I throw it and it feels right, there's no thinking involved and it's on target." And she realized she had found her sport. Yih loves having learned to punch and block: "Boxing gave me a sense of self-confidence I never had before," she says. "You can defend yourself physically if need be." But more important, she thrives on having a workout with a strong mental aspect. "You have to think and use your body—if you're not focused it won't work. There's nothing like doing something physical that requires the brain to call on everything in you."

Boxing might look like just a handful of punches and some blocks, but Yih says she never stops learning. "You work on perfecting your moves and combinations. Steve might say jab, jab, then right cross, then left hook, then duck, then move around and a few body shots." At first, her moves were hesitant, but she learned that speed is essential. "Steve isn't going to baby you. If I don't duck fast enough, he whacks my head with the focus pads and my bandana will go flying." That's as close to getting hit that Yih ever wants to get, but she trains with the dedication of a competitive fighter, learning complex combinations and strategy. "It's like playing chess," she says. "Any time you challenge yourself to learn something new, you're using more brain cells—making yourself smarter and staving off senility."

TACKLE THE TRUTH

Boxing is the most dangerous sport	No one will claim that getting punched is safe. But unless you go pro, you shouldn't be in grave danger. Amateur boxers wear headgear for a little protection, and their goal is to score points, not necessarily a knockout. Also, the ringside doctor can stop the fight any time there's a risk of serious injury. If those safety measures aren't enough for you, stick to cardio boxing, shadowboxing, punching bags, and other training that doesn't involve getting hit. You'll get a great workout that's as safe or safer than other sports.
You have to be aggressive to be a fighter	Good boxers are often graceful and quick, seeking to avoid punches as much as deliver them. A good trainer will work with your strengths, whether you're strong, quick or good at strategy—as long as you're willing to work hard. There are many different personalities that do well in the ring. And when you step into the ring, you might find it's a good way to release pent up frustrations.
Boxing coaches are abusive	Part of the process of becoming a boxer is getting tough, physically and mentally. A coach will goad you to do more, even it if takes taunting. He'll boss you around, more pushy than polite, until you're resilient. Not for you? Try cardio-boxing, where the teacher may be more gruff than in step class, but not as tough as in a boxing gym.

GET MORE FROM YOUR SPORT

Boxing requires body awareness, balance, and coordination, which is why dancers sometimes excel at the sport. Tennis, basketball, street hockey, and soccer are good crosstraining for boxing; they build stamina, awareness, and fast feet, especially because these sports require sideways (lateral) movement as in boxing. Tennis is the best fit because it uses a similar stance and cross-the-body swing plus precise timing and strategy.

The twisting motions in boxing require core strength. Yoga and pilates are perfect for developing a strong center, balance, and body awareness. Also, the flexibility you get from these exercises are vital to counter the effect of the explosive moves in boxing, which tend to produce short, tight muscles (being muscle-bound will restrict your ability to punch and move). Swimming and rock climbing are also useful sports for elongating your muscles. If you lift weights or do calisthenics, be careful to stretch sufficiently to maintain your flexibility or improve it.

Unless you go to Vegas to compete or watch the pros, boxing isn't much of a traveling sport. There are boxing camps in almost every state, from Bear Mountain in California to the Catskills in New York. But these centers are oriented toward fighters with extensive training. "It would be very unkind to go to one if you didn't know what you were doing," warns Lee.

Watching experienced fighters can be informative, because each will have a different style, from the force of Mike Tyson to the grace of Muhammad Ali. There are plenty of fights on television and free clips online to provide basic boxing education. You can also jump-start your knowledge and conditioning with a training video such as *Everlast Boxing Workout —Beginner* (available on www.EverlastBoxing. com under "cardio and aerobic boxing").

RESOURCES

➡ **www.balazsboxing.com**, a gear purveyor site, has an instructional section called "In the Gym." Look for "Boxing Basics" to learn the steps for wrapping your hands, throwing punches and hitting the bags.

➡ **www.boxinggyms.com** has a state-by-state listing of boxing gyms, tips for picking a gym and a trainer, plus a helpful section with advice on various aspects of the sport.

➡ *The Ultimate Boxer* by Christy Halbert, Ph.D., a trainer who has worked with women on the U.S. National team, covers everything from the boxer's stance to expectations in training and tips for success in competition.

➡ *Workouts from Boxing's Greatest Champs: Get in Shape with Muhammad Ali, Fernando Vargas, Roy Jones Jr., and Other Legends* by Gary Todd provides interesting insight into the differences between the weight classes in boxing, because each boxer wants to be at the top physical condition possible without slipping up into the next category (where there are bigger, presumably stronger, boxers).

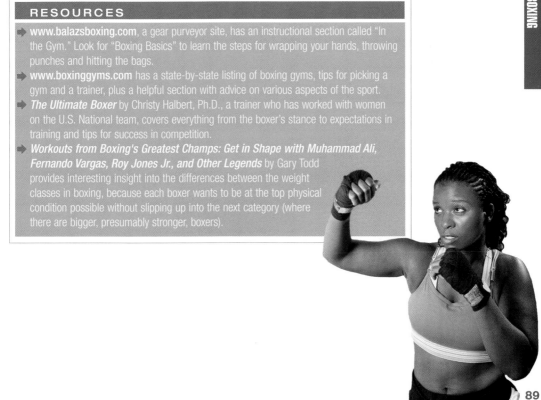

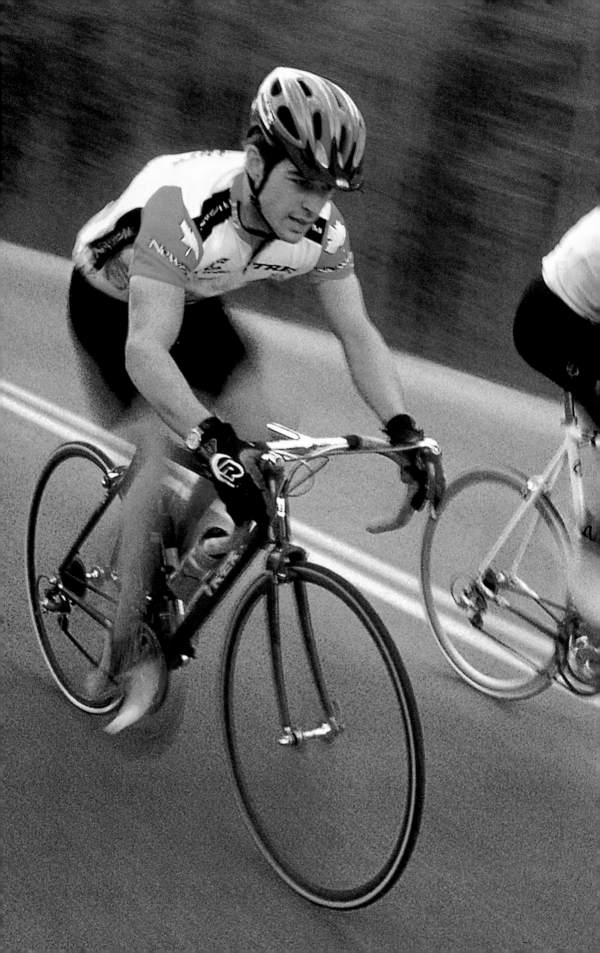

8

CYCLING

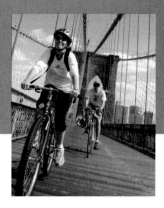

YOU'LL LOVE THIS SPORT IF YOU:
- want to improve your balance, cardiovascular fitness, and lower-body strength
- want a quick learning curve to mastery of an activity
- enjoy setting your own pace, whether slow or fast
- enjoy a versatile sport; you can practice outdoors in good weather and indoors at any time
- enjoy exploring; cycling is a great way to sightsee
- want to be so distracted by scenery that you won't realize you're exercising
- want a sport you can do with family, friends, or alone
- want to compete
- want a sport you can do on vacation
- enjoy gear options

YOU MIGHT NOT LOVE THIS SPORT IF YOU:
- can't do three things at once: steer, pedal, and brake, for example
- hate having your feet off the ground
- don't like maintaining gear or the possibility of a flat tire

There is an oft-cited adage, "It's a skill you don't forget, like riding a bike." But the simple view of cycling as a one-trick sport belies the exciting variety open to cyclists, from bombing downhill on a mountain bike to touring the south of France with stops at vineyards along the way. And there's a form to fit every lifestyle and personality, whether you want to tool around town with the kids or compete against the pack. Indeed, the basic techniques are the same, no matter which style of the sport you adopt; but at advanced levels, there are specialized maneuvers and tactics for safety, comfort, and competitive advantage.

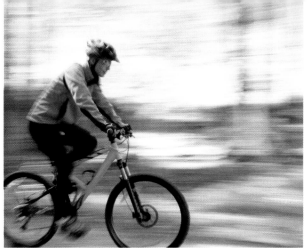

Learning to stay balanced on two wheels probably won't take long for any adult who didn't learn as a child, and it's well worth the effort. Cycling is a low-impact sport that allows for long bouts of heart-healthy exercise. You can go for a leisurely outing and enjoy the scenery while working off breakfast, or increase the pace to a fast, sweaty ride that triples the calorie burn—equal to running a ten-minute mile but without the painful pounding on your joints. Riding develops stamina and balance, plus strong thigh and butt muscles—especially if you tackle hills. The sport also conveys mental benefits from spending time outdoors in fresh air while exercising, which can greatly reduce depression, fatigue, anxiety, and boredom. Whether on roads or trails, cycling offers an opportunity to explore new places, covering greater distances than you could on foot but getting less noise and pollution, better views, and a fitness bonus that all are lacking when you drive.

For those who thrive on speed and competition, there are several good matches in cycling. For example, road racers can reach speeds of up to 45 miles per hour as they sprint for the finish line, with 25 miles per hour considered a fairly easy pace. In these events, teams of racers typically work together, employing complex strategies of pacing and position, because the rider taking the lead suffers the most wind resistance while those following on his tail, called *drafting*, conserve energy. Using this technique, road racers move in a pack, at close proximity and high speeds. These races often cover 50 to 100 miles and may stretch up to five hours, yet top-level riders don't stop for water, food, bathroom breaks, equipment malfunctions, or clothing adjustments as weather conditions change. They may get sustenance and gear help from a team car riding behind, and there are feed zones to grab an energy snack when you're on the go.

The high-tech bikes used by today's racers have little in common with models of an earlier vintage. The first bikes, circa 1790, were wooden planks with wheels, no pedals, and no steering mechanism. Fifty years later, the predominant style was the penny farthing, which had a huge front wheel (the bike was aptly nicknamed a "bone shaker" because of the effect of hard wheels on cobblestones). In 1885, the Rover safety bicycle came along, which had wheels of the same size and brakes. This maneuverable bike was responsible for the surge in the sport's popularity, earning it a place in the first modern Olympics held in Athens in 1896.

At the turn of the 20th century, cycling was a richman's sport, and a separate patent office was opened just to handle bicycle inventions. Today, on the banked tracks of the velodrome where indoor races are held, bikes may be made from carbon-fiber technology

SCORE

Road-cycling calorie counts have been determined for a variety of paces, shown in the chart below. Use the chart to estimate the energy burn from other styles of cycling, assuming that mountain biking means cycling up a lot of hills, which will burn more calories than the average road ride.

Miles/hour	Effort	Calories/hour*	Calories/hour/lb
10-11.9	Slow, light cruise	300	2
12-13.9	Moderate leisure ride	420	2.8
14-15.9	Racing or vigorous ride	540	3.6
16-19	Racing, not drafting	660	4.4
> 19	Racing, drafting	660	4.4
> 20	Racing, not drafting	900	6

* 150-lb person

and have spoke-free disc wheels and new proportions for improved aerodynamics. Unique bikes adapted to the terrain are used in each type of organized cycling race—road, track, mountain, and cyclocross—with each category appealing to completely different personalities.

Road races can be a short loop (usually less than one mile) with lots of corners and perfect for sprinters, or a much longer point-to-point race that covers varying and often hilly terrain. Another event, called the *time trial*, pits the individual racer against the clock as riders race over a set course one by one, each competing for the fastest time. A *stage race*, like the Tour de France, combines different styles of road races over several days or weeks of competition, with each stage having a separate start and finish on that day.

Roller-coaster fans tend to love track racing. The feeling of a fast turn around a banked track has been compared to the rush of the drop from the top of an amusement park ride. Track racers combine sprint ability with tactics, such as rising high on the bank to stage an attack. Like road racing, there are various events, from short sprints to team events, with riders taking turns in the fray. Speed is king here and track bikes have no brakes!

The relative newcomer, mountain biking, has two main styles: endurance events over obstacle-laden natural courses; or downhill tracks that have similarities to downhill ski racing. You can mountain bike along gentle hard-packed fire roads through the woods, or fly down single-track paths no wider than one tire, with frequent challenges, such as roots, rocks, trees, and rivulets.

The fourth type of competition is not an Olympic sport—at least not yet. In winter, there's a type of race called *cyclocross*, which involves fast loops around streets, and off-road tracks with obstacles to force riders to dismount, toss their bikes on their shoulders, and run over and around obstacles before hopping back in the saddle. Cyclocross races are a wild experience, with riders expecting bumps, bruises, and bike damage, but the races are great fun and provide unparalleled training for any type of racing.

Thanks to innovations designed to shave seconds off the time of top competitors, everyday riders now have better bikes, too. Recreational bicycles have gotten lighter, sleeker, and less expensive over the last few decades. Helmets, padded shorts, plus well-designed saddles all make the sport more comfortable and safer. And improved stationary bikes and Spinning classes allow for training, when and where outdoor conditions are not conducive to a ride (although a cyclocross rider would disagree!). You can even get a

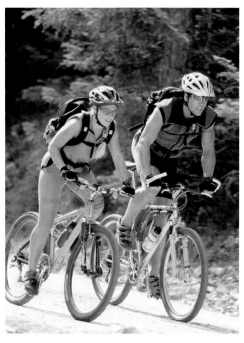

device called a *wind trainer* that easily attaches to the rear axle of your regular bike, temporarily converting it into a stationary cycle. And a variety of creations make it easier to cycle as a family, such as tandem bikes specially designed to allow one rider to do more work than the others, small carts that attach behind a bike for toting a couple of kids (or pets), and a device that creates a temporary tandem for an older child to pedal behind an adult.

GEARING UP

Buying a bike today means choosing from such categories as road, mountain, comfort, fitness, hybrid, and others. Road bikes are designed for speed and distance, with thin, hard tires and low handlebars (a crouched rider suffers less wind resistance). Off-road styles have heavier, more durable frames, fat tires that grip the ground, and require a more upright rider position.

Most beginners do well with a comfort, fitness, or hybrid bike, which offer the best combination of road and mountain components for comfort and safety without the cost of the full performance benefits. For example, the tires are a compromise between the thin ones on racing bikes (which tip easily and provide no shock absorption) and the fat ones on mountain bikes (which stick to the ground creating drag), so you feel stable and able to maneuver. Expect to pay $200 to $300 for an entry-level bicycle, and a little more for added gears, an ergonomic saddle, and other features.

Renting a bike is a viable option for your first rides, but be sure to take a look at the equipment to determine if it looks overly worn or obviously damaged. Proper maintenance is vital, because you don't want brakes that fail or tires that are on their last bit of tread and will easily go flat. Take the same precautions if you opt for a used bike (see *Getting Bargains on Gear*, page 207, for ideas on finding them). There are plenty of high-quality secondhand bikes on the market, but if you're not well-versed in bicycle mechanics and fit, have your new ride checked at a bike shop—if possible, before you buy. And always test ride a bike before making a purchase. Bikes that have identical specifications but are made by different companies can feel completely different when you're riding, and you won't enjoy the ride if you're not comfortable.

In addition to the various styles, bikes come in different sizes plus men's and women's models. Some bikes that say they are made for women simply come in pink with a smaller-size frame. Unfortunately,

women don't always fit well on bikes that are simply scaled-down men's models; they need additional adaptations, which you can now find on many better brands. For example, smaller hands need smaller brake levers so they aren't uncomfortably far from the handlebars, as well as a shorter distance from the seat to the handlebars to accommodate a shorter torso. (Tall women may find these

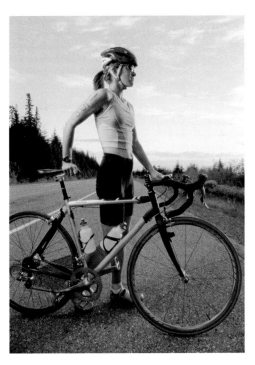

women's bikes too small.) If you've had trouble with bike fit in the past, work with a bike shop to get a better-fitting model and make adjustments. These bikes don't have to be pricey—the biggest expense, after all, is getting gear you won't use.

When buying a bike you'll ride mostly on paved surfaces, you should have one to two inches of clearance over the top tube when standing flat-footed. For an off-road bike, riders often prefer three to six inches of space so that when you need to jump down off the pedals, you don't crash into the bar, considering that sometimes the ground where your feet land is lower than the tires.

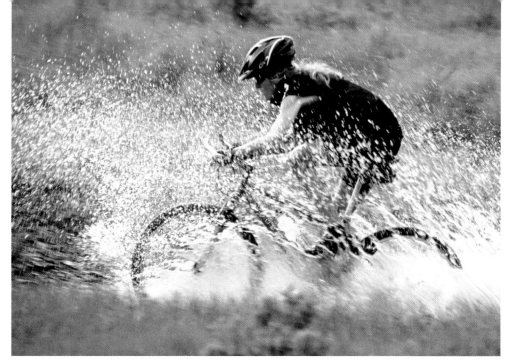

After choosing the right bike, your next vital piece of equipment is a helmet. Thanks to congestion or ground conditions, you're likely to fall at some point. But almost all head injuries are preventable by wearing a properly fitted helmet. They are light and vent well when riding, plus they're inexpensive (especially compared to the cost of a head injury). Choose one that fits snugly so it doesn't shift easily but is not too tight. It should be worn low on your forehead—sitting just above your eyebrows—to protect the front of your brain. The straps should come down in front and back of your ears, flat and snug. And the chin strap should tuck in near where your jaw meets your neck so it can be secure without limiting your ability to open your mouth. When adjusted properly, the helmet should not wobble when you shake your head vigorously.

Your helmet should be approved by the Consumer Products Safety Commission (CPSC), which will be listed on the label inside the helmet and on the box. Never buy a used helmet because damage cannot always be seen. For the same reason, if you fall and hit your head, you must replace your helmet. They are designed to absorb the impact of the fall, which means they don't work twice.

When you head out on a ride, pack a small bicycle repair toolkit, a spare-tire tube, and a portable pump. Of course it's best to learn to use these items, but bring them along even if you don't know what to do, because someone else might be able to help. There are handy, inexpensive wedge-shaped bags that hang under the seat to hold these items. Also tuck in a small first-aid kit holding adhesive bandages, duct tape, and medical information, plus some money for emergencies. And stick a label with personal identification information inside your helmet in case you are somehow separated from your bike.

If you'll be going farther than a few blocks, bring along a water bottle as well. For long summer rides, freeze a half-bottle of water the night before, then top it off with liquid, or fill the bottle with a mix of ice and water so you'll have cold water all day. Also, pack snacks you can munch as you ride and keep them handy. Wear sunscreen and sunglasses that wrap around your face to keep wind and bugs out of your eyes. Leave the iPod home because it's unsafe if you can't hear other riders or cars.

For any ride of thirty minutes or more, you may want padded gloves as well as extra padding between you and the saddle. You can opt for a padded seat, seat cover, shorts liner, or shorts. For long rides, try an ergonomic seat combined with shorts padded with old-fashioned leather (chamois) or easy-maintenance gel or synthetics in whatever style you like— from skin-tight road racing silhouettes to looser versions designed for recreational and off-road riding.

CYCLING

You can ride in any comfortable clothes, but be wary of pant legs and shoelaces that might get caught in the gears as you pedal. Shorts or close-fitting pants are good choices. For sneaker laces, tuck them into the shoes on the side with the chain. Loose shirts and jackets may flap in the wind as you ride, which can be annoying, so opt for a slimmer silhouette up top, too.

YOUR FIRST TIME

The first step in preparing for any ride is to double check the weather and look over your bike. Make sure the brakes and gears are in working order and the tires are properly inflated. Give your helmet an inspection for cracks or wear.

If you don't know how to ride, head to a flat location with no traffic and see if you can balance and coast, with some pointers from a friend. The slower you go, the more you wobble, so leave room to pedal in a straight line at a consistent pace before needing to hit the brakes and put your foot down. It's fairly easy from there.

Experienced riders who are ready to take up fitness riding or racing can simply head off on a ride with little or no preparation, but it's far more rewarding to plan ahead for a ride that you'll enjoy from start to finish. Whether you're interested in burning calories or training to compete, start with short excursions to test your equipment, assess your stamina, and build confidence. Contact your local parks and recreation department and check for books and Web sites that outline trails and roads most suitable for riding. If you come up empty-handed, consider testing intended road routes in a car first, to measure the distance and look for trouble spots. Scope out good places to pull over for meals and pit stops. For off-road riding, start with marked trails in well-traveled parks so you'll have company in case you run into trouble. Bringing your own buddies is safer and more fun, so if you can, ride with friends. No mat-ter how many of you ride together, leave information with someone about your route and expected return time.

Many riders don't bother using hand signals, but it's useful to learn them for signaling to cars and fellow riders. Point to the left or right with a straight arm to indicate you'll be turning in that direction. Another way to indicate a right turn is to lift your left hand up in the air, elbow out at shoulder height. A straight arm pointing diagonally down means the rider is slowing. When the elbow is straight out with the hand down, the rider is stopping.

As you ride, note any spots in your body that feel uncomfortable. Try to keep your shoulders down and back, away from your ears, to prevent stiffness and soreness. Vary your position on the handlebars to avoid pressure spots. Every so often, firm your abdominals, flex your elbows, and lower your nose slightly toward the handlebars to gently stretch your neck as you ride. For added intensity—and to give your bottom a break—stand and pedal from time to time using a high gear. When you're ascending hills, try to switch to a low gear and remain seated for efficiency. But if you can't make it to the top in a seated position, go ahead and rise off the saddle to get more leverage on the pedals. And don't be shy about getting off and walking if you're wobbling or exhausted.

Practice braking before you'll need to use the skill. If you're moving fast and grab hard with the front brake, the one typically controlled with the left hand, you may flip head over heels. Learn to favor the rear brake, which is safer, but try to use both for best results.

Also, practice the art of banking, or leaning into a turn. If you have sufficient speed as you approach a curve, stop pedaling, bring the inside knee up, and lower the outside pedal until that leg is almost straight, applying weight on that foot. Lean your torso toward the handlebars and slightly into the raised knee. Your body position will help the bike lean into the turn on the edge of the tires, which is more efficient and effective.

As you pull out of the turn, start to pedal and bring your torso up.

Banking is more essential in racing and mountain biking than in a leisurely roll down the road, but you'll feel more mastery of the sport if you do it for any type of ride. Whatever terrain you're on, practice pulling up on the handlebars to pop over small obstacles. Off-road, you'll be happy to have this skill when you need to avoid a small stream, say, or larger branch or root. But even on paved surfaces, there will be debris, sewer grates, and sometimes a curb to mount. Keep in mind that sand and gravel may shift under your tires, and try not to turn sharply unless you are prepared to skid. And any soft surface can mire your tires enough to force you to step down. If your pedals have cages (straps or metal pieces that hold your feet), drop your heels to facilitate slipping out easily should the need arise. (More advanced riders generally use clipless pedals in which the cyclists' shoe clicks in like a ski binding—and releases if the heel is twisted to the side.)

Mountain biking down bouncy slopes will leave you with a sore behind if you attempt to stay seated. Unfortunately, standing can make you feel uncontrolled. The compromise is to set the pedals even, parallel to the ground, with your knees slightly bent, and hug the saddle lightly with your thighs, your rear raised to a safe height. Grasp the handlebars with a wide grip, holding firmly but lightly, and using your elbows as shock absorbers so the vibrations don't shoot up your arms. Keep at least two fingers on the brake levers for quick stops. In this position, the bike can buck beneath you without bouncing you akimbo.

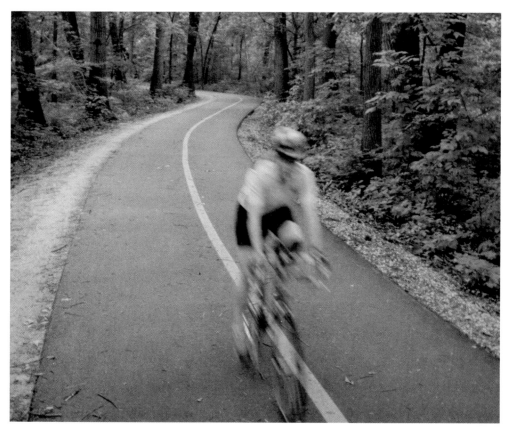

SECRETS TO SUCCESS

No matter which form of cycling you choose, if you want to use the sport as a significant part of your fitness plan, you'll be spending a lot of time "in the saddle." "Consistency is the biggest key to getting stronger and faster on a bicycle," says Chris Carmichael, a renowned cycling coach who has trained Olympians as well as Lance Armstrong. "And your perform-ance and results are going to improve as you gain more experience, in training as well as racing." Be sure to select options to continue your fitness or race training when the weather isn't conducive to out-door riding.

If you're ready to road race, it won't take long to get good at this sport. "As a beginner, you can be ready to enter your first race in as few as four months," Carmichael says. "And you'll do fairly well in it if you can devote eight hours a week, broken up in three to six rides." Prepping for your first *century* (a 100-mile ride) takes less time, because speed is not as essential. "You can prepare in about three months, riding as little as six hours a week." But cycling in any form takes dedication in order to see gains in per-formance. The biggest challenge is getting comfortable in a crowd of cyclists and

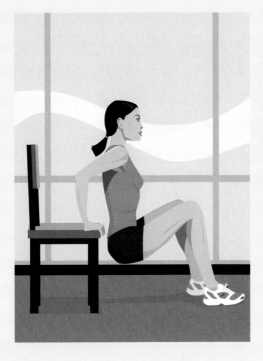

chair dips

Sit on the edge of a chair with your hands grasping the front edge, on either side of your butt. Extend your feet out in front. Put your weight onto your hands, lift your butt off the chair, and shift it forward. Slowly bend your elbows to lower your butt toward the ground until your upper arms are parallel to the floor (or as close as you can get without pain in the front of your shoulder). Use the muscles in your arms and shoulders to press back up until your arms are straight, but don't lock your elbows. Do 3 sets of 10 to 12 repetitions, resting 1 minute between sets.

learning how to draft. But that skill, too, comes simply with practice and some good instruction.

Mountain biking requires a looser style, more movement in the saddle, and adaptation to terrain. You're likely to fall a few times as you learn the skills, but the challenge is part of the fun—and falling on the dirt can be less painful than on pavement. This type of riding is less buttoned down, with a looser style of clothing as well as a more laid-back attitude than road riding. You'll catch yourself breaking into big grins as you learn to bunny hop over small obstacles. You'll feel like a kid bounding around a playground and splashing in puddles. The best way to learn these techniques is to have someone show them to you.

For any type of riding, you'll develop strong leg muscles while you're on the bike. What can make the experience more pleasurable is to work on your core muscles, plus arm and shoulder strength, so you're more comfortable leaning over the handlebars. Try these pre-ride training moves:

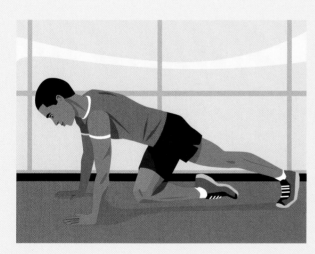

plank and twist

Start lying facedown on the floor. Place your feet hip-distance apart, toes on the floor. Prop your head and chest up by bringing your hands under your shoulders, fingers spread wide. Press your shoulders down away from your ears and push through your palms into the floor. Press your hips up off the floor until there's a straight line from head to heels. Hold the plank position for 30 seconds, then lower to the floor and rest for 30 to 60 seconds. Repeat 5 times. Work up to holding for 60 seconds. Next add a twist: Get into plank position. Inhale. On the exhale, bring your right knee toward your left shoulder as far as you can without losing balance. Return to start. Repeat with the left knee to complete 1 repetition. Repeat 3 times, building up to 5.

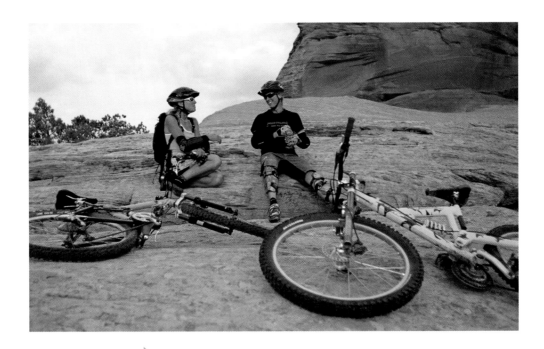

Rita Cohen, 65

Growing up in the Bronx, Rita Cohen didn't do much riding—and the little she did left her with powerful negative memories. "I was excited to get my first two-wheeler, but it didn't have brakes, so I had to jump off to stop," she recalls. One day, she got spooked by a car, tipped over, and gashed her leg. "I got a bad cut on my knee, and it bled a lot; I still have the scar." The emotional scar was worse, leaving Cohen uninterested and fearful of riding, especially near cars. When she outgrew the brakeless bike she didn't get another. But about fifteen years ago, with her kids in college and newly married to an avid cyclist, Cohen saw an ad for a local bike shop holding its annual second-hand sale. There's nothing she likes better than a bargain, so she decided it was time to get a bike. About a hundred bikes stood roped off in a parking lot while shoppers scoped the perimeter like vultures appraising their prey. At the appointed hour, the ropes

came down and the people pounced. Cohen's choice was easy because she wanted a woman's style, and there weren't many options. She picked out an aqua Schwinn with knobby tires for $20.

Setting the seat too low, so her feet could touch the ground, Cohen began riding around her neighborhood to gain confidence. A few weeks later, she felt a rush of accomplishment after completing a one-mile loop with her daughter.

Over the next five years, Cohen slowly added distance to her rides. Then she and her husband decided to join a cycling group that they'd heard about from friends. One member of the group was in her 80s and had had two hip replacements. "I couldn't keep up with her," Cohen recalls of that first ride, which covered 30 miles. The group cycled at a leisurely pace, about 12 miles per hour, including many breaks and a long lunch. Another club member, a restaurant critic, chose the post-ride meal destination—and everyone enjoyed the rewards of an exercise-primed appetite. Cohen was ecstatic to celebrate her accomplishment over dinner. And she and her husband

became regular riders with the group, logging hundreds of miles every summer.

A few years ago, back pain made cycling difficult, and Cohen's doctor told her she had osteoarthritis in her spine. Tempted to give up her bike, she attended a program at Canyon Ranch that emphasized healthy activity. "One of the experts said you can become immobilized or take the pills and keep moving," she recalls. Now she takes doses of ibuprofen the day of the ride and has no trouble.

Today, Cohen still prefers to cycle where there's little traffic, and she tends to lag at the back of the group, but she has more confidence and has upgraded to a better bike. (She bought it new, but with a big discount, of course.) Sometimes the group takes rides she calls "shorter"—only 25 miles. "You get back to the parking lot and want to keep going," Cohen says. "You feel high, it's a gorgeous day, and you want to do more—to enjoy the camaraderie, the scenery and the feeling of being out in nature."

CYCLING

TACKLE THE TRUTH

I'll get huge thighs from cycling

Riding a bike works the legs more than other parts of the body, but you'd have to log a lot of miles and push up major hills using high gears to build big gams. If that starts to happen, you can back off with other forms of training. But it's far more likely that recreational riding will tone your legs and butt, making them less jiggly. And if you slim down by burning calories on your rides, your legs will look trim.

Cycling will hurt my butt

Getting sore in the saddle is a common deterrent for new riders, but your body will adapt quickly. Hasten the process by getting a gender-specific saddle that reduces pressure spots, and get it adjusted to the right height and angle. Wear padded bike shorts, even for short rides (no underwear because extra fabric bunches up). And wiggle around: Rock your hips, round your back, stand in the pedals—anything to give your butt a rest. If you're mountain biking, be sure to stand as you bounce downhill.

I don't want to ride because it's dangerous to go in traffic

It takes confidence to share the road with cars and trucks when you're on just a bike. And parked cars can be even more dangerous if the occupants don't look before opening doors. But with a little planning you can find bike paths and off-road rides that avoid these problems. One great option: Look for rail trails—old railroad tracks that have been converted to wide recreational paths.

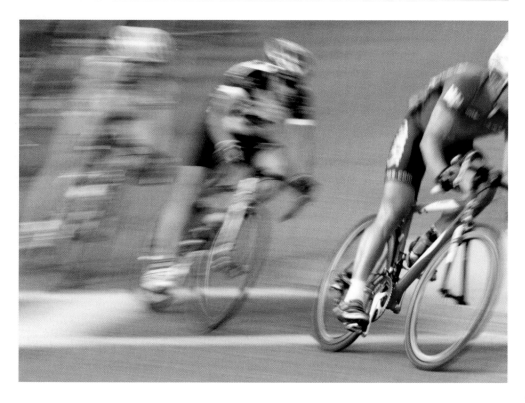

CYCLING

GET MORE FROM YOUR SPORT

If you love cycling because you like to spend time outdoors close to nature and because of the camaraderie, try also taking up hiking, in-line skating, trail running, snowshoeing, and cross-country skiing as alternate sports. Even rock climbing and SCUBA diving might be a good fit. But if it's speed that you adore, opt for speed-skating, snowboarding, downhill skiing, or rowing. Kayaking works for either personality—nature lover or speed freak—because you can take leisurely paddles over the pond or head for the rapids.

Serious bike racers usually log plenty of training miles plus time in the weight room. To hone your cycling skills while participating in other sports, you can't beat the balance, aerobic, and leg-strength gains from any form of skating. Consider yoga and pilates to round out your program, build core strength, and maintain flexible muscles. Many cyclists get into triathlons after taking up running and swimming as crosstraining pursuits.

When you're ready to take your skills to the next level, consider signing up for an organized ride—they're not just for racers. As a recreational cyclist, you can ride in noncompetitive events such as New York's Five Boro Bike Tour (www.bikenewyork.org). Or sign up for a charity ride such as the American Diabetes Association's Tour de Cure, which takes place in eighty-four locations across the country; it has optional distances from 15 to 100 miles and required fundraising starts as low as $150 (www.tour.diabetes.org). When you can manage 35 miles a day, you can even sign up for a three-day road riding camp for beginners in Massachusetts (www.ridenoho. com) or any number of multiday tours in the U.S. and overseas with an adventure-travel outfitter (see *Sport and Adventure Vacations*, page 103).

There are plenty of races and training camps for cyclists who do want to compete. Coach Chris Carmichael runs cycling and triathlon camps, and even one for cyclocross in Colorado and California (www.trainright. com). Camps for advanced riders often include sports-psychology sessions and in-depth concepts in physiology. Two other popular camps are AthletiCamps (www.athleticamps.com) and triathlon training camps with Joe Friel, author of *The Cyclist's Training Bible* (www.ultrafit.com).

RESOURCES

➡ **www.usacycling.org/cycling101/** offers basic information on the types of cycling, plus a glossary of terms.

➡ **www.bicycling.com** is the Web presence for *Bicycling* magazine, which covers road and off-road riding and racing. Online, you'll find gear reviews, tips and drills, links to events, and plenty more.

➡ **www.giantforwomen.com** is a site from Giant Bicycles designed to help women get into biking—with blogs from female riders, bike maintenance and riding destination tips, and help finding riding partners.

➡ **www.adv-cycling.org** is the home of the Adventure Cycling Association, a nonprofit that encourages riders. The site provides links to events and a place to read (or create) postings to find fellow riders.

➡ **www.velonews.com** is a bike-racing site with useful information in the tech and training sections.

➡ *Bicycle Repair Manual* by Chris Sidwells has clear explanations and helpful photos so you can keep your bike in top shape—or put it back together if something shakes loose on a ride far from home. The book is an updated guide covering everything you might need to know about, from tires to brakes to gears.

➡ *The Ultimate Ride* by Chris Carmichael is not just a racing book for the likes of Carmichael's elite athletes. The pages are packed with insights for road riders at any level, from fitness cycling to racing, including exercises and training programs to help you meet your goals.

➡ *Mountain Bike Magazine's Complete Guide to Mountain Biking Skills*, written by the magazine's editors, covers tips and techniques in a light yet informative tone. This book explains indispensable maneuvers for anyone going off-road, whether you'll cruise easy hiking paths or bounce down single-track trails.

Sport and Adventure Vacations

When you've gotten your sports routine humming along and feel more fit, consider heading out on an adventure. There's nothing like stepping out of your comfort zone to test your skills and fitness level. And it's great fun to reward yourself for all that hard work of training in your chosen activity. Every sport in the world offers exciting getaways to exotic destinations. In addition to the typical (and fun!) 30-mile-a-day bike rides and rafting trips, you can study yoga in India or travel to Asia for an immersion in martial arts.

When you're choosing an adventure vacation, the descriptions all sound wonderful. To help you narrow down the field, first explore the companies. Below, a few questions you should ask:

* Is the company insured and bonded?
* How long has the company been in business.
* How many times have they traveled to the country you're interested in?
* Do they know the lodging and gear options well?
* Do the guides speak the local languages?
* What qualifications do the guides have (CPR and instructor training, etc.)?
* What are the procedures in case of a medical or weather emergency?

For your first trip, try to go with a well-established company that has tested the itinerary numerous times and has a local support system that can easily manage lost luggage, broken gear and other hassles. You also might not want to gamble on a new venture that could go out of business, leaving you stranded.

Many trip packagers offer extensive information about what to expect on each day of the trip, based on prior excursions. Get as much detail as you can, paying attention to any additional fees, such as entrance charges for sightseeing destinations, airport transfers, meals that aren't included, and other extras that can hike up the cost. As in real-estate ads, read between the lines: "authentic" may mean roughing it; "free time" means you're on your own, with no guide; "tours" and "transfers" could be crowded bus rides. For example, an independent trip titled "Thai Cultural Experience" from Intrepid Traveler includes a chance to meditate with Buddhist monks, get a traditional Thai massage, and learn to cook a classic meal. But you should note that the trip is not a group trip but a detailed itinerary for individual travelers; and the authentic home-stay at a house on a canal involves a rustic boat ride and sleeping on a mat. This type of trip works well if you know what to expect, but it isn't for everyone.

Once you've selected your destination and guide company, ask for suggestions on how to prepare physically for the trip. Many outfitters provide guidance to help you get into shape for a different altitude, or simply for all the mileage you'll cover each day. Of course, if you have special needs such as dietary restrictions or an extra-tall bicycle, be sure to get a firm commitment that your request can be met before sending in your deposit.

Some top companies offering active getaways include:

* www.Adventure-Life.com
* www.AustinLehman.com
* www.Backroads.com
* www.ButterfieldandRobinson.com
* www.EquestrianVacations.com
* www.GapAdventures.com
* www.IntrepidTravel.com
* www.MTSobek.com
* www.PowderQuest.com
* www.Randonnee.com

To find more options, head to the outdoor enthusiast site **www.gorptravel.com**.

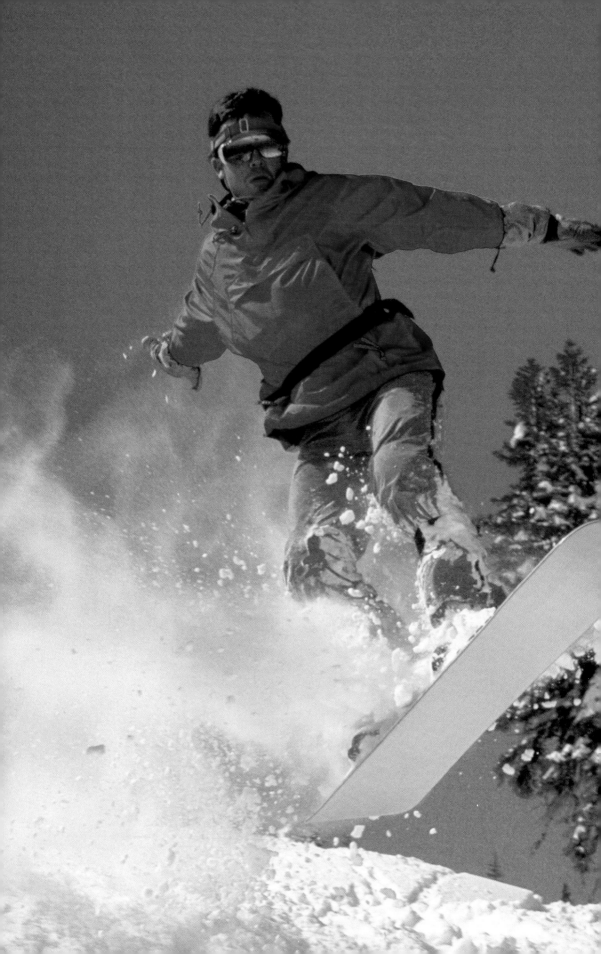

9

DOWNHILL
SKIING AND SNOWBOARDING

YOU'LL LOVE THESE SPORTS IF YOU:
- like to combine cardio with strength, agility, and balance
- want a thigh-and-butt toning workout
- enjoy speed
- want to play outdoors during the winter; enjoy beautiful scenery
- want a sport that's so much fun you'll forget you're exercising
- enjoy sport vacations and weekend getaways
- prefer a sport that can be solitary or enjoyed with a group

YOU MIGHT NOT LOVE THESE SPORTS IF YOU:
- need instant success
- hate waiting—equipment rental and lift lines can be long
- are terribly afraid of heights—chairlifts and scenic spots are often high up
- have chronic knee or back pain
- hate acquiring and carrying gear
- are sensitive to cold or don't like to bundle up

If you've ever taken a sled out to enjoy freshly fallen snow, you know the rush of flying downhill. That pleasure is enhanced when, instead of trudging back up, you can ride a lift or gondola to the top. Skiing and snowboarding are wonderful ways to spend an entire day exercising without a moment of boredom.

The pleasure of spending a winter's day outdoors is physically and mentally refreshing and rewarding. These downhill sports offer a combination of breathtaking views, companionship, and the calming, almost meditative effect of a graceful, repetitive sport. If you have a competitive personality, you can set tough goals for yourself and challenge your

DOWNHILL

buddy to a race or train for any number of events. And while the skills can be frustratingly elusive at times, you rarely see a scowl among the faces of people on the hill—some shivering, perhaps, but most people ski and ride because it's incredible fun. Downhill sports are naturally social: You'll meet people on the chairlift, at the terrain park, or at *après-ski* activities that often include cocktails and music. But if you prefer solitude, you can head off the groomed trails to practice some peaceful turns through the trees and simply skip the evening get-togethers in favor of a well-deserved rest by the fire.

The calorie burn and fitness benefits from four to six hours of skiing or snowboarding are hard to match. But if your body isn't prepared, the extended workout can mean sore muscles and fatigue. The antidote is simple: a moderate approach to the first day on the mountain and, if possible, a little physical preparation. Both sports use a lot more leg muscle than most people develop from their ordinary pursuits. Overly tired legs can lead to a loss of control and injury, so you want to plan your last run when you're still fresh enough to make it to the bottom in fair form. A downhill day will also tax your lung capacity as you wind your way down the trails, using muscles from head to toe to stay on your feet and head in the right direction. In addition to leg strength and stamina, both sports require balance and maneuvering ability, which are derived from agility and strength in the core muscles.

Snowboarding, with your feet in a fixed position on a single platform, is a lot like skateboarding or surfing on the snow, whereas downhill skiing has some overlap with ice skating or in-line skating. All these sports share the need to balance on the edges of your gear. To get a feel for edging, stand with your feet shoulder-width apart, knees slightly

SCORE
If you weigh 150 pounds, you'll burn about 425 calories in an hour of skiing or snowboarding. (To calculate your hourly burn rate, multiply your weight in pounds by 2.8.)

bent. Next, press your hips to the left, rolling your weight onto the left side of both feet, leaning your torso and head to the right for balance. That's an exaggeration of the classic posture for edging on downhill skis in order to carve a turn—similar to that horizontal position a downhill ski racer uses. In both sports, you use the long edges of the gear, but because the stance is different in each, the techniques are not the same. For skiing, you use the inside and outside edges of your feet, whereas snowboarding is more about leaning into your toes and heels. Whatever the direction, the skill of edging requires body awareness, balance, and core strength. If you lack these three characteristics before you take up the sport, you'll develop them by the time you've reached the intermediate level.

The learning curve is fairly steep in both sports, with a few key skills needed to stay on your feet and then plenty more to master in your quest of excellence on the mountain. Snowboarding is tough for a few days but then gets a lot easier. Skiing, on the other hand, is simpler to start but can take much longer to master. Pick the one that suits your personality better.

Unless you live near the mountains, you'll probably have limited access for practice. But if you hit the slopes at least once every few months, you will see progress, because you won't forget much from one session to the next. Over the summer, you may lose ground a bit, but you'll quickly pick it back up when the next season starts. If you're looking for a family sport, kids often take to skiing and snowboarding more easily than adults, thanks to their lower center of gravity and greater flexibility. Some children are ready for lessons as early as three years of age, while others do better when they're a little older. Look for a mountain resort with a well-developed children's teaching program to get youngsters off to a good start.

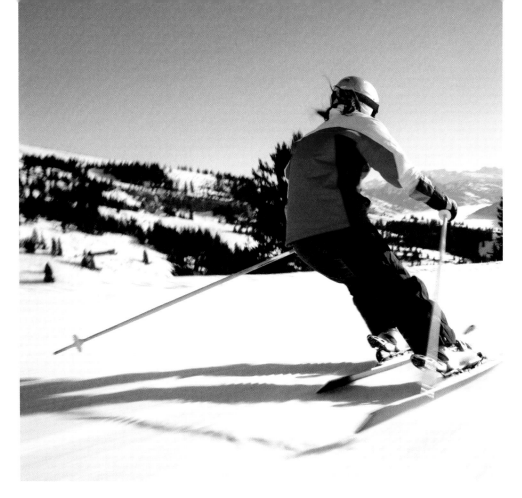

SKIING

It's no surprise that skiing began in cold climates as a form of transportation. The sport is thought to have originated in Norway about 5,000 years ago with hunters. And the Norwegians held the first modern alpine ski competition during the 1850s, after the invention of the first full bindings helped skis stay on athletes' feet. Skiing became an Olympic sport in 1924 with *slalom* racing (the downhill course with flags called *gates*) and ski-jumping events. Today, there are ten Olympic alpine competitions and three ski-jumping events.

In Europe, skiing became a recreational sport at resorts hoping to extend their seasons to include winter activities—and thus attracted a wealthy following. The first skiers had to hike uphill carrying their gear. The first rudimentary lifts were installed in the early 1900s, but the big change came in 1936 when Jim Curran, a railroad engineer, designed the first chairlift based on a similar machine he'd invented for loading bananas into boats. But the equipment itself remained fairly primitive—waxed wooden skis, bamboo poles, and leather boots—until the invention of buckle-closed plastic boots, step-in bindings, and metal poles in the 1950s. As skis and equipment continued to improve, Americans invented *freestyle* skiing, a combination of downhill with acrobatics such as jumps and flips.

Meanwhile, snowmaking, grooming, and detachable chairlifts (which are much easier to get on and off), made the sport less frightening for beginners. And then came *shaped* skis (also called *parabolic*, *hourglass*, and *sidecut*), which made it easier to learn because the sidecut shape is far easier to control and turn. These skis turn with so little effort, in fact, that experienced skiers had trouble switching to them—but even they converted, and today you won't see many "straight" recreational skis on the slopes or in the shops.

DOWNHILL

GEARING UP

When you're ready to try skiing, it's best to rent skis, boots, and poles for the first few outings at least, if not for the whole first season. Rental equipment will help you discern what you like and dislike as you decide whether you want to stick with the sport. If you can, skip renting at the ski resort's concession and head to a ski shop: The price will be better, the gear will be of higher quality, the waiting in line will be shorter, and you'll get more expert attention in fitting the skis (which is vital for safety and success). If possible, try to demo the current season's skis so you get the latest technologies. A few shops also demo boots, which is a great way to test out different brands to try different fits and features.

If you have time, get your gear the night before your first foray onto the mountain so you can avoid the morning crowds. No matter where you rent or buy, the salesperson will select your poles and skis based on your height, weight, and skiing ability (don't improve the numbers if you want the right fit). The bindings will be adjusted so they stay attached to the boots while you ski but release properly in dangerous conditions, which helps protect your knees and legs from injury if the ski has twisted out of control.

Ski boots are awkward—big and bulky, hard to walk in and often difficult to put on and take off. When you stand upright, your toes will be crammed against the front of the boot. The proper ski stance is a slight crouch, which draws your foot back toward the boot's heel. To test boot fit, wear the socks you'll ski in, buckle the boots, and get into the ski stance. Lean from side to side as far as you can without falling, step side to side and do other moves that will mimic your action on the hill. Spend more than a few minutes testing the fit to be sure it's snug enough to let you firmly control the ski but not too tight, because restricted circulation will leave your feet cramped and cold. Proper-fitting boots make such a profound difference in your ability to ski that you'll probably want to invest in a pair by the end of your first season.

Any decent ski pole will work as long as the size is right. To test it, turn the pole upside down so the handle is on the ground, then grasp it just below the *basket* (the plastic ring). If the pole is the correct size, your elbow will be bent at a right angle. Make sure the straps are intact—you'll find them useful so you can "drop" a pole and have it come along instead of needing to go back uphill to get it.

Decent ski garb can make your day much more comfortable. Dress in layers, because you'll heat up on downhill runs. However, the lift rides can be long and cold, so you'll want to zip up. In addition to a secure hat and

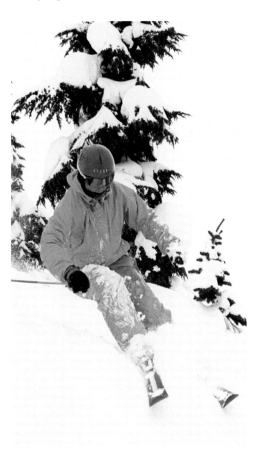

water-resistant gloves, ski pants and a parka, and socks that come up higher than the ski boots, it can help to wear a neck gaiter and goggles. Sunglasses with safety lenses can work in the best weather, but most days you'll want goggles to protect your eyes from snow, wind, glare, and debris. For your first pair of goggles, try yellow or amber lenses because they work in most conditions and aren't so dark that you'll be squinting in the shadows. Other helpful gear are: water; lip balm; tissues; quarters for locker rental; a strap designed to tote boots; dry socks; and cozy boots for après ski, and a bag to carry it all.

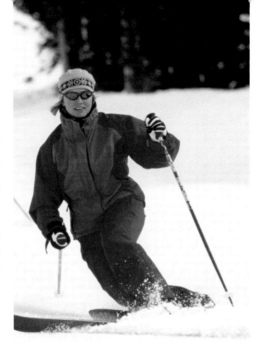

YOUR FIRST TIME

Your first goal is to walk as little as possible in your boots or skis, so take care of any errands that require walking, such as buying a lift ticket, arranging lessons, stopping in the restroom, grabbing a snack, and so on before putting on your boots. Then, find a comfortable seat where you can put on your ski boots, stash your shoes, and make any necessary adjustments to your clothing. Don't put your goggles over your eyes until you're out in the cold, or they will fog up. Leave at least a half hour to accomplish all these items.

Skiing is one of those sports in which a good first lesson can make a world of difference in your future enjoyment. Group ski lessons are cost-effective, and many resorts run introductory rental, lesson, and lodging packages for beginners at a reduced price. Your ski instructor will first teach you to adjust your boots, get in and out of your bindings, and get up after a fall without sliding downhill. Next, you'll get pointers, while standing still, about shifting your weight to get a sense of balance and positioning your skis with the tips together and tails spread, which is called a *wedge* or *snowplow*. You'll do your first sliding in this ski position—and may spend the entire first lesson practicing it. Skiing in a wedge position uses a lot of thigh-muscle strength, which is tiring, but you will be able to ski slowly and maintain control. You can also use the snowplow to turn and stop simply by pressing harder on one or both skis. The instructor will explain how to link turns

together and follow the downward slope of the mountain, called the *fall line*. The lesson will include tips for walking uphill so you can ski down from there or get to a tow or lift to take you farther uphill. You may also get instruction on riding the lift and, more important, getting off (which is prime time for your first fall, if you haven't already had one). By the end of your first lesson, you should be able to glide, stop, and turn to ski down a beginner run, also called the *bunny slope*.

When you've mastered the initial skills of sliding and turning with control using the snowplow, it's time to bring your skis to parallel. This shift can be a slow process, which some skiers never fully accomplish. Parallel skis move faster downhill, but they are also easier to maneuver—and the position requires far less leg strength. To carve a turn on parallel parabolic skis, you simply roll both skis slightly to the side and the edges dig in. To ski slowly, you can carve wide turns that traverse back and forth across the trail instead of heading straight down. And to stop, simply continue a turn until you're facing slightly uphill and the skis will halt (don't go too far uphill or you can slide backward).

DOWNHILL

109

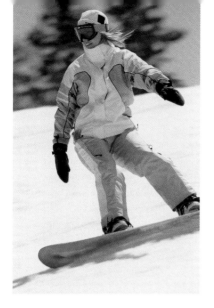
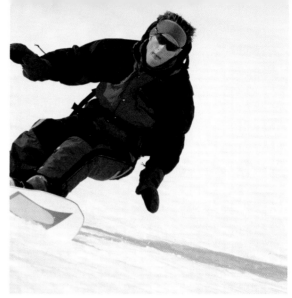

SNOWBOARDING

The first snow-surfing board to be sold commercially was the Snurfer, introduced in the 1960s. The thin wooden board—similar to a skateboard but without wheels—had studs to hold your shoes in place and a string attached to the front for steering. Snowboarding, as we know it today, started in Vermont in the 1970s. Jake Burton Carpenter, founder of Burton Snowboards, started building wooden snowboards with rubber loops for bindings. The first snowboard competitions were held in Vermont during the late '70s and early '80s. The best-known event, the U.S. Open, is now headquartered at Stratton Mountain, which was one of the first large mountains to welcome riders. The sport's reputation in the early days wasn't helped by the stereotypical image of teen troublemakers complete with baggy clothes and irreverent attitudes. Skiers complained that riders scraped off the snow and whizzed by with little concern for safety, and many resorts did not allow snowboarders on the trails.

Although snowboarding has grown quickly in popularity and acceptance over the last two decades, there remain four "ski-only" resorts in the U.S.: Alta and Deer Valley in Utah, Taos in New Mexico, and Mad River Glen in Vermont. Anyplace else, you're likely to see businessmen and women, moms, dads, and some grandparents shredding along with the kids. There are now two styles of snowboarding: *freeriding* and *freestyle*. Freeriding is the type done on ski trails and other slopes, carving turns like a surfer on the waves. Freestyle involves tricks and jumps most often done in a terrain park with numerous obstacles. Most of the freestyle tricks are borrowed from skateboarding, including riding rails and the most popular, the *half-pipe*. Within freestyle, there are also competitions called *boardercross*, a spin-off of motocross racing that involves the same concept: an obstacle-dotted track over which a number of riders race. Giant slalom and half-pipe competitions were added to the Olympic program in Japan in 1998 and boardercross joined in 2006 in Turino.

GEARING UP

Each style of snowboarding comes with its own gear. But most beginners use freeriding boards with soft boots because they are the most versatile for any conditions on the mountain and also do a fair job in the terrain park. If you want to focus on tricks after you've learned the basics, you'll want a freestyle board, which is shorter and more maneuverable than freeriding versions, and better suited for riding with either foot forward (freeriders tend to stick to one stance). Snowboard slalom racers use longer, stiffer boards, hard boots, and plate bindings—more similar to ski gear than other snowboard setups.

As with skiing, it's wise to rent, not purchase, gear for your first few days on the slopes to help determine the type that works best for you and whether or not you love the sport enough to stick with it. And keep in mind that equipment is continually improving, so if you won't make it to the mountain more than a few times the first year, it can pay to wait until the next season to get outfitted with the latest designs. When you rent gear, you'll need to determine where the bindings are set—which foot should be in front, how far

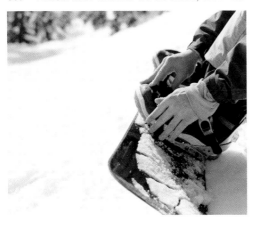

apart and at what angle the feet should be on the board. Snowboard bindings are easy to adjust and many combinations work, so ask the shop to explain how to arrange your bindings and other options you can consider if you aren't comfortable. The most important factor is which foot rides in front. Every person has a dominant side, just as we're left- or right-handed. Your balance and ability will be dramatically reduced if you end up with the wrong foot in front. There are several off-snow tests to determine which setup is best. Here's an easy one: Stand with your feet side by side, a stable distance apart. Have a friend give you a gentle shove from behind. Note which foot automatically slides forward to keep you from falling—that's the foot to put in front on the board. If it's your left foot, you ride *regular*, and if it's your right foot, you ride *goofy*.

Beginners do best with shorter boards, which are easier to control. Check the size by standing the board on end in front of you. For your first day, choose a board that is at least as high as your collarbone but doesn't come above your chin. The width of the board should be not much bigger than your boots in your bindings (so you need to know the angle of the bindings first). A board that's too fat will be hard to control, and one that's too thin will let your toes or heels drag in the snow and toss you over.

Snowboard boots may look a lot like hiking boots, but they're not interchangeable. The boots you use to snowboard are designed to fit snugly into the bindings, to have stiff sides for support, to be waterproof, and to be warmer than the average hiking boot. You can rent boots as a package with your board.

Although snowboarders have their own style, ski gear will work just fine for your first few forays, if you happen to own it already. Dress in layers and avoid anything restrictive. Be sure to have waterproof gloves and pants of good quality because you will be falling a lot; riders spend more time sitting in the snow than skiers as they adjust bindings or rest. Goggles are helpful, too. Beginners should also consider wrist guards (like the ones from in-line skating) and helmets to protect the most vulnerable spots on the first days of almost-guaranteed falls. Tuck in as much as possible—gloves inside jacket cuffs, for example—to keep the snow out.

YOUR FIRST TIME

Technically, snowboarding is easier to learn than skiing, although it might not feel that way the first few days. Many new riders opt out of lessons; after all, this is a sport with a nontraditional culture. But if you can afford it, an instructor is a nice advantage, if only to help you to your feet or provide feedback on what just happened after a fall.

The challenges begin immediately. Just learning to walk with one foot buckled into the binding, the other stepping alongside the board, is tricky. Next, try *skating*, which is like skateboarding in that you push off on the ground then step on to glide, resting the back foot on the *stomp pad* that's affixed to the board between the bindings. You'll need to skate off the lift, so it's a key skill.

When you can balance on the immobile board, walk, and skate, it's time to try sliding. First, you need to select a direction: Facing downhill is called *heelside* because the back edge of your board faces the mountain. This is a good position for beginners because the first backward falls (called "catching a heelside edge") are a little gentler, just like sitting down hard. Unfortunately, the downhill view is intimidating, and if you're alone, it can be almost impossible to get into this position. Turn around and face uphill, called *toeside*, and the backward fall involves whipping all the way downhill before crashing into the slope. On the plus side, to get started facing uphill you simply kneel in the snow and push off with your hands. If you don't have a friend or instructor to help you, toeside might be your only option.

When you've picked your position, tip your front foot ever-so-slightly downhill to start the slide. To stop, pull up gently on the front foot to return to the start position (perpendicular to the hill). Don't turn around; simply try the same slide with your other foot leading. Move back and forth across the hill, slowly making your way down, in a pattern called a *falling leaf*. Practice until you can do the falling leaf toeside and heelside.

Next, head up the lift and try a turn or two on the way down by sliding a little straighter downhill, then lift the front toes, curving to the side to stop perpendicular to the hill. Repeat the turn until it's comfortable in both directions, then string them together in an alternating pattern, and *voilà*, you're snowboarding.

Three is the magic number in this sport. Most people pick up the basic skills of the sport after a disheartening three days of falling. The fat board is a stable platform when still, but any shift in balance is likely to make you catch an edge for a quick flip to the ground. Beginners repeat this pattern over and over, often as a result of hesitancy when concerned

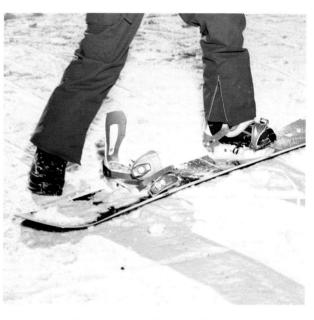

about going too fast, which naturally induces you to lean back—and, wham, you're down. The first two days, you spend a lot of time sitting in the snow and pushing back up to standing, which can be tough on the wrists and arms. Somehow, miraculously, on the third day most beginners suddenly get a feel for the edges of the board and succeed at steering it downhill for a successful short run.

One possible shortcut: Burton Snowboards has developed a Learn to Ride program designed to make the first day less painful. It uses boards with slight curves along the sides so you're less likely to catch an edge and fall. They also offer women-specific training and classes for kids. The program claims to have most riders linking turns by the end of the first day and is available at many ski resorts.

TACKLE THE TRUTH

Skiing and snowboarding are very dangerous sports

No sport is perfectly safe, but the reputation of skiing and snowboarding as dangerous sports is exaggerated. A fall is likely to be little more than cold and uncomfortable, especially if the snow is soft powder. You're most likely to jam a thumb, get a bruise as you bounce, or strain a muscle that's not used to the exertion.

The most common serious ski injury isn't the infamous ACL tear in the knee joint, but rather damage to the nearby MCL that can usually be treated with a knee brace and a period of physical therapy. Most snowboard injuries are sustained from falling on the first day out. The main site of damage is the wrist because of the natural tendency to extend the arms to soften a fall (it's healthier to tuck your arms). Some people wear in-line skating wrist guards for the first few sessions to protect the area. And you can wear a helmet if you fear a bad fall.

You have to be rich to take up downhill skiing or snowboarding

A top-notch mountain vacation can cost thousands. But if your budget is more modest, there are ways to bring down the costs. Small mountains offer less expensive lift tickets and lodging options, or look for discounts for mid-week and after lunch access or combination deals of lifts, lodging, lessons, and gear. Some hearty athletes even forgo the lift tickets entirely and do backcountry versions of the sports, where you hike up carrying your gear, then glide down—talk about a workout! You can even test out your affinity for the sport close to home on a sledding hill or golf course with gently sloping terrain. Some town recreation departments and athletic clubs organize ski trips that include transportation and tickets. Often, these are day trips that cut out the cost of lodging, and they may offer group lessons at a discount. For gear bargain ideas, check out *Getting Bargains on Gear*, page 103.

You're going to freeze

Snow sports often mean enduring cooler temperatures (although some days out West can be balmy, with people skiing in shorts). But even when the thermometer registers below zero, you can stay comfortable on the slopes if you dress wisely, thanks to advances in technical clothing. For example, you can eliminate cold toes with little instant-heater packs you can stuff into your boots. For more ideas on keeping warm, read *Staying Warm and Safe in the Cold*, page 197.

DOWNHILL

SECRETS TO SUCCESS

One intimidating aspect of skiing and snowboarding which is not a myth: You are going to fall. But you can minimize the negative consequences and make it just another part of an exciting day. "If you're not falling, you're not learning," says Jan Griscom, a trainer at the Sports Center at Chelsea Piers and a former ski instructor. Even though you want to stay safe and in control, part of the joy of these sports is learning new skills, which requires practicing moves a little beyond your abilities—and that means falling. What you don't want to do is career out of control, but instead just push yourself a little. Start by learning how to fall well and get up safely, so you can spend less time fearing the inevitable.

After the first three days, you'll do much less falling in snowboarding than skiing. "You can pick up a little snowboarding in one weekend because there's a rhythm to it," says Griscom. "In two lessons, I've seen people being able to get down some intermediate trails." As your skills improve in either sport, you fall less—and you generally get somewhat used to it. Still, adults tend to fear falling, and that trepidation creates one of the most ironic situations: When you feel nervous, the natural tendency is to stiffen up and lean back. But these two moves almost guarantee a fall. Instead, if you face down the mountain and go with the movement, you'll be far more likely to stay on your feet. Of course, if this posture means speeding along at 30 miles per hour, it's not a good plan. The compromise: Bend your knees to lower your cen-

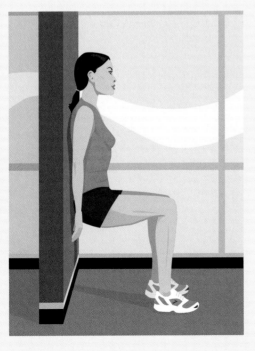

wall sits

Stand with your back to a wall, leaning against it. Keeping your feet slightly more than hip-distance apart, walk your feet away from the wall and allow your body to slide down. Keep going until your thighs are parallel to the floor (if that's too hard, go as far as you can). Make sure your knees don't jut out beyond your toes—if they do, shift your feet out farther. Try not to use your hands against the wall for help. Hold the position for 30 seconds, building up to 3 minutes.

DOWNHILL

ter of gravity and firm your abs as you point your skis or snowboard to traverse the slope slightly downhill but mostly sideways. For snowboarding, face the direction of travel and lean into your turns. For skiing, face downhill, lean your body slightly forward from the ankles so your weight is on the balls of your feet, and let the skis travel to the side while the body counterbalances. Moving sideways will be slower than bombing straight downhill, but your balance and posture will remain in the most stable orientation.

The bent-knee position requires thigh muscle strength, and can be hard to maintain for hours on the slopes. Just having a big plank or two attached to your feet is tiring, too. Muscle endurance is the key to fresh legs. If you have time for pre-season training, fifteen reps on the leg press isn't the best way to prepare for five minutes moving down the mountain. Instead, do longer sets with lighter weights to get the muscles ready for the challenge. "Work on one leg at a time to build even strength," advises Griscom. And do some lateral moves such as side lunges and sideways hops, because this type of movement isn't part of our daily activities but is necessary on the slopes. The same goes for abdominal work— focus on building endurance and the ability to use muscles for twisting from side to side, targeting the obliques more than the central abs. Try these exercises:

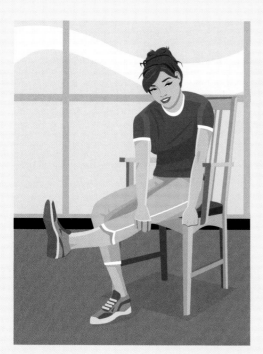

chair obliques

Sit on the front edge of a stable chair, feet flat on the floor. Lift your left leg straight in front, level with the seat, and hold it in place. Keeping your head in line with your spine, lean back from the hips as far as you comfortably can. Rock forward rapidly, punching your right arm across your left leg as far as you can (don't move your left leg). Lean back, lower your left leg, and quickly repeat on the opposite side to complete 1 rep. Start with 10 reps. Build up to 3 minutes.

DOWNHILL

Kristin Lawson, 26

The first time she tried snowboarding, about two years ago, Kristin Lawson did not have a good time. She signed up for a lesson because her younger brother wanted to go. "I spent four hours on my butt. I couldn't even stand up with my feet strapped in," recalls the avid skier from Burlington, Vermont. "I returned the snowboard and put my skis back on." She knew from friends that the sport had a painful but fast learning curve, but her prior experience made her hesitant to try again. "As an adult, we're not used to falling down," she says. Plus the body takes longer to recover from the effects of the pounding.

Recently, however, Lawson was practically forced to give snowboarding a second chance. She works at the Boys and Girls Club in Burlington, which participates in the Chill program run by Burton Snowboards; the program allows disadvantaged kids to try snowboarding in six weekly sessions at Bolton Valley resort. And Lawson's club sends ten kids each year. "Someone from the Boys and Girls Club went every year, but this year there wasn't anyone to go, so I volunteered."

During the one-hour lesson, the instructors taught the group how to use the step-in bindings and the safe way to fall—hands tucked in, letting the body absorb the impact. Then, with just one foot strapped in, they learned how to skate along flats and climbed a small hill to practice sliding down. Lawson had only fallen a few times by the end of the lesson. Feeling bolder, she hiked to the top of the bunny slope, strapped in the second foot, and practiced sliding short distances and stopping. "In the next two hours, I fell at least 100 times," says Lawson. "I had to keep telling myself to get up and try again. Falling, rolling over so you can stand back up—it's exhausting. But once I got comfortable falling, that made a big difference." By the end of the session she was able to slide a few feet down the mountain.

The success that day left Lawson excited about the following weeks, but the weather the next two times did not cooperate. "It was icy," recalls Lawson. "I flew over backward and bounced a few times on my tailbone and head; I was glad I had the helmet on." Tempted to go inside and cry, she struggled to stay strong. "Chill has a theme each week," says Lawson. "I thought they sounded cheesy and that I'd have to pretend it was worthwhile." But the topic for week two was "persistence," and she didn't have any trouble persuading herself or her group that the discussion was valuable.

Week four was about "courage"—and Lawson needed a lot after her experiences on the icy slopes. She was rewarded by making it down the easiest run twice. By the last week—the topic was "pride"—Lawson was linking turns and feeling excited and in control on the board. "I'm not competitive at all; but it's been good for me to prove to myself that I could do it. And it's been amazing watching the kids grow and learn."

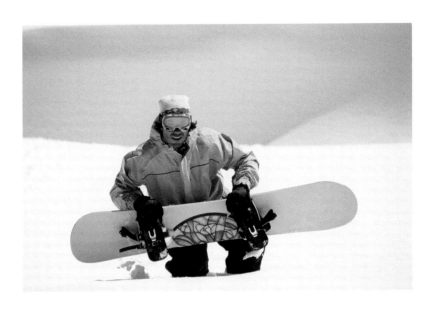

GET MORE FROM YOUR SPORT

Skiers and snowboarders who start as adults can end up as instructors and competitors if they take to the sport easily or dedicate some serious time to learning. Whether you just want to tool around down the slopes or aspire to a trophy, there are plenty of other sports that can give you an edge. Any type of dance can enhance your downhill rhythm, leg and lung stamina, and balance. Skating hones the same skills plus provides a useful sense of edging, especially if you do slalom turns. The leg and stamina workouts from bike riding, boxing, jumping rope, volleyball, and other court sports can also translate to a better day on the mountain. Swimming can improve coordination, timing, and the pacing of breathing. Even the elliptical trainers with arms or cross-country ski machines can be terrific ski and snowboard prep.

If you love skiing and want to take up more sports, waterskiing, in-line skating, and ice skating are the most similar. Snowshoeing and cross-country skiing are great options for mountain activities. Horseback riding, hiking, and mountain biking are fun ways to enjoy the slopes in warmer weather.

Snowboarders can do off-season training on a skateboard, surfboard, or wakeboard. Other top picks for riders: mountain biking, in-line skating, and trail running. If you love the terrain park, try kayaking and rafting, gymnastics, bicycle motocross, and rock climbing.

Most skiers and riders enjoy traveling to different mountains to experience a variety of terrain—and views. When planning a trip, look for features you'll use such as terrain at your level, excellent instruction, and equipment-demo days. In general, Western resorts have more natural powder and longer seasons than those in the East, but all mountains have something fun to offer with each having its own style, from kid-friendly Sugarbush in Maine to the history-steeped Stowe in Vermont and the extended season at Arapahoe Basin in Colorado. Keep in mind that many of the smaller resorts provide expert instruction, easy trails, and less crowding.

If you want to go to a ski or snowboard camp, there are excellent programs that provide intensive courses with hours of instruction, meals, lodging, and often top gear. Rank beginners can sign up for a novice camp or try one open to all levels. Some programs are for women only, with an emphasis on the physiological and psychological differences in gear, techniques, and learning styles. Other camps are designed for helping intermediates and advanced athletes improve even more or focus on specific skills such as terrain-park tricks or moguls.

RESOURCES

➡ **www.skimag.com**, *Ski* magazine's Web site, is a useful resource for tips on technique and for finding resorts and lodging.

➡ **www.abc-of-skiing.com** offers an array of topics, from gear info to destinations to a glossary of jargon.

➡ *Learn Downhill Skiing in a Weekend* by Konrad Bartelski and Robin Neillands will teach you the jargon and concepts before your first lesson—and deliver a refresher course before your next one.

➡ *The New Guide to Skiing* by French ski instructor Martin Heckelman is packed with precise photos and clear instructions for mastering shaped skis and progressing from novice to solid skier in any conditions.

➡ **www.abc-of-snowboarding.com**, the sister site to the ski version, is also packed with info on travel, gear, and more.

➡ **www.powderroom.net** is designed specifically for female riders (and wannabe riders), but the basic info is useful for any beginner. Check out the "Your first snowboard lesson" article in particular.

➡ *Complete Snowboarder* by Jeff Bennett, Scott Downey, and Charles Arnell covers the gear, the styles and the tips to get you started or take your skills to the next level.

DOWNHILL

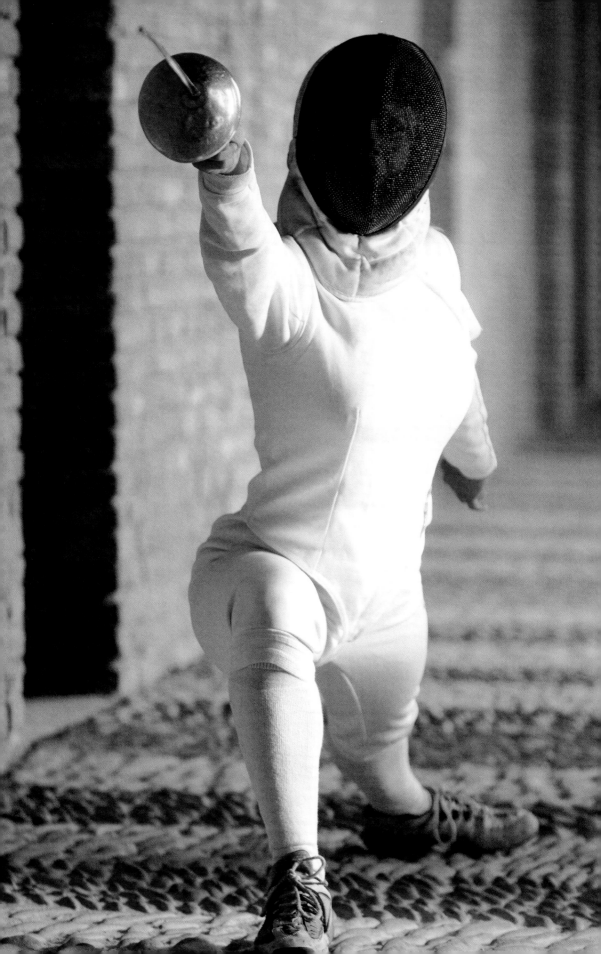

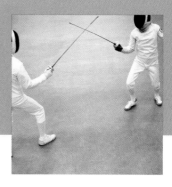

10

FENCING

FENCING

YOU'LL LOVE THIS SPORT IF YOU:
- like to combine cardio with strength, agility, balance, and flexibility
- want a workout that gives you a great butt
- love a sport that combines strategy, precision, and a sense of history
- prefer sports that require so much mental focus you'll forget you're exercising
- want to compete individually
- prefer a sport in which it's common to be an adult beginner

YOU MIGHT NOT LOVE THIS SPORT IF YOU:
- prefer to do things your own way rather than following the rules
- hate losing
- don't like physical contact with an opponent
- need to feel like part of a team
- have knee or back pain on a regular basis
- prefer to set your own schedule rather than rely on an opponent

To many people, fencing means Zorro, the Three Musketeers, and Errol Flynn—all flashing swords and seemingly effortless footwork. Fencers, of course, know better. The reality is long hours spent mastering the intricacies of the sport and not so much slashing as precise, directed moves. Yet those swashbucklers of the screen are part of the sport's rich history and lore. Fencing evolved from the sword-wielding duels fought in the 17th century, before guns became popular. Back then, studying the skills of swordplay was a matter of life or death. Today, when a sword worn on the hip is seen only in Hollywood or at Halloween, such bouts are reserved for fencing *salles* (that's "rooms" in French) and tournaments.

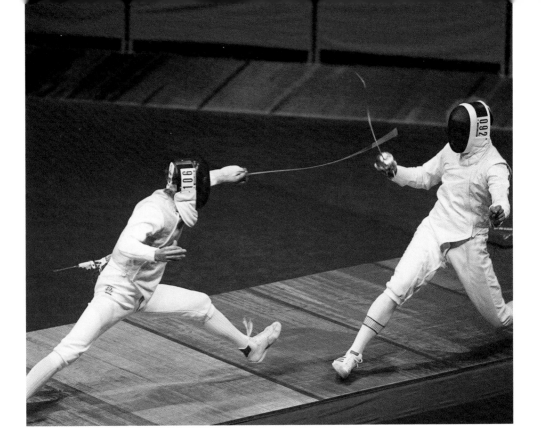

The sport of fencing has similarities to the close combat of martial arts, the strategy of chess, and the poise of dance, with steps as choreographed as ballet. Unlike boxing or wrestling, fencing is scored by a touch to the target area on the opponent without the likelihood of harm. To that end, fencing is a formal sport, in which etiquette and politeness play a strong role. Although it's a fight, you won't get hurt.

A fencing bout is conducted on a strip or *piste*, a surface such as wood or metal (or sometimes just tape marks on the floor) that is 1.5 meters by 14 meters, which is about 5 feet by 46 feet. Each fencer takes his or her position on a starting line marked 2 meters from the center. They salute each other and the director. The action begins with a sign from the referee, who officiates at the bout in French. Fencers wear a protective white uniform and mask. The weapon used in competition may have a body cord coming from the weapon's *guard* (which is near the hand) that then runs along the inside of the fencer's sleeve, then out the back of the jacket, to a reel that attaches to an electronic scoring machine. The movements in fencing require such speed that without the machine it can be a difficult to know if a touch was scored.

Most styles of fencing have a *right of way* that designates the offensive player from the defensive one, which is based on who initiated the action; only the offensive player can score a touch. However, as soon as the defensive fencer has deflected an attack with a move called a *parry*—often a simple flick of the weapon to the side executed by rolling the wrist—the roles switch and he or she can then score in the next second. A fencer can also score a touch by driving the opponent off the back edge of the strip.

There are three styles of fencing, each using a different weapon. *Sabre* fencing uses a curved blade reminiscent of a cavalry weapon, and the target area includes any part of the body above the waist. Sabre is the only form of fencing that allows hits with the side of the weapon as well as the tip. In a tournament, sabre fencers must wear a metal vest or *lamé* that covers the target area, and a hit is registered via the electronic scoring device when touched by the weapon. The mask is also designed to register a hit. Right of way is observed in sabre fencing. *Épée* (pronounced "EHP-pay," which is French for "sword") derives from dueling, and here a long, stiff blade is used. In this style, the entire body represents a target, but only the point of the weapon can make a score. There is no right of way in épée; both fencers can land a touch at almost the same time. The third style, *foil*, is the most popular form of fencing. The weapon used in this style is a variation on the swords used for dueling practice by nobility. They are smaller, lighter, and more flexible than the épée. Only the tip of the weapon can score a touch, and the target area is the entire torso, front and back. Foil fencers can score with a lighter hit than in épée. Like sabre, foil fencing observes the right of way and fencers wear a lamé that indicates when the touch is in the target area.

Many tournaments use a *round robin* process in which the fencers are divided into pools and everyone within the pool fences against everyone else. At the end of the round, all the fencers in the tournament are ranked. At that point, the bouts switch to direct elimination in which you either win and continue or lose and are replaced. A bout continues until a designated number of touches are scored by one fencer or the time runs out. In round robin bouts, the goal is typically five touches. For direct elimination, bouts are generally divided into three periods, each lasting three minutes with a minute of rest between, and the fencers work toward fifteen touches to win. At the end of a bout, the fencers salute each other, shake unweaponed hands and say something pleasant to each other.

The classic fencing stance is a semisquat, akin to a plié in ballet. The moves strengthen the quadriceps and gluteal muscles because you are constantly lunging and stepping. Great thighs and a firm butt are the classic sign of a fencer's body. Core strength and balance are important factors in staying steady on the strip, where one must be ready to attack or retreat without falling. Once you've mastered the basics, the fast pace of the sport makes it a good aerobic workout that can leave you dripping in sweat. Some fencers are very athletic, bounding and bouncing on the strip. The speed of fencing will improve your agility, reflexes, and hand/eye coordination. Possibly it is fast footwork that can determine the winner.

Fencing requires focus. You have to plan and move quickly so you don't get hit. You must remain alert, because even a moment's distraction will allow your opponent to score. Fencing bout after bout in a tournament is certainly exhausting, but even a few hours of fencing practice can leave you spent. This is not a sport in which the athletes tend to go out for a beer afterward, although tournaments can be social. Most fencers belong to a fencing club that offers instruction and fellow fencers to practice with. A few people from the same club may attend a tournament together—at which point they suddenly become opponents rather than friends. The shifting nature of these interactions can be a challenge for your mental focus as you strive to score against someone you know and like. But there are advantages to learning an opponent's fencing style in order to capitalize on weaknesses or subtle variations in his or her technique that will allow you to score a touch. *En garde!*

SCORE

If you weigh 150 pounds, you'll burn about 300 calories in an hour of fencing. (To calculate your hourly burn rate, multiply your weight in pounds by two.)

GEARING UP

If you sign up for lessons at a fencing salle, there's a good chance they'll provide the gear you need, from the mask to the blade. A fencing uniform is white: You wear one glove on the fencing hand, a thick white jacket with a strap that goes between your legs, and a zipper up the back. The complete uniform worn by competitive fencers includes white knickers and tall white socks. For protection, you'll wear a mask with a mesh front. An underarm plastron covers half of the fencing arm. Women will wear a sturdy plastic breastplate under the jacket for extra protection. You'll need a weapon—most fencers have several, including an electronic weapon used during competitions. For sabre and foil fencing, you'll also need the lamé. There are special fencing shoes designed with traction specific to the sport (including on a metal piste), which protects against twisted ankles and provides extra durability in the spot that wears out if you drag your trailing foot on the ground instead of lifting it off cleanly. The fencing salle where you take lessons can provide advice for gear purchases, when the time comes. To start, dress in comfortable gym clothing (nothing too loose or it might get snagged) and sneakers, and borrow the jacket, mask, and blade.

YOUR FIRST TIME

The inaugural fencing lesson is guaranteed to make you feel awkward. You suit up in an outfit that's a little like something an old-fashioned undersea explorer would have worn—the antithesis of a dashing swashbuckler. First, without a weapon, you learn the basic footwork. Your lead foot—the right if you're right-handed—points along the strip, while your trailing foot is turned out to the side. To advance, you step-together, step-together, holding your weapon arm out in front, your other arm behind you, hand up and elbow down. To retreat, you step-together, step-together in reverse. (It feels like it would be a lot faster just to run away!) For the attack, you advance until you're a short distance from your opponent, then, at the same time, lunge forward and thrust the weapon. These three basic moves are plenty to learn the first time, and they will feel completely unnatural. Surprisingly, over several weeks of practice, the moves start to feel more comfortable.

The early maneuvers you'll learn may not seem athletic, but take a minute to watch more advanced fencers and you'll see that the sport is very active, with plenty of quick forward and backward motion, ducking, and

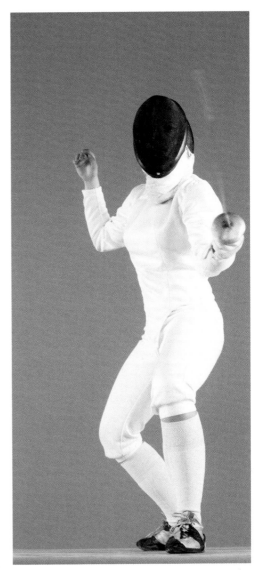

leaping attacks. As a beginner, executing the slow steps over and over will leave your legs quivering and weapon arm feeling weak because your body isn't used to moving in this pattern. Even though the weapons don't weigh much (a practice foil weighs less than a pound), holding it and your arm up for extended periods can be taxing. There's not much we do in daily life, or in other sports, in which you have to hold one arm out for long durations, and your muscles just aren't trained to do it.

Try to stretch before your fencing lesson so your muscles are ready for action. Many classes are held after work, so it's rare for fencers to stick around to stretch afterward. But doing at least a few limbering moves at the end can help avoid stiffness as your muscles cool down and relax.

When you line up on the strip against an opponent for the first time, be prepared to feel mentally overwhelmed. There's a lot of concentration involved, but the main shock to the psyche is the act of being touched with a weapon. Even though you know you're safe, you will have a visceral reaction that can be taxing. With practice, you get used to the experience.

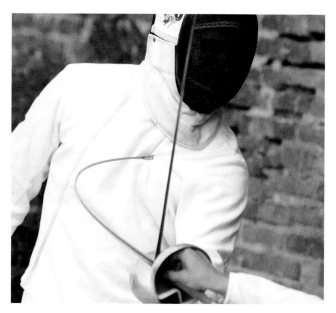

You may have seen him on television, but these days you're more likely to find him on the piste than on the evening news. Veteran WABC anchorman John Johnson was always fascinated by fencing. He dabbled in the sport a bit during his college years, but his school did not offer fencing, and he felt his parents would not approve of time spent away from his extra-full load of classes and the job that provided him with pocket money. So Johnson paid for his own equipment and lessons without their knowledge. There wasn't much extra time or cash, so he had to give it up before long, dedicating himself to studies, and later, his career.

Almost fifty years later, he had a chance encounter with a trainer at his gym who happened to do the same form of fencing he had learned as a teen: a traditional style of foil. They began to practice together, and Johnson felt his love for the sport return as he repeated the moves on the strip. His opponent, a veteran female competitor, was a shy, polite woman off the piste but became an "exacting rapier" behind the mask, Johnson says. She needed someone to parry and thrust with, and Johnson rose to the challenge.

Johnson and the trainer fence a few days a week now. He is quick and has long arms, giving him a natural advantage. His attack is strong, forcing defensive action from his opponent. For her part, having studied for many years, she is a facile coach, astute and knowledgeable. "My fencing skills have soared," he says. Now, his goal is to compete in a Masters Open event.

"I don't like mindless exercise," says Johnson. The discipline and concentration keep him focused. An avid chess player, he loves the strategic aspects of fencing, as well as its physical components. And with his television career no longer taking center stage (he retired to care for his ailing father), Johnson has more time to fence, as well as to pursue his interest in writing and painting. "It's a beautiful and thoughtful sport that fits into my whole artistic psyche," he says of fencing. But that doesn't mean it's easy. "Your body is flexed and ready to spring like a cat when the opportunity arises," he says. "Every time I take the mask off, I'm dripping." He was worried that at his age he'd have trouble with the sport's physical demands and at first hesitated to take up the foil again. But while his knees do give him some trouble, he's found that he can fence as well as he'd hoped. "It's a great exercise at any age," he says.

FENCING

SECRETS TO SUCCESS

"You won't learn fencing in a week," says Sharone Huey, a competitive fencer who teaches basic fencing fitness classes at the Sports Center at Chelsea Piers. "But after a month, you will start to pick it up and feel the tempo." After just a few months of dedicated practice, some people are ready to compete, although they can expect faster, more fluid opponents to win. Seeing as few American kids take up fencing, tournaments are packed with people who came to the sport as an adult. For you to get the most out of your first lessons, Huey suggests trying to go during the day or early evening before the fencing salle gets crowded. In the evening, the room is frequently filled with pairs in combat, plenty of noise, and distractions. Once you've mastered the basics, do seek the busy times, because you'll need to bout in such conditions at a tournament.

In fencing, you could adopt the motto "Less is more." Don't rush in to attack but rather size up the situation first. Try not to wander all over the strip or wave your weapon about wildly. Conserve energy. Fight smart. Fencing is a sport of finesse.

To progress quickly in fencing ability, build up endurance in your weapon arm,

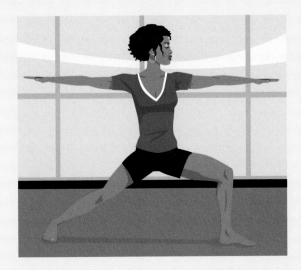

warrior II

Stand with your legs as wide as you comfortably can. Rotate your left foot so the toes face out then angle your right toes in slightly. Lift your head high and press your shoulders down away from your ears. Lift both arms to shoulder height, pressing out through the fingertips, palms facing down. Bend your left knee into a lunge (the knee should be aligned over your toes), shifting your hips and torso forward but maintaining an erect, strong posture. Tuck your pelvis slightly, press into your right heel, and try to lower your left thigh parallel to the ground. Turn your head to gaze out over your left fingers without shifting your torso and hips. Breathe deeply and hold the position as long as you can, keeping energy flowing through your thighs and arms. Return to an erect posture. Then repeat the sequence on your other side.

practice footwork and lunging, lunging, and again, lunging. It's also helpful to firm up your core muscles to attain balance and good posture. You should also stretch to stay supple. Yoga poses can be helpful for building strength in the legs and arms. Try these exercises to improve your abilities on the piste:

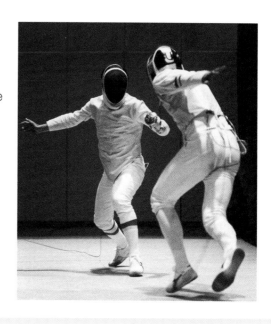

down dog extended

From your hands and knees, extend your legs straight back so you are balanced on your toes in a plank position with your hands on the ground directly below your shoulders, fingers spread, body in a straight line from the top of head to heels, feet shoulder-width apart. Walk your feet forward while raising your butt as high in the air as you can and pointing your head downward to form an inverted V. Press your shoulders down, away from your ears, and draw your thighs toward your chest while trying to keep your heels down. Now lift one leg to form a straight line from head to heel, without allowing your hips to twist. Hold for 1 breath. Lower and repeat with the other leg. Keep alternating legs for as long as you can.

TACKLE THE TRUTH

Fencing is an aggressive sport, and you have to be aggressive to do it

Although fencing is a combat sport with a history of to-the-death matches, a strong tradition of etiquette insures good sportsmanship and polite behavior, such as not striking outside the target area or storming off the strip after a loss. The best fencers stay calm and use more skill and precision than they do brute force or aggression. Even shy people can excel at fencing, because the scripted moves and masked bouts can provide a means of self-expression. Fencers gain an advantage through mental prowess as much as physical ability; and when the latter skill stands out, it's more likely to be speed and agility that provide the advantage rather than power.

Being able to size up your opponent and find openings to strike is key to success on the strip. Also, you must plan an attack and, after your opponent deflects your weapon, plan a counterattack or defense maneuver. You are constantly thinking and formulating your strategy in the course of the bout.

You'll get stabbed or hurt when fencing

You won't actually get stabbed while fencing. As a matter of fact, the protective gear and blunt weapons make this sport one of the safest. The typical ailments from fencing are sprained ankles, blisters, and bruises.

A firm but light touch registers as a hit, so there's no need for a piercing blow. And your opponent won't want to strike harder than necessary because a strong move might throw him off balance and because every fencing bout can be exhausting. Because you might be completing many bouts in a single day, conserving energy is a good strategy.

You have to be young and thin to fence

Fencing is a sport for all ages, sizes, and shapes. Tournaments are divided by sex, level, and age, with a special veteran's designation for those forty years and older; some fencers still compete in their eighties. As long as you can step and hold a weapon, you can continue to fence. And while heavier fencers may not be as light on their feet, they can make up for any deficit in physical ability by mastering the strategy of the sport. Also, thin people aren't always the quickest. Some big fencers can be surprisingly speedy.

FENCING

GET MORE FROM YOUR SPORT

Practicing fencing is fun, but most people don't aspire to fence in front of a mirror. The goal is to bout, and usually to bout in a tournament. It can be intimidating to consider matching up against dozens of fencers in one day, and it certainly is exhausting, but stick to your studies and you'll get there. Find a fencing instructor whom you respect and who can explain the moves and strategies in an understandable way. Or seek a mentor who will coax you out of any hesitation and into fluid moves. Stick around the salle to watch your fellow fencers, but only follow one fencer with your eyes at a time. You will learn how she adds her own variations to the standard moves, and you may glean some of her strategy.

Any martial art will have some similarities to fencing, as do boxing and wrestling. A step or boxing aerobics class will provide excellent cross-training for fencing. Any activity that increases your stamina will improve your fencing abilities. Try ballet, pilates, and yoga training.

Tournaments provide ample opportunity to combine fencing and travel. They are held all over the world, from Italy to Japan, and you can attend with your fencing club or as an individual fencer. There are also clubs sprinkled all over the U.S. that offer classes, plus summer camps for learning advanced skills. Check fencing Web sites to find the latest information on locations.

RESOURCES

➡ **www.usfencing.org** is the site for the official American fencing group that organizes tournaments and ranks athletes. The basic information on the Web site is useful, and it offers a link where a prospective fencer can find local instruction.

➡ **www.fencing.net** is a site with a wide array of information, from weapon care to footwork drills. The message boards provide a forum for getting questions answered.

➡ *Fencing: Techniques of Foil, Sabre and Epée* by Brian Pitman covers the modernized version (not old-fashioned classic technique) of all three styles of fencing. It's especially useful for helping the beginner learn about and choose from all three.

➡ *Fencing: Steps to Success* by Olympian and instructor Elaine Cheris covers maneuvers and drills for beginners. Simple line drawings clearly illustrate how to execute basic moves.

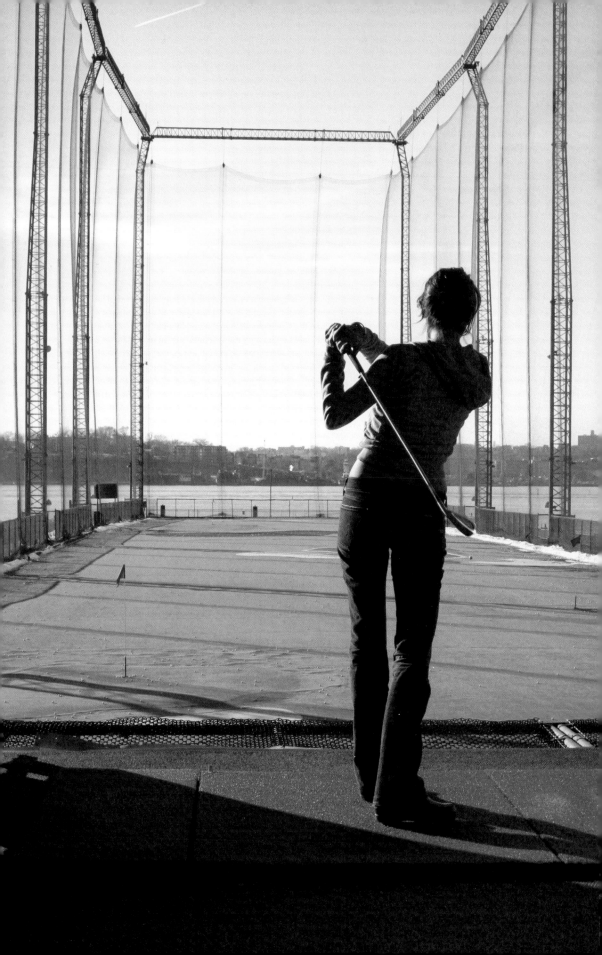

11

GOLF

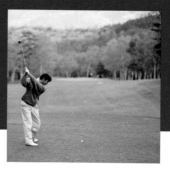

YOU'LL LOVE THIS SPORT IF YOU:
- want to develop strong legs and a toned core
- need a mental challenge in addition to a physical one
- want a sport that provides a lifetime of learning
- enjoy being outdoors in beautiful locations
- enjoy variety; you can putt at home or play eighteen holes in St. Lucia
- want a gentle cardio activity you can do for hours
- enjoy spending time with others and participating in social activities

YOU MIGHT NOT LOVE THIS SPORT IF YOU:
- are impatient or quickly become frustrated or angry; the game can be infuriatingly complex, progression can be slow, and skills can be subtle and difficult to master
- don't have chunks of time; a round of golf takes hours to play
- have a chronic injury such as knee or low-back pain; the golf swing may exacerbate your problem (although you can learn how to work around such conditions and still play)

Golf is addictive. There you are, standing still, the ball motionless. You swing…and who knows what will happen? It's amazingly difficult to hit a golf ball straight down a fairway. You think you're doing everything just right, but the ball veers off into the woods or plunks into the pond. You think you've done exactly the same stroke as last time, but zoom, the ball flies 150 yards toward the hole. Players get frustrated, but anyone with an ounce of perseverance comes back to try to do better the next time—perhaps with a few trips to the driving range and the practice green in between.

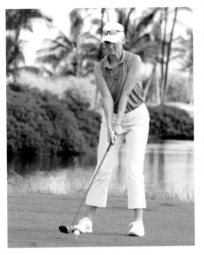
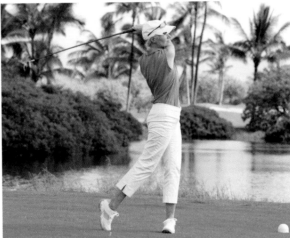

The sport can be an excuse for a long walk in a beautiful park. But the game itself can also be rewarding once you've learned the basic skills. It feels satisfying when everything clicks into place for a successful shot. Plus, a golfer is never bored, because there's so much to learn—from a *chip shot* with a *wedge* (a short lofting shot with an angled club), to precision putting, to understanding how a handicap works. Even when your game is advanced, there's always more you can learn to bring down your score or keep trying for the ever-elusive hole-in-one.

There aren't a lot of self-taught golfers, for good reason. The game can feel overwhelmingly complex to a beginner, but the fundamentals of the golf swing can be learned in one good lesson (after that, you can spend years getting better at it). The first few skills are, perhaps, the most awkward physically. The motion of the swing is not a natural body movement, and nobody would grip a club the right way without instruction. Reading about the sport is helpful, but you need a knowledgeable teacher to place your hands on

the club correctly and watch as you swing. After a few hundred repetitions and corrections, the golf swing will start to flow in a smooth motion, allowing you to begin working on technique to send the ball where you want it to go. Also, you will need to learn the rules and etiquette of the golf course.

Many people don't think of golf as a taxing sport physically, and the professional players certainly make the game look easy. But golf is more of a workout than just a long rambling walk—although the 4 to 5 miles of walking eighteen holes is decent exercise on its own. You also have the option of carrying a bag full of clubs, which can be quite heavy. During play, there's plenty of up and down movement of the body, so by the end of a round you've done a good series of squats and lunges. At the start of each hole, you bend down to put your tee in the ground and the ball on the tee. After a shot you first have to find your ball, which can mean some time spent wandering around, and then you might need to crouch to view the line to the flag to assess how to proceed.

SCORE

If you weigh 150 pounds, you'll burn about 270 calories in an hour of golf while carrying your clubs, 240 calories in an hour if you pull your clubs and 150 calories in an hour if you ride in an electric cart. (To calculate your hourly burn rate, multiply your weight in pounds by 1.8 if you carry your clubs, by 1.6 if you pull your clubs and by one if you ride in a cart.)

Then there's repair work: replacing *divots* of grass flung up by your club, raking a *bunker* of sand after you hit out of it, lifting the *dent* (also called a divot) in the green where your ball has landed. Golf can be akin to doing a little gardening. The swing can be very energetic, too. A solid swing uses the entire body: Once you've set your feet and club in position, you must swing the club back, lifting the front heel as you twist your trunk and raise both arms. Next, you swing the club down, bringing the entire torso around as you lower the front heel and then swing through, bringing the arms up to the front, continuing the torso twist and raising the rear heel. With all that activity, postgame sore muscles are no surprise. Of course, if you're not physically able to stay on your feet and carry your bag for four hours of walking the course, you can also ride in a cart or hire a caddy, making the game much less energetic. Or you can split the difference by pushing your clubs in a wheeled bag or fancy motorized cart while you walk.

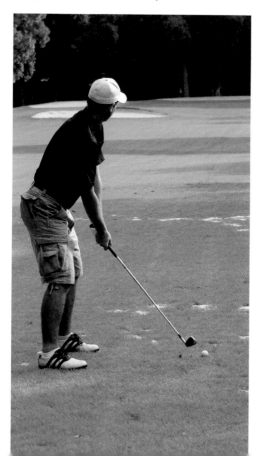

On the golf course, you play in a foursome. You can sign up for a tee time with three friends, or volunteer to be slotted in with others. If you find that you don't enjoy the company of your companions, you'll have plenty of chance to head off alone after your ball and skip the socializing. But spending four hours on a course with strangers who share your love for the game can be a great way to make new friends.

Golf has a strong mental component as well. You must make strategic decisions about which clubs to play and how hard to hit, and you have to evaluate the wind and terrain, and more. As you play, you spend hours in a state of concentration that resembles a walking meditation. Although some people find the game frustrating, others gain a sense of relaxation from the combination of beautiful environment, physical exertion, and mental focus.

Although golf has a dedicated following in more than one hundred countries, it is currently not on the Olympic program. Golf was played in the Olympics in 1900 and 1904, but it has not returned since, despite some effort from organizers. Even without the ultimate competition, there are plenty of tournaments all over the world. In the United States, there are three main governing bodies for golf: The United States Golf Association (USGA) oversees the rules and handicap system. The Professional Golfers' Association (PGA) supervises tournaments for top players, certifies instructors, and provides information about courses, travel, and more. The Ladies' Professional Golf Association (LPGA) is a similar group for female players. All three of these organizations cater to serious golfers, but they can provide basic information that is useful for a beginner as well—especially about rules, etiquette, and finding instruction. You'll also find instructional videos on the PGA and LPGA Web sites (www.pga.com and www.lpga.com).

GEARING UP

You can spend a lot of money getting outfitted to play golf, but you can also start on a shoestring. Many courses rent clubs, which is a great way to test out the game. If you decide to buy your own, consider starting with used clubs. Golfers are frequently upgrading their gear, so high-quality used items aren't too difficult to come by. You can find information about local dealers who stock used clubs through the PGA Web site's Trade In section. You'll only need a small selection of clubs to get started, not the full twelve-club set or the maximum of fourteen. Golf clubs are numbered, with higher numbered clubs meaning higher *loft* (the angle of the head to the ground) and usually having shorter shafts. There are *woods*, which produce long, low shots that can go great distances. These clubs are no longer made of wood, and unfortunately they are the most difficult to hit accurately. *Irons* are shorter, with more angle to the head, and are used for high-lift and short distances. The *pitching wedge* is a short iron used for *chipping* or popping the ball up to go just a few yards. Finally, there's the *putter*. A standard set of clubs has three woods, eight irons, and a putter. As a beginner, you can get by with a wood or two and a few irons, a pitching wedge, and a putter. The first time you play, use just four clubs: a three iron, seven iron, wedge, and putter.

Purchasing a set of clubs, either used or new, does warrant getting some expert advice from a specialty store or pro shop (some sporting goods stores may have seasoned salespeople but at many the staff may not be knowledgeable enough to help you select the proper clubs). First, you need to be sure the length is correct so that you connect with the ball when you swing properly. If you are quite short or tall, inquire if you might benefit from clubs that are not the standard length (which are designed for average-height folks). Then there's the *lie* of the club: This is the position when you hold the club correctly and the center of the bottom rests on the ground. If the tip or heel of the club is grounded, your

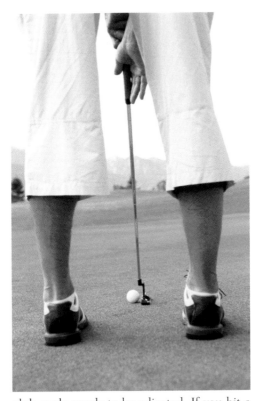

club angle needs to be adjusted. If you hit a perfect shot but the heel of the club hits the ground, your ball will veer to the left (if you're right handed), and a tip-grounded club will send your shots to the right. You also need proper stiffness in the shaft. The club actually bends as you swing down toward the ball, and how much it bends is called the *flex*. There are five flex ratings, so be sure to get the right one by discussing your level of play with the pro where you shop.

Next, you'll need golf balls. This part is much easier. You can purchase used golf balls in a variety of places, from eBay to golf-course pro shops. In theory, you play one ball from the first tee to the end. Beginners tend to lose balls in the woods and water, so don't invest in brand-new, brand-name balls that are just going to get lost around the course. Mark your balls with a permanent marker so you can identify them if they land near other players'. When your game becomes more advanced, you can learn about minor differences in golf balls and develop a preference for a particular type. You'll also need some tees. A small towel is nice to tote along for cleaning your clubs so they work properly—water or dirt on the club face changes the flight of the ball. (For the same reason, dew-soaked grass in the early morning makes for a tougher game because your clubs are constantly wet.) Bring a second towel to keep your hands dry.

A golf bag is the other essential piece of gear. Even if you only use a few clubs, a golf bag will hold the clubs, balls, pencil, and scorecard, a drink (you'll be out walking for four hours!), umbrella, towels, and other necessities. You can choose between a bag designed to be carried or one that is meant to be put on a golf cart (these tend to be bulkier). Some carry bags have a built-in kickstand device so you don't have to place it flat on the ground. Whichever type of bag you choose, look for one that is sturdy but light and feels comfortable on your shoulder (even a cart bag will need to be carried to and from your trunk). Avoid purchasing the least expensive bag you can find if you think it might not stand up to the abuse it will get on the course and in your car. It's best to buy a bag at the same time that you buy clubs since you'll have plenty to tote around. But if you want to wait to purchase your main bag until after you've gotten more of a feel for the game, consider the inexpensive options of a used bag or small travel golf bag in the interim.

Golf shoes are not a requirement for a beginner. Any pair of decent sneakers or walking shoes will carry you over the course. But a golf glove is worth purchasing right away to help your sweaty hands grip your club. Other golf-specific togs are optional. A comfortable pair of shorts or pants and a collared shirt and ball cap will serve admirably. Courses have dress codes, so leave the jeans, T-shirts, and sandals at home.

For comfort, also bring bug spray, sunscreen, Band-Aids for blisters, and a snack. Turn off your cell phone. And bring a coin to mark where your ball is when it's in the path of a fellow player's shot. Toss a light sweater or jacket in your golf bag in case the weather turns cool.

YOUR FIRST TIME

Some people do start golf by heading out for nine holes, but that approach is asking for frustration, because it's part of golf etiquette to keep pace and not delay the foursome behind you—which is a challenge as you try to learn the stance, the swing, the strategy, the rules, which club to use, and so on. It's far

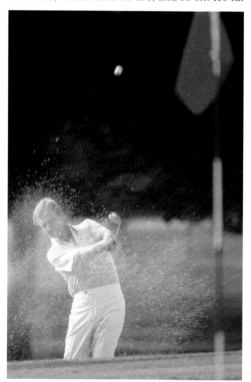

more effective to tackle one step at a time. First, learn how to hit by scheduling a lesson at a course or driving range. No matter who is teaching you—a friend or a PGA winner—an effective lesson requires good communication. If you have trouble understanding the explanations you're given, the instructor might not be a good fit. Try again with someone else before giving up on the sport. Good players are not always the best teachers. You

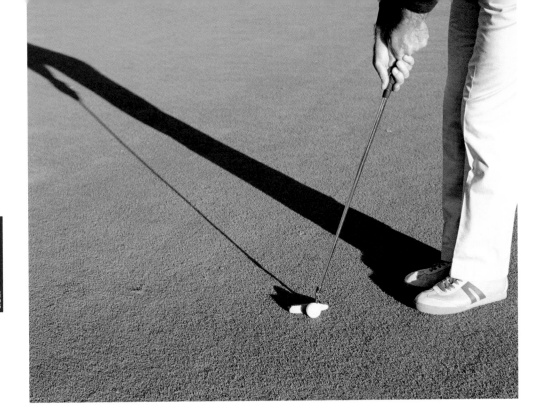

need to learn from someone who can be clear while describing the subtle suggestions for adjusting your technique. A lesson should produce noticeable results within an hour. Golf clinics are a wonderful way to begin the sport or to improve your game. These programs range from once a week at a local course to a multiday getaway to a golfing destination. Playing consistently without taking weeks between sessions is important as you try to get the feel for golf.

Your inaugural experience will start with instructions about holding the club properly. Next, you'll learn to address the ball, meaning how to stand before taking a shot. After that, you'll learn the proper steps to the swing. Then you'll take some practice swings away from the tee. You can be well into your first lesson before attempting to connect a club with a ball—and chances are good that your first swing will be a complete miss. Most new golfers lift up their arms and club as they swing, topping the ball or swinging right over it.

Once you've learned the swing, you'll need to practice. Going to a driving range and hitting is the best way to repeat the motions until they feel fluid and you develop a sense of where your shots will go. Take your time

between swings to think about what you did and how it felt, realign your body, check your grip, and visualize the next swing. It can take years to develop a proper swing with consistent results, and some people never get there, so go easy on yourself and try not to take the game too seriously. Start with shorter clubs such as an eight or nine iron or a wedge, because these are easier to hit with. Leave the long woods in the bag until your abilities match their complexity. After you've practiced a few times, consider videotaping a lesson or using a simulator. These training tools help you see what you're doing and analyze the results. If you can afford this type of lesson, take one because it can be difficult even for an adept athlete to understand the unique movements of the perfect golf swing.

Putting is a completely different but equally important set of skills. You can practice at home on the lawn or on a carpet, using a cup placed on its side as a target hole. Golf courses and driving ranges often have practice greens where you can try out your putting skills and further hone them.

When you're itching to do more but the weather is uncooperative, try reading a few beginners' golf books to learn the rules, jargon, and etiquette. Ben Hogan's *Five Lessons*

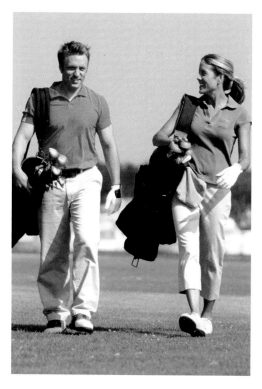

is a good choice for your first read. Try not to get bogged down reading about tips and technique pointers. The game is loaded with nuances, which is what makes it a lifelong pursuit, and you can't learn it all by studying for a weekend or two.

After you've practiced enough to develop a serviceable swing and decent putting skills, it's time to head for the course. Be sure to go with an experienced friend, instructor, or caddy because the rules and etiquette of the game are complex. You'll probably also want assistance in selecting clubs. Don't try to keep score the first few times you play. This sport generally requires a bit of struggle and repetition, trial and error, and practice. Simply making it around nine holes is a successful first attempt, and that includes not playing every hole fully; the first few times you head out, don't feel badly about picking up your ball and skipping a few hits to keep pace, giving up after a few putts, or dropping a new ball if yours goes off into the woods.

ATHLETE IN ACTION

Ivy Balnarine, 33

"I'm not athletic," says Ivy Balnarine. "In school, the most I would do is play dodgeball, and I'd often say I was hurt so I didn't have to play." Golf didn't come easily either. "I thought you had to be tall, athletic, have muscles, maybe have a background in baseball," says the marketing professional from New York. But she learned that it was a game that anyone can do—even a Latina with a penchant for shopping, not sports. "Four years ago, I went to a clinic," she says. "I was very surprised that I liked it."

Balnarine watched how others executed their swings, and got pointers from a boyfriend. She then took lessons once a week and worked on her swing in front of the mirror without a club. "There's so much to remember: keep your head down, plant your feet, turn your shoulders," says Balnarine. "I tried to hold my stomach in because I heard people talking about the core. I have to constantly remind myself of everything." But her instructors were patient, and she practiced. "It's just repetition and getting comfortable with the movement," she says. "I didn't worry about making contact with the ball; I focused on getting the swing correct."

When she felt she had a decent swing, Balnarine signed up for a golf outing. "You don't have to be great to hit on a course," she says. "I didn't do well; I didn't keep score, but I met new people and had a lot of fun." She practices at a driving range all winter, and makes one outing each summer. "I still haven't graduated to keeping score, but I'll get there eventually," she says. The game has taught her perseverance. "I'm stubborn, and I want to keep trying. The next hole is a new opportunity each time." Balnarine is patient with her progress. "I think I can do this sport for life," she says. "It's an elegant sport and a social activity, too."

SECRETS TO SUCCESS

One of the appealing aspects of golf is that anyone can play, says Tom Sutter, Head Pro, Class A PGA, Golf Academy at Chelsea Piers. The game is easily adapted to your abilities and skill level at any age—and whether you choose to putt or drive, you'll continue learning. After mastering the swing, you'll find the hardest part of golf is the etiquette, and you can do damage without doing much. For example, the player the farthest from the hole plays first, so a beginner can unknowingly keep an entire foursome waiting. The fundamentals are easy: Don't cause distractions, disturbances, or delays. Outbursts of anger are inappropriate on the course (but mild expressions of exasperation are quite common). Be quiet when others are hitting, stay out of the

way, and keep up the pace—if it's taking you ten strokes to complete a par-3 hole, pick up your ball and move on. If your ball can't be found in five minutes, give up and drop another one. Yell "fore" if your ball might hit another golfer.

Repair any damage you create in the grass and sand, and especially on the putting green, where even tiny dents from a falling ball might require remedy. Players are not allowed to damage living objects such as trees, and some parts of a course are off-limits to carts—stay on the path. Skip the cart if you can. The shortest distance between you and your ball may not be drivable territory, so you'll play a faster game on foot.

Serious players head to the course early in the morning and spend four to

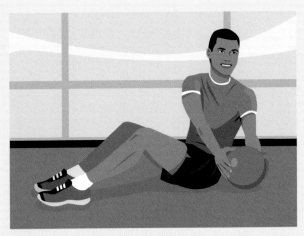

medicine ball twist

Sit on the ground with your knees bent, feet flat on the floor. Hold a medicine ball in both hands in front of your torso. Lean back slightly, keeping your feet on the floor, back erect and head up. Twist your torso to the left, reach out with your arms, and try to touch the medicine ball to the floor as far from your knees as you can. Return to center and repeat to the right. Do 10 to 20 repetitions to each side. Build up to 3 sets of 30 reps.

five hours playing. The first time you go, tee off at four or five o'clock. At this hour, the best players are gone because they can't start at five and expect to play eighteen holes. But you can get your fill in the two or three hours before dark. Most public courses offer a twilight discount.

When you become a serious player, the rules get more complex. For example, players have handicaps and courses have separate handicaps. A player can calculate her own handicap for a particular course, allowing her to compete with better players by deducting a number of strokes from her final score. But don't worry about these intricacies of the game until you have played for a while.

In the meantime, you can do a few things to improve your game, namely stretching and core strengthening. Pre-golf stretching is essential, whether you're at the range or heading for a course. The swing requires a lot of torque: your feet face the ball, your hips turn 45 degrees and your shoulders turn 90 degrees (think owl's neck!). You need to be limber to do it. Hold a club with one hand at each end and twist your body gently as far as you can to each side.

Core strength is helpful in keeping your swing centered (and in preventing back pain). A few twisting abdominal moves a few times a week can be extremely useful. Try these:

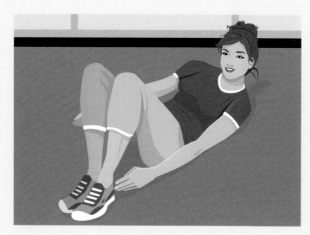

oblique reach

Lie on the ground with your knees bent, feet flat on the floor, knees and feet together, arms at your sides. Contract your abs by drawing your navel toward the floor. Exhale and lift just your head and shoulders off the floor (your shoulder blades remain in contact; the arch in your lower back will naturally flatten along the floor). Hold this slight crunch, inhale, and reach your left hand toward your left ankle by moving your torso along the floor to the side. Try to swat at your ankle. Return to center, exhaling, but do not lower the crunch. Repeat to the right. Do 10 reps to each side. Build up to 3 sets of 30 reps.

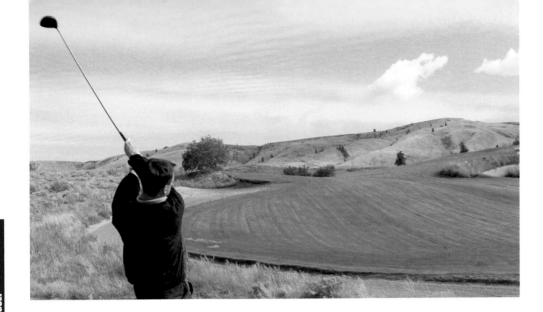

TACKLE THE TRUTH

Golf is an extremely expensive sport

You can spend as much as you want playing golf. If you want to enjoy the game at the elite level, you can drop many thousands of dollars on clubs, renting a cart, joining a country club, and vacationing in Pebble Beach, Phoenix, and Palm Desert. But you can also play a rewarding round of golf using a small collection of rented or second-hand clubs at the local municipal course. For top dollar, highly credentialed pros can provide lessons to help you progress in the sport. But you can also sign up for sessions with talented teachers who aren't as expensive, get pointers from friends or others in your foursome, or even look for classes at colleges and parks. Also, watch for events such as the LPGA one-day clinics, which take place from Boston to San Jose to introduce women to the game while raising money for charity. Check www.PlayGolfAmerica. com for more beginners' opportunities.

You have to be an early riser to play golf

Early weekend tee times are coveted because a round of golf takes hours—so if you start later in the day, you will have trouble fitting a second activity into the afternoon. And the midday sun is hotter if you are out on the fairway. There's also the challenge of scheduling lunch. If you can work around those obstacles, you'll find plenty of time to play after the early birds have gone home to nap.

You can't play golf with your kids

Country clubs usually won't allow children on the course until after 2 P.M., but there's plenty for kids to do on municipal courses, driving ranges, and practice greens. Kids as young as three can start enjoying golf with a small plastic set of clubs at home. And once your kids are preteens, take them along to caddy for you, keep score and hit a few shots when the next foursome is not right on your tail. There are college scholarships for top golfers, so get the kids started early.

GET MORE FROM YOUR SPORT

If you love golf, consider taking up billiards and boxing. Billiards has a number of similarities: hitting balls into holes using a stick, and needing to understand spin, direction, and speed to do it well. The mental aspects of the game will appeal to the same personalities as those who like golf. Boxing also involves strategy, but surprisingly the overlap with golf is more physical. The twisting torso moves of a boxing punch have a lot in common with the golf swing. The bobbing legs and crouches used to avoid punches feel the same as the up and down of teeing the ball and crouching to evaluate a shot. Balance and core strength are also important aspects of both sports, as is choosing the right weapon (club or punch).

To play sports that might make you a better golfer, go for balance and core work. Dance, yoga, ballet, and pilates are all helpful for understanding how the body moves, as well as in developing strong abdominals and improving your stance.

Golf is one of the easiest sports to take on vacation. You can play gorgeous courses with unique scenery and challenges all over the world. There are quality schools at many popular destinations, so it's easy to plan a vacation by selecting where you'd like to travel and then finding a clinic, from Miami to Maui. Many golf destinations offer a variety of golf schools plus plenty of family activities. Log on to the PGA Web site, www.pga.com, for a good start locating top schools.

RESOURCES

➡ **www.pga.com** has information about professional players and tournaments, equipment, rules, and getting started in golf.

➡ **www.lpga.com** is similar to the PGA site, but focuses on golf for women.

➡ **www.usga.org** is the governing body for golf rules in the U.S., and their site offers an overview of the game plus an excellent description of course etiquette.

➡ **www.OnlineGolfClinic.com** offers a thorough introduction to the game, the gear, tips, and travel oriented toward beginners.

➡ *Five Lessons: The Modern Fundamentals of Golf* by Ben Hogan is a timeless classic with clear explanations of the swing, grip, and game that makes it the perfect primer for a novice.

➡ *The Plane Truth for Golfers* is written by respected instructor Jim Hardy. The book explains his premise that there are two types of golf swings—a one-plane version and a two-plane style. He helps you select the right swing and execute it well.

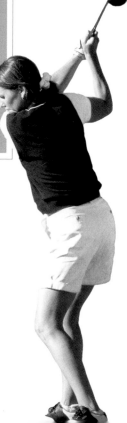

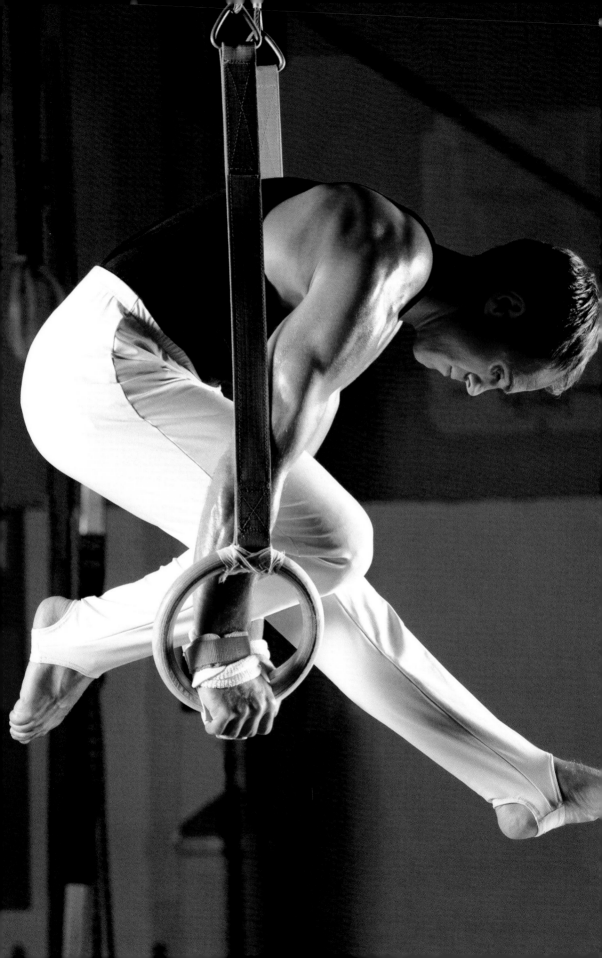

12

GYMNASTICS

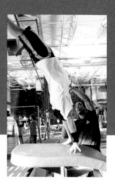

YOU'LL LOVE THIS SPORT IF YOU:
- want to improve your flexibility, stamina, and strength—from head to toe
- thrive on learning new skills and pushing your limits
- want to have so much fun you don't even know you're exercising
- look for camaraderie and social engagement in activities

YOU MIGHT NOT LOVE THIS SPORT IF YOU:
- are impatient; it can take thousands of repetitions to learn one new skill
- need to be the best in class—sometimes it's not the most athletic person who excels
- don't like to take direction; gymnastics requires coaching and supervision
- are an analytical thinker; gymnasts learn new moves by imitation, not dissection
- have physical limitations such as back and knee injuries
- are afraid of falling or heights

Because there's such a variety of skills and pieces of apparatus on which to work, taking up gymnastics can feel more like joining a three-ring circus than starting a single sport. It has been practiced for centuries, but unlike the current style, the early form of gymnastics was used as physical training for battle. Some of the skills practiced back then, such as rope climbing and club swinging, were on the roster of the first modern Olympics in Athens in 1896; current favorites such as the uneven bars and high bar didn't appear until later. Today, gymnastics skills range from tumbling on the ground to flying through the air, bouncing, bounding and balancing—and it all adds up to a workout that hits every muscle in the body, large and small. Practicing the moves is hard work, both mentally and physically, but the experience is so much fun that you'll barely realize you're exercising.

There aren't many sports for adults that bring out the kid in you the way gymnastics does. Gymnasts tend to be supportive, cheering each other on and celebrating one another's accomplishments. The typical gym is filled with laughter and smiles. Of course, it's not all a lark. The sport requires discipline, patience, and perseverance as you wait your turn, listen to the coach's instructions and fall, flail, and fail for months—maybe even years—working on a specific move, until one day it suddenly comes together.

Whether on the uneven bars, balance beam, or floor exercise, gymnasts train their bodies to use speed and momentum to flip or twist through an entire gravity-defying move and then stop precisely, changing direction for the next move or ending a routine by landing on two feet in a wobble-free dismount. That kind of control requires strength in the entire body. Even people who take pilates and lift weights regularly will get sore muscles from this sport—and get stronger as they practice it. Gymnastics is one of the best all-around sports, working every muscle from head to toe, including a bunch you won't know you have until you awaken to find them aching the morning after your first class. In addition to taxing the usual large muscles you use for other activities, such as the quadriceps, the glutes, and the abs, gymnastics targets the tiny muscles that work hard to stabilize your body as you move. This full-body muscle recruitment explains why gymnasts are in such amazing shape even though they rarely hit the weight room. When you tumble, you're lifting your entire body weight, which is heavier than any dumbbells you heft at the gym.

Running, jumping, and swinging your body are intense aerobic exercise. And the pace of a gymnastics workout can leave you panting, which is the sign of an effective cardio session. The actual amount of aerobic conditioning you undergo is up to you, because you can step out of rotation for a break rather than try another pass at a tumble, adding more as your stamina improves.

The combo of muscle work and cardio can translate into serious weight loss if you practice frequently and don't increase how much you eat. And the workout can inspire you to stick to your diet. Gymnasts tend to try to get lean and stay that way, because it's harder to do the moves with more weight to maneuver.

A bonus for Baby Boomers: Despite the padding of mats and the spring-loaded floor, the impact you get from gymnastics will keep your bones strong. And because bone-building is site-specific (for example, runners may have strong leg bones but often weak ones in their arms), gymnastics is unique in the benefits it offers for the upper body. There aren't many sports, after all, in which you often walk on your hands. Also, gymnastics training will improve your ability to balance, reducing the risk of falls—and balance starts to falter as early as age fifty.

In competition, judging is based on elements such as the level of challenge, precision, and creative interpretation of the routine plus the execution of required moves. Points are deducted for every slight break in form, with each piece of apparatus having different standards. On the rings, for example, it is important for the body not to shake and the rings to remain as still as possible, but on the vault, points are awarded for height, distance, and explosive force with a *stuck* landing—that is, a balanced landing that doesn't require an extra step to avoid falling over. Bonus points can be awarded for particularly challenging moves.

Competitors typically begin training as children. Most adults who take up gymnastics are content to master new tricks rather than aspire to a place on the medals podium. Although you probably won't compete, you'll

SCORE

If you weigh 150 pounds, you'll burn 280 calories by doing an hour of gymnastics. (To calculate your hourly burn rate, multiply 1.89 by your weight in pounds.)

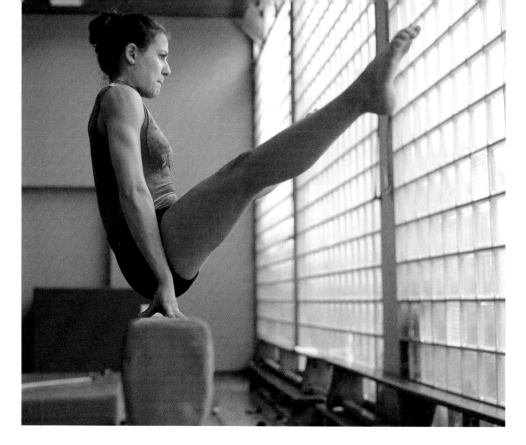

strive for the same qualities as an Olympian as you practice each move in class. And you'll feel like you've won the gold the first time you complete a back handspring. Even the most reserved adults get giddy from that addictive rush of success, which keeps them coming back again and again. The never-ending challenge of gymnastics is the perfect antidote to gym ennui, because you will always learn new skills and improve your abilities.

Some gyms cater only to kids or competitors, so call before you go. To find a location that has an established program for folks old enough to vote, log on to www.adultgymnastics.com and click on the "classes" link.

If you are nervous or unsure about taking up gymnastics, call ahead to ask if you can watch a class or attend one trial session before signing up for a full semester. Find out if the gym has an open-house night for prospective students.

GEARING UP

You don't need to buy a single thing to take up gymnastics. No expensive gear or fancy sneakers are required, nor are protective padding or high-tech outfits.

Wear any form of comfortable clothes that are not restrictive. Keep in mind that you'll be upside-down part of the time, so loose togs can be revealing. Slim-fitting tanks, leotards, shorts, and leggings are good choices, because the instructors need to grasp you firmly without loose fabric getting in the way, and you won't want your clothes flapping about as you try to execute precise moves. But when you're first starting out, shorts and a T-shirt should suffice. You'll practice barefoot (so perhaps a pre-class pedicure is in order).

YOUR FIRST TIME

When you're ready to begin gymnastics, don't go it alone. Sign up for a class: You'll need professional instruction to be safe and learn the skills. Some sessions are held in adult gyms, but many take place in the same space used for kids—often because parents, jealous of how much fun the tots have in tumbling class, clamor for their own time on the mats and trampolines. Beginner classes don't necessarily match the elements of Olympic competition, the trampolines being an example. Each gym sets its own curriculum, some

143

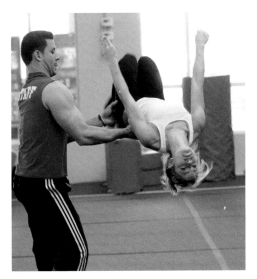

such as cartwheels, handstands, front walkovers, and flips. To practice a move, students have to line up and wait their turn. Advanced students will run toward the mat where an instructor is ready to spot them, helping them execute the move and avoid mistakes that could be dangerous. You might start by walking forward to do a slower move or running to try something simple. The process helps you learn the pacing so you can initiate the move in just the right place—not too far from the spotter and mat, but not running onto the soft surface before leaping. As you progress, you'll take on tougher skills, from cartwheels to flips. You try the skill, land on the mat (if you're lucky, on your feet), then walk off to get back in line for the next try. Some gyms have a pit filled with foam cubes so you can practice a move in the air with a soft landing (and then struggle with large clownlike steps to get out again).

In a class that includes equipment, you might walk on a *balance beam*, try maneuvers on the *uneven bars* or *high bar*, swing and hold poses on the *rings*, or walk your hands down the *parallel bars* while swinging your feet. For the *vault*, there's often a springboard to help convert the forward running motion into a leap high enough to land on top with your hands or feet. Eventually, you'll learn to push off and land.

Although the atmosphere may be lighthearted and filled with laughter, there's intense work being done in gymnastics class.

offering tumbling plus every piece of apparatus, while others focus on one aspect such as floor exercise skills. If you have your heart set on soaring on the uneven bars or vault, ask in advance to make sure it's included in the program.

If you have a choice between class times, keep in mind that weekday classes tend to be less crowded because more adults are stuck at work and can't make it to the gym. In a smaller class, you'll get more individual attention but less rest, because your turn will come around faster. Larger classes, often held on weekends and evenings, will be more likely to have other participants at your level by virtue of having more students. You'll watch more and do less in a packed class. Check the student-teacher ratio to be sure you're getting the instruction you need.

When you enter the class, music may be playing in the background to add to the boisterous mood—or the tone may be quiet and studious. Most classes start with a group warm-up session to get muscles moving for greater flexibility. Once you're sweating somewhat, you can start learning the skills. If the floor is spring-loaded, bodies will bounce high off the ground as they run, leap, and twist in the air. You may start by working on a forward roll while classmates perform moves

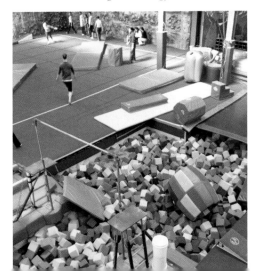

Students struggle to make small improvements as they repeat a sequence again and again. The bodies tend to be all shapes and sizes, some firm and fit, others more jiggly. Strong, skilled instructors make sure everyone makes progress and feels successful. Most important, however, they act as spotters, helping students move safely and standing ready to prevent mishaps.

Gymnastics classes are structured. To stay safe, you must follow directions and wait your turn so you can be spotted by an instructor. Classes may split into groups according to ability to work on different drills. In one area, advanced students may be combining moves into tumbling runs. Elsewhere, beginners may be learning one aspect of the skill with hands-on instruction, sometimes using a prop such as a large bolster or a harness (a thick belt with ropes attached to pulleys overhead so the instructor can help hoist and support your body while standing out of the way).

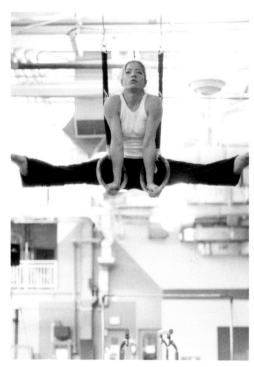

ATHLETE IN ACTION

Debbie Gleicher, 29

"I think it's like *real* gymnastics," Debbie Gleicher, then 26, told her friend about the class they planned to take at the Field House at Chelsea Piers. But they tried it anyway. "I could just manage a forward roll, and my friend could barely do that," says Gleicher. "It was pretty mortifying. And I couldn't even walk the next day." Debbie's embarrassment was compounded by feeling out of shape. "I was twenty pounds heavier then. And to spot beginners, they grab your waist," she says, cringing. But she was not deterred. Gymnastics class became a Thursday night ritual for Gleicher and her friend.

"We laughed so hard," she says. When she started, her legs would shake from fatigue by the end of the session, but after three months, she could take class two days in a row without pain. "Then I got obsessed because I wanted to do a front handspring," says Gleicher. When she did, she was ecstatic—and became hooked on doing more. "I started going three times a week, practicing at the beach, standing on my head," she says. In little over a year, she did a back handspring. "Now I can do front flips, back flips, and bounders, which are like a front handspring off two feet. With a spotter I can run and do a series of three moves on the tumbling track."

Gleicher played sports such as soccer as a kid, but finds gymnastics unlike other activities. "You get excited about the smallest gain, like holding a handstand five seconds longer," she explains, because you're doing it with just your own body. Comparing it to her prior gym regimen of running, Spinning, and cardio machines, Gleicher says: "I like it because there are no mirrors. I enjoy going—I don't stress about getting there. I've made friends in class and we hang out when we're not in class," adding, "Gymnastics attracts people who want to try something different."

And then there's the workout. The class not only helped Gleicher sweat off the pounds; it inspired her to adjust her eating to lose weight. "The lighter you are in gymnastics, the better you'll be," she says. "So that was extra motivation."

Now, she enjoys watching new people come to class. "People come who can't do anything, and I say to myself, 'That was me.' "

SECRETS TO SUCCESS

You don't have to be in shape before you begin. You'll work on strength, stamina, and flexibility in class, so don't worry if your nickname isn't Gumby. But beware of overdoing it that first time, warns Peter Kormann, the first man to win an Olympic medal in gymnastics for the U.S., who runs programs for all ages at the Field House at Chelsea Piers. Chances are good that you'll be having so much fun you won't realize how hard you're pushing your body. It's not uncommon to wake up unable to move the day after your first class. If you want to avoid extreme aches, do a little less than you think your body can handle.

Show up at your first class early and talk to the instructors beforehand so you can let them know about your abilities (or lack thereof!), concerns, and goals. They'll keep an eye on you and might suggest that you take it easy to avoid overtaxing your body the first time. They'll certainly keep you safe.

Students learn at vastly different paces, so it's almost impossible to predict how long it will take to master the basics. Go at your own speed and stick to it and you can expect to pick up about twelve tricks in total. "The average person can learn somersaults, cartwheels, handstands, front and back handsprings, and some skills on the bar and balance beam," says Kormann.

If you want to progress quickly, consider adding some gymnastics-inspired workouts between classes. If your first class leaves you breathless, do jumping

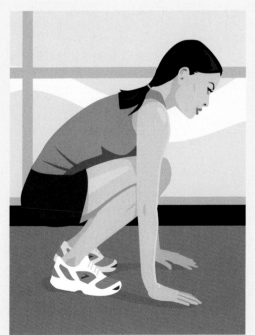

crouching ankle stretch

Start on your hands and knees. Bring your left knee toward your chest, placing your left toes on the ground under your body. Repeat with the right leg until you are in a deep crouch with your weight on your legs and just your fingertips touching down for balance. Try to align your feet parallel to each other and press your heels toward the ground. Hold for 10 deep breaths.

workouts to build up your stamina so you can do more in each class before tiring. Try jumping rope or jumping jacks. In class, you'll do bursts of activity, then again wait your turn, which is similar to aerobic interval training with its alternating spurts of high intensity work and slower recovery sections. Try a burst of thirty to sixty seconds of jumping rope followed by marching in place for the next thirty to sixty seconds. Keep alternating for as long as you can, pushing yourself to your top intensity for the jumping sections.

One of the biggest surprises in taking up gymnastics is the pressure the moves put on your wrists and ankles. You can prepare these joints in advance by doing some exercises. If there's time, do these moves for a week or so before your first class. After class, once any soreness has subsided, do ankle and wrist strengtheners every other day until your next gymnastics session. Any exercise in which you wobble will work the ankles, so skipping and balancing on one leg are helpful. Also, try sitting down and "writing" the alphabet in the air with your toes. For the wrists, try push-ups holding yourself in plank position, doing wrist curls with a dumbbell, or rotating your wrists in every direction as far as you can to stretch them. If you do yoga, practice poses such as down dog, cobra, up dog, tree pose, and royal dancer. Also, try these moves to stretch, warm up, and firm your abs:

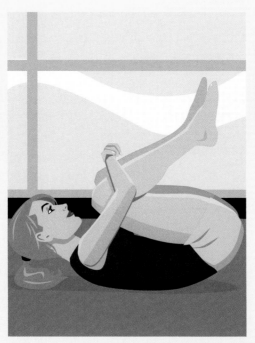

rolling abs

Lie on your back on the floor. Hug your knees toward your chest, wrapping both arms around them. Keeping your head tucked in, rock gently, building force until you can roll from your shoulders to your hips in a controlled motion. Continue for 1 minute, then rest. Repeat 3 times.

TACKLE THE TRUTH

There's no point in trying gymnastics if you're not short, strong, and supple

It's not always the petite powerhouses who excel at gymnastics. Sometimes the least athletic-looking students learn the moves the fastest because gymnastics requires mimicking others (rather than analyzing each move).

It's true that extra body weight makes the movement more challenging, and being flexible and strong is helpful. But that's not a reason to avoid the sport. You can improve in these areas with practice. A longer learning curve just means more excitement when you master each new twist and tumble.

You have to be young to take up gymnastics

True, kids have a few advantages in the sport. It may be easier to learn new tricks when you're young in both body and mind and can imitate movements without trying to think them through—a factor that can hamper some adults. Young bodies typically bounce back faster when they fall, and children may have less fear. But adults benefit from experience, perseverance, and patience. If you're inflexible or have injuries, you might have to work a little harder and wait a little longer for each success, but a good instructor can teach an old dog new tricks. Even seniors take gymnastics classes.

Some of the advantages kids have in gymnastics endure if you tried it as a kid and come back to it after a few decades. Starting fresh during your thirties, forties, or even later is more challenging. But even if you've never done a cartwheel in your life, the sport is well worth the effort.

Contorting your body on some piece of gymnastics equipment will land you in the hospital

Some people pass on gymnastics because they assume the sport has a high rate of injuries. Small aches and pains, such as a jammed finger or sprained ankle, can certainly be part of the sport. But if you work within your abilities and team up with a good instructor, you won't get hurt. If you don't wait for a spotter, fail to follow directions, or try a reckless maneuver, however, you could get injured—but in any case, those behaviors aren't allowed in class. Pushing yourself too hard and showing off are risky as well, and it's up to you to know your limits (although your instructors will be watching out for you, too). If you are concerned about getting injured or have a physical limitation, talk to the instructors before class.

GET MORE FROM YOUR SPORT

If you love gymnastics, there are a few sports that complement it well. Because gymnastics uses all the muscles in your body, almost any activity that makes you stronger or more flexible will help improve your performance. To take your gymnastics practice to the next level, you can try sports that closely match its physical demands, such as wrestling, which uses your body in a variety of positions with explosive force. Pilates, yoga, dance, and any kind of skating will improve your balance, flexibility, strength, and rhythm, all of which will help you perform better on the mats and apparatus. Golf and yoga help develop strength and flexibility in your wrists. Diving into a swimming pool can be a great way to practice skills and improve your strength, flexibility, and stamina.

Because gymnastics is a full-body sport, it doesn't leave any gaps in the fitness benefits you get in class. If you attend class frequently, you won't need to augment your workouts with other training. That being said, cross-training is always wise for preventing repetitive-strain injuries and adding variety to your regimen. So go ahead and shake up the schedule with some other sports—just to keep it safe and satisfying. Swimming is an excellent choice if you want to give your body a break from the impact while still using muscles from head to toe—and it's another sport that provides more physical challenge than you'd expect.

If you'd like to capitalize on your newfound flexibility, strength, balance, and ability to bounce, consider a circus class or camp where you can fly on the trapeze and walk a tightrope. Flying-trapeze classes are sprinkled around the country, mostly in big cities. Near Washington, D.C., you can sign up for a single class on a summer weekend at Circus Arts Workshop. In Chicago, the Flying Gaonas Gym specializes in the flying trapeze and also teaches general circus skills. You can study Chinese Acrobatics, trapeze, and other skills at Circus Center in San Francisco. If you have a kid to team up with, head for northern Vermont, where Circus Smirkus offers a family camp covering acrobatics, aerial skills, juggling, and other sports. Circus Minimus, a New York group, offers sessions in Circus Yoga for the Family at centers across the U.S. Circus Yoga combines acrobatics, juggling, and other skills with yoga focus. Skilled gymnasts can apply to the National Circus School in Montreal, where the Cirque de Soleil acrobats train. There are plenty more adult options for circus classes and camps in the U.S. and overseas, from Beijing to New Zealand. For a list of links, go to: http://dmoz.org/Arts/ Performing_Arts/ Circus/Schools/.

RESOURCES

➡ **www.USA-gymnastics.org** is the official site of the national organization, which oversees competitions in the U.S. You can learn more about the sport and be inspired by televised events (a guide is listed on the site).

➡ **www.AdultGymnastics.com** is a portal for sharing information, finding classes and posting questions about taking up the sport as an adult.

➡ *Superguides: Gymnastics* by Joan Jackman is a book geared toward kids. But the clear instructions, easy-to-understand illustrations, and background information are helpful for any beginner.

➡ *The Best Book of Gymnastics* by Christine Morley covers the basics of learning each move and piece of equipment, competition, and scoring, plus mental aspects such as teamwork.

➡ *I Can Do Gymnastics* by USA Gymnastics is geared toward intermediate athletes who want to learn more about the sport.

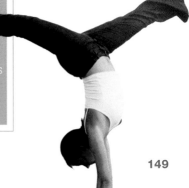

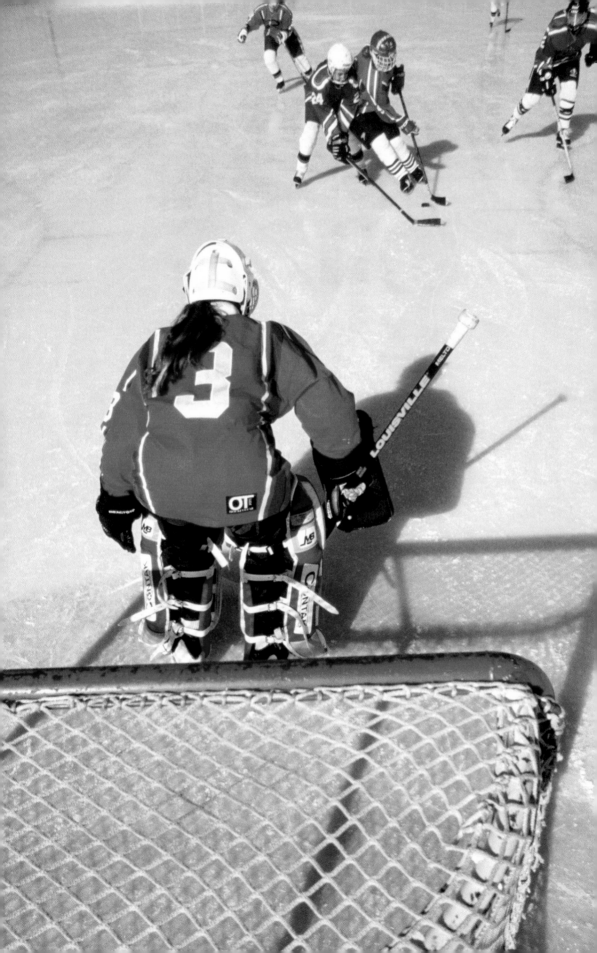

13

HOCKEY

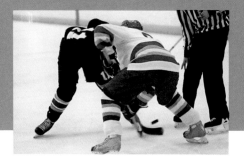

YOU'LL LOVE THIS SPORT IF YOU:
• want to improve your balance, flexibility, cardiovascular fitness, and strength
• love strategy—need a mental challenge in addition to a physical one
• thrive on learning new skills and pushing your limits
• love speed and competition
• want to be so engaged that you don't know you're exercising
• enjoy a versatile sport that you can do outdoors during winter, or play indoors any time
• enjoy team sports, camaraderie, and social activities
• like to have a set role because you play a specific position on the team

YOU MIGHT NOT LOVE THIS SPORT IF YOU:
• never want to risk an injury. Even in non-checking leagues, there are collisions
• already have a chronic injury such as knee or low-back pain; the bent-over posture
  you adopt to get the stick on the ground might exacerbate your problem
• prefer to set your own schedule rather than rely on teammates

The word "hockey" typically brings to mind images of the National Hockey League (NHL): Men in bulky pads, zipping over the ice almost too fast for the eye to follow, banging into each other, getting into fights, and being sent off the ice for penalties. Fortunately, the sport is much more than pure aggression. First, note that most recreational leagues do not allow *checking* (intentional hitting), which makes for a less combative and more skilled game. The skating versions of hockey include ice hockey, in-line hockey, and pond hockey. Hockey on foot is divided into field hockey (played on grass), street hockey (played outdoors on a hard surface), dekhockey (played in a rink with a plastic surface), and ball hockey (played in a rink with a harder surface, usually cement). For a complete departure from the classic sport, there's even underwater hockey in which the players wear swim fins, mask, and snorkel, and use knock-hockey-style sticks held in one hand.

Hockey is traditionally thought of as a men's sport, with field hockey as the women's version. But even field hockey first came to the Olympics as a men's game, debuting in 1908. It took another seventy-two years for women's field hockey to get a spot in the Olympic games. Ice hockey is a popular sport in the Winter Olympics, with the men's game making the roster in 1920 and the women's game added in 1998. Meanwhile, women's and mixed hockey teams have been growing fast on a recreational level.

In leagues all over the U.S., you'll find expatriot Canadians on the team. What baseball is to the U.S., hockey is to Canada—both a national sport and a national passion. The sport was first played in Canada in 1880 and is named for the French word for a shepherd's crook, *hocquet*. Hockey's U.S. debut was in New York in 1896, and the area is still one of the national centers for the sport. American towns that host NHL teams, such as Dallas, Atlanta, and St. Paul, Minnesota, tend to have strong hockey programs for kids and adults. Teams from both the U.S. and Canada compete in the NHL.

The action in hockey goes by in a flash, making it difficult for novices to follow the game. It's easier to understand the strategies if you watch players who don't have the added speed provided by skates, such as those playing street or field hockey. All forms of hockey are similar to the game of soccer: There are two teams, each having offensive and defensive players and a goalie. The object is to get the *puck*, or ball, into the opposite goal. The game is played in periods, with three twenty-minute periods in ice hockey and two periods for many of the other forms of the sport. There are penalties for fouls, some of which result in a *foul shot*—when a player is given a shot at the goal with only the goalie playing defense.

SCORE

If you weigh 150 pounds, you'll burn about 420 calories in an hour of hockey—noting that much of that time is not spent playing but sitting on the bench. (To calculate your hourly burn rate, multiply 2.8 by your weight in pounds.)

Most hockey games begin with six players per team. There's a goalie to defend the net, two defense players who help prevent scoring on the goal, and three forward offense players, two wings, and one center. Later in the game, there can be fewer than six players fielded for a team if someone is in the penalty box. Teams can have up to twenty members, allowing players to switch in and out either to rest or for strategic adjustments. Adult teams are often fairly small, with just a few additional players on the bench. Often, the goalie plays the entire game.

If hockey players didn't switch out of the game periodically they would drop from exhaustion. Playing hockey is physically demanding. Without skates, it's akin to a fast-paced basketball or soccer game (and these sports also use substitutes). On skates, the experience is even faster and more energetic. All forms of the game involve sprints and skirmishes, taxing the body's aerobic system to generate speed and placing demands on the musculature for maneuvering and quick stops. Flexibility helps you extend to reach the puck with your stick. And, of course, balance is key to skating styles. Agility and stamina are advantages in hockey—and if you don't have them before you take up the sport, you'll develop them as you play.

From a muscle-toning perspective, hockey is a full-body sport. Bending to place the stick on the ground uses the back, butt, legs, and abs. Stick work develops strength in the shoulders, arms, and upper back. And running or skating focuses on the muscles of the legs and butt.

You can play hockey at any age, with kids as young as four playing in Mite ice-hockey leagues. Kids' leagues are divided by age, while adult leagues may have age or skill designations, depending on the pool of available players (more players allow for more speci-

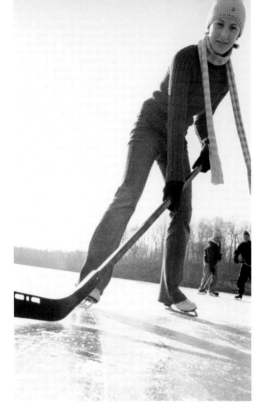

GEARING UP

Hockey played on foot requires very little gear. For street hockey, you can walk into almost any sporting goods store and purchase a stick and puck or ball. If you have a flat surface to play on, buy a street-hockey puck; if there are obstacles, such as small debris and cracks, get a street-hockey ball. Field-hockey sticks may be a bit harder to find but can easily be ordered over the Internet. Hard-plastic shin guards will prevent injuries when the ball or stick strikes the legs, and tall socks are usually worn.

Once you add skates, the gear collection increases—and not just because of the skates themselves, but you also add a lot of protective-wear. For roller hockey or ice hockey, expect to spend $700 to $1,000 to get the basics—pads, clothes, skates, and stick—if you're buying them new. You'll need elbow pads, gloves, a helmet, shoulder pads, hockey pants with pads (or a separate padded girdle and pants), shin guards, a garter belt to hold up special socks, and a jersey that will fit over it all. Guys also need a protector cup. Some players also wear a

ficity). For example, the U.S.A. Adult Hockey Classic ice-hockey competitions have divisions for novice, intermediate, advanced, over-30, over-40, and women's teams.

Like basketball, you can play hockey in a pickup game if what you want is sporadic or recreational play. Leagues are competitive, but they generally have room for adult beginners. Hockey players tend to be encouraging and social, helping novices learn new skills so they can enjoy the sport. Plenty of players take up hockey as adults, so there's no barrier to progressing to the top levels, although it can take years to master the game. There are competitions all year long, both across the U.S. and overseas. The first U.S. pond-hockey championships began in 2006. In pond hockey, several rinks are cleared on one lake, with skate-through warming huts and beer huts erected right on the ice.

For all types of hockey, players tend to form tight-knit bonds because the game demands close teamwork. There can be a scoring star in the group; but even so, success is almost always a matter of working together, and frequently the assistance is vital to making the goal. Another reason players tend to bond is that hockey isn't an easy sport to start out with; it requires an investment in gear and dedication to master the skills.

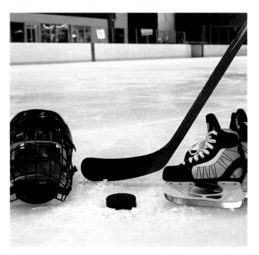

mouth guard. When you purchase gear, don't buy anything if it isn't a good fit. Have a knowledgeable friend, seasoned teammate, or knowledgeable salesperson help you make selections. You will skate better if your gear fits because you'll be more comfortable.

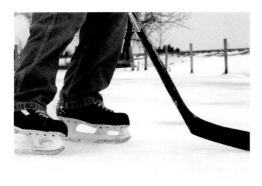

In addition to the outfit, you'll need a stick and skates—and a bag to carry it all in. Skates are the single biggest expense, but don't skimp. Ill-fitting skates can hamper a player's performance markedly. Make sure your skates are comfortable but snug so that every slight movement of your body is conveyed to the blade. The boot should hold your heel firmly in place but leave your toes room to wiggle a little. Top brands of ice hockey skates include CCM, Nike, Bauer, and Easton. For roller hockey, you can purchase hockey-specific in-line skates from companies such as CCM, Bauer, and Mission.

You can try to keep the cost down by buying used gear, but be sure it fits well, because you want to be able to move as freely as possible under all that padding. Also, the pads can't be washed, and you will sweat—a fact that makes used gear a little less appealing. Because gear can't be washed, it's vital to hang it out to dry after each skating session. A product called a hockey tree is designed to prop up the gear to air-dry; it looks like an overgrown coat rack with branches sticking out in all directions and at various levels. You can enhance drying by pointing a fan at your gear.

YOUR FIRST TIME

Everyone wants to get out there and shoot a *slap shot*, that classic power move that sends the puck flying into the goal. Go ahead and try one if you like—but they are much harder

than they look, so don't be surprised if you miss the puck entirely. When you watch a game, you'll see that players rarely take slap shots but instead do a lot of passing and maneuvering.

To learn the game, start by picking up a stick and getting a feel for moving a ball or puck around on the ground. Even if you plan to play on skates, it's easiest to gain a few skills first without them. This makes the game a little slower, plus you're less likely to get tripped up by your feet. Next, find a friend with whom you can practice passing back and forth and shooting a few attempts at a designated goal, which is 6 feet wide and 4 feet high.

At the same time, practice your skating skills without the hockey stick. The sport requires precision skating ability because you

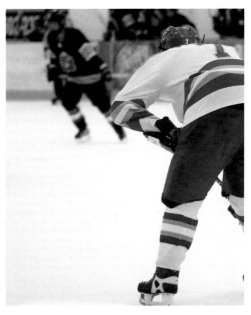

can't be thinking about your feet while trying to watch your opponents, keep track of teammates, and manage the puck. And to play well, you have to be able to skate away from your opponents, which is why great skaters can be better players than the ones who have great aim.

If you want to play ice hockey, it's best to master skating basics using figure skates before switching to the hockey style. Figure skates are easier for novices because they have more blade in contact with the ice (hockey blades curve up at the front and back), and a toe pick allows you to push off easily. When you're very comfortable with your ability on figure skates, the switch to hockey skates will be fairly easy. If your budget is limited and you prefer not to buy both types of skates, rent figure skates. It's tempting to skip this step, and guys often dislike the idea of figure skating. But the time you invest to learn the right skills will pay off in much better skating after the switch, making you a better hockey player.

The transition from skill drills to a game at full speed will be overwhelming. Before you're ready to play your first game on skates, get a feel for being out there with other skaters. Try a small skirmish with a friend or two to experience the sensation of another player rushing at you, sometimes colliding by accident. Also, try reading a basic book about the game, such as *Hockey for Dummies*. Most aspects of hockey need to be learned from experience, but it's helpful to have some idea of the positions, plays, and penalties.

When you're ready to put skates, stick, and puck together, be prepared to be dazed. Trying to master any one aspect—stick handling, following the puck, skating, off-sides and strategy, knowing when to enter and exit the game—would be enough for a new player. Doing them all at once is guaranteed to be more than you can manage the first time. But stick with it, because it gets easier, and it's a lot of fun. You certainly won't be bored with this sport.

ATHLETE IN ACTION

Keith Champagne, 51

"I was in my forties and thought the point of no return was coming up, so I had better find a fitness activity that I loved," recalls Keith Champagne. The son of Depression-era parents, Champagne grew up in Louisiana, where sports seemed to be only for rich kids and skating wasn't popular. "I had never skated and thought it would be fun to try," he says. As an adult living in New York, he signed up for ice-skating classes and enjoyed that enough to keep going for a few years. "But I didn't like the solo aspect of figure skating," says Champagne. "I met people who were playing hockey, and they were extremely supportive." He signed up for hockey prep classes, which included skating and stick-handling skills. Hockey turned out to be the fitness activity he was seeking: Five years later, he plays every week and is the managing director of the New York City Gay Hockey Association.

Champagne was ready to play on a league when he had decent stick and skating skills, but he wasn't able to truly learn the game until he was in it. "I learned on the ice," he says. "It was scary—and you don't want to make a fool of yourself. The first four times, I can't say I had a lot of fun." But when you sign up for a team, you have to show up for the season, so he kept going back, and by the end of the first month he had gotten a little better. He notes that people who learn to play as kids have an advantage, but many of them don't have polished skating skills, which is where an older novice can gain an edge.

But for Champagne, the game is not just about the skills. In his nonchecking league he has teammates as varied as a woman in her late 50s and another woman who is not yet of legal drinking age. He loves the camaraderie of the sport. It's a group you'd never expect to find in the same room, yet they've bonded. "Hockey isn't something I saw myself doing," he says. "My family is shocked." But not only does he play and train for hockey regularly; the sport got him back into the gym, where he does conditioning workouts, including pilates. "I was not a sports person ever, but people looked like they were having a great time," he says. And now Champagne is one of those people, trim and fit, who encourages the beginners on the ice like a veteran player.

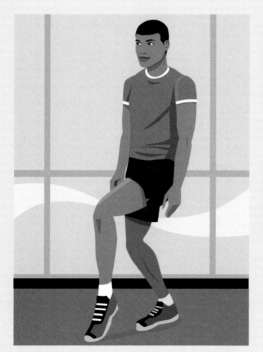

Coach's Corner

SECRETS TO SUCCESS

During a hockey game, you should never find yourself standing still, says Jim Bugenhagen, director of ice hockey at Sky Rink at Chelsea Piers. You're constantly making adjustments to your position so you're in the right place to receive a pass or block a shot. Also, it's easier to maneuver quickly if you are already in motion. On ice, moving all the time will keep you from getting cold. If you're not in shape before you take up the sport, you will be before long. It's terrific exercise. "You play intensely, full out, for short periods of time. That pattern requires stamina," says Bugenhagen.

When you join a league, you'll probably play once a week. And if the league is well organized, you'll be well matched with players close to your level. To advance in this sport, it helps to play in tournaments where you will be exposed to better players and play many games in just a few days. When you see a new trick you'd like to try, you'll get a chance to do so in your next game.

Another way to pick up skills is to watch good players. Professional games on television aren't as informative as watching them up close, on site. Follow a specific person, not the puck, and you will learn a lot from how he moves, as well as his mistakes and effective maneuvers.

Everyone wants to be out in front making the goals, of course. If you get the chance, play both offense and defense, because doing both helps provide an overall comprehension of the game. Defensive players do get to make goals

one-legged squats

Stand with your legs a little less than shoulder-width apart, with your weight on your right leg. Bend your right knee slightly and slide your left foot forward a few inches, toes touching the ground. Keeping your shoulders back, head up, and abs firm, bend your right knee as far as you comfortably can, as though you were about to sit in a chair. Allow your erect upper body to tilt forward for balance. Press down through your right heel and squeeze your glutes as you return to standing. Finish reps, then switch legs and repeat. Start with 5 reps on each side. Build up to 3 sets of 15 reps.

from time to time, and the positions near the goal are a great place to watch the action while you're learning. Knowing how to be in the right position for a pass or an assist is more valuable than constantly trying to score.

If you're able to squeeze in gym workouts alongside training and playing, try stamina-building cardio intervals. Using any form of aerobic exercise (running, cycling, etc.), complete a warm-up and then alternate between sprints and recovery periods of equal length, lasting thirty seconds to two minutes. For the sprints, push yourself as hard as you can. For the recovery, do the same exercise at a pace that's light enough to catch your breath; don't stop completely. If you can, keep a water bottle handy for a sip. Do five to twenty intervals in a row and end your workout with a cool-down period. To progress, add more intervals, make them longer, or do the sprints at a faster pace.

If you do strength workouts in the gym, try working one side of the body at a time. Hockey players hunch over the stick in one position, which can cause imbalances in the muscles. Also, we all have a naturally stronger side—for example, one foot tends to lead when you walk up the stairs. To be a better player and prevent injuries, try to balance out your body by lifting weights with one arm or one leg and then switching to be sure the other side is just as strong. To do one-sided strength work at home, try these moves:

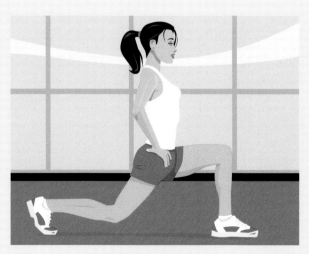

reverse lunges

Stand with your legs shoulder-width apart, shoulders back, abs firm, head up, and hands on your hips. Step back as far as you comfortably can with your right foot, right heel up, left knee aligned above your left foot. Bend your right knee and lower it toward the ground, keeping your torso as erect as possible. Squeeze your glutes as you return to the start position. Repeat on the opposite side to complete 1 rep. Start with 5 reps. Build up to 3 sets of 15 reps.

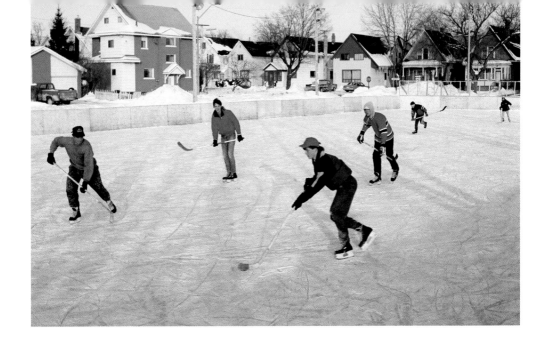

TACKLE THE TRUTH

You have to be aggressive to play hockey

Hockey has gotten a bad name from a tradition of fisticuffs in the NHL. On an amateur level, even in the most competitive leagues, it's not a brutal game, but one of finesse and skill. Sure, there will be accidental collisions, and there are leagues that allow checking. The game is fast, and you won't do well if you hesitate, but you don't need a raging temper to play. The people who get emotional and excited don't do as well, because they lose control. The best players stay cool and execute complex skills and strategies.

Hockey is a dangerous sport. Getting hurt is guaranteed

You are more likely to get injured playing hockey than, say, swimming—but most hockey injuries are minor (strains, cuts, and bruises). Well-fitted gear offers excellent protection from serious damage. The pads make a fall on the ice less damaging than it is for a figure skater, for example. Look for a non-checking league and be aware of other players when you're on the ice so as to avoid a collision. If you're so concerned about getting hurt that you might skip the sport, consider tending goal. It seems counterintuitive, but in the position in which you're the target of the puck, you're less likely to get hurt because collisions with other players are uncommon.

Only men play hockey

Women play a lot more than just field hockey these days. There are hockey teams that are for women only and some mixed teams, too. You don't need to be big to play the sport—some top scorers are the smaller, quicker players. Anyone who can handle a stick can play hockey. The sport is not for wimps, though. Hockey is competitive and part of the game includes posturing, or slandering your opponents. It's all in good fun, but if you have a thin skin, you might not enjoy it.

GET MORE FROM YOUR SPORT

If you like one type of hockey, consider trying the other forms. You can work on some of the common skills and strategies by switching from roller to ice, and so on. In addition, consider other team sports played on a field with two goals: soccer, basketball, football, and lacrosse, for example. Each of these activities can improve your strategic ability and teamwork.

A variety of sports provide useful cross-training to improve specific aspects of your hockey game. You can improve your hand/eye coordination for better puck handling by taking up golf, fencing, or tennis. Work on your aim with archery or almost any sport that involves a ball, from baseball to dodgeball. Any time you spend on skates will tone the muscles and hone the skills you use when you play (see *Skating*, page 183, for more ideas about sports that can make you a better skater). For general improvements in stamina, any aerobic activity works, but sports such as cycling, which focuses on leg muscles, are particularly useful for hockey players.

People who enjoy hockey tend to like challenging sports that take years to master. If you're in that category you may want to consider gymnastics, rock climbing, boxing, or martial arts.

There aren't hockey-playing vacations per se, but you can take a trip to a hockey skills camp. Keep in mind, this is not generally a bring-the-family getaway, unless your kids are enrolled in camp, too. Because ice time is expensive and in high demand, you will not get much extra practice time at home, so the chance to play day after day in camp helps you progress much faster than weekly games in a league. Some camps are intense hockey-only experiences, while others offer more of a vacation feeling. Heartland Hockey offers a nice combo: weekend camps for adults in Florida that combines coaching by former NHL player and Olympian Steve Jensen with off-ice activities such as water skiing and mini-golf (www.HeartlandHockey.com). To find more, go to www.USAHockeyMagazine.com and click "hockey camps".

RESOURCES

➡ **www.LifetimeHockey.com** is a site about nonchecking hockey for adults. You'll find basic information, such as the twelve plays you need to know, as well as a glossary of hockey jargon. They even have pages about building your own hockey tree to air out your gear after games.

➡ **www.USAHockey.com** is the main site for information about competitions. You'll find links to disabled-hockey programs and almost anything else you need to know. The official rulebook is online, which can be a helpful read for a beginner.

➡ *Complete Hockey Instruction* by Dave Chambers, Ph.D., a former NHL coach, covers all aspects of the sport, from skating skills to strategy.

➡ *The Hockey Handbook* by Lloyd Percival is a classic introduction to the game. The 1997 version updates the 1951 original with newer training techniques.

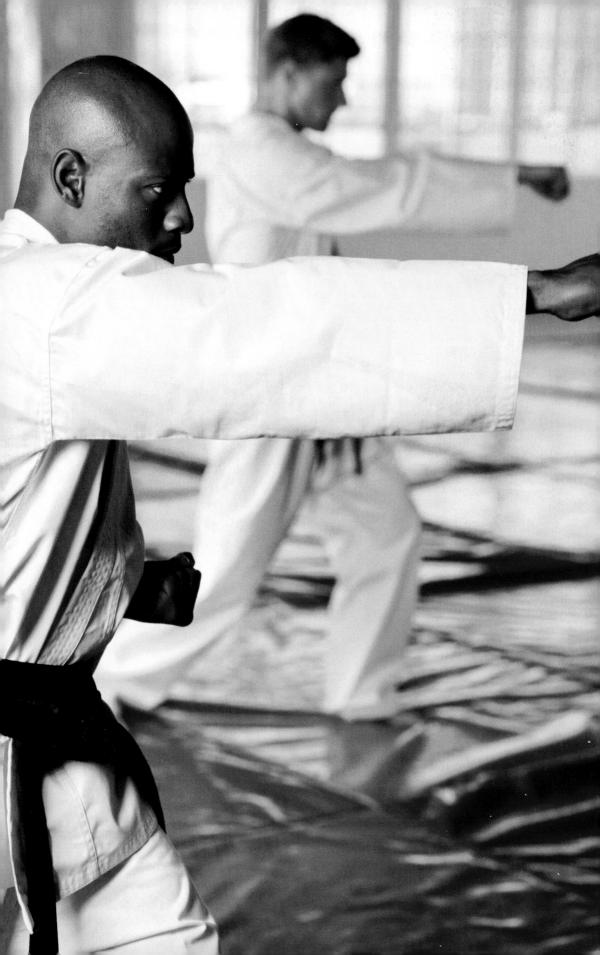

14

MARTIAL ARTS

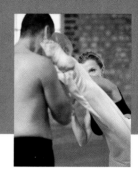

MARTIAL ARTS

YOU'LL LOVE THIS SPORT IF YOU:
- want to build flexible strength, balance, and an injury-resistant body
- need a way to reduce stress
- thrive on learning new skills, like to achieve new levels of mastery
- need a sport that challenges the mind as well as the body
- enjoy working with an instructor
- like having a code of conduct
- revel in competition
- prefer activities you can share with your children

YOU MIGHT NOT LOVE THIS SPORT IF YOU:
- are impatient; these activities require practice and are not easy to master
- don't like being told what to do
- are uncomfortable if a teacher delves into life lessons
- need social interaction as you practice; classes do not encourage conversation

For many Americans, taking up the martial arts begins as a way to get in shape or as an alternate gym routine rather than a sport per se. It's easy to see why: Martial arts practitioners tend to be firm and fit. These activities build strength, flexibility, balance, and agility, working every muscle from head to toe as you improve your stamina. Kicks, chops, and twisting evasive maneuvers tone your muscles as you move, resulting in a fluid strength that makes daily activities seem much easier. Perhaps more important, martial arts require and instill discipline. If you've had trouble sticking to regular workouts or staying on a diet, you may have success through martial arts. The traditional teachings call for discipline and respect from the student for both the practice and the teacher (who is often called the master or *sensei*). You'll experience some aspect of this formality even if you begin your training in a less strict environment such as a gym class, because safety requires that you follow certain rules.

The longer you stick with martial arts, however, the more hooked you'll become on them as a rigorous sport. At heart, the martial arts are exactly what the name implies—preparation for battle. Each form originally began as training for soldiers and self-defense maneuvers for civilians (who were often protecting themselves from the soldiers). Some of the disciplines date back thousands of years, spreading from India and China to Thailand, Indonesia, Japan, and Korea—and, later, the United States and the rest of the world. Over the centuries, different styles evolved, taking on the aspects of each local culture. Stricter forms involve training that resembles military boot camp, while some of the softer styles are moving meditations with similarities to yoga.

Whichever style you pick, from t'ai chi to tae kwondo, kendo to karate, you will cultivate confidence as you develop mastery over your body and mind to execute the moves properly. Over time, you will learn to measure the force you need to achieve the necessary effect and feel that you can protect yourself from any threat. You'll work hard, push past your previous physical and mental limits, learn to take criticism, and build character. You will improve your ability to focus, reduce stress, and enjoy the camaraderie of your fellow students before and after classes.

The most highly trained martial artists sometimes seem to defy the laws of gravity and the frailties of the human body. While their abilities may be exaggerated in mythology and lore—and especially in kung fu movies—the disciplined channeling of body,

SCORE

A 150-pound person who spends an hour practicing the harder martial arts—such as judo, jujitsu, kickboxing, karate and tae kwondo—will burn about 540 calories (or 3.6 times your weight). For the softer forms such as t'ai chi, the same person will burn about 180 calories per hour (or 1.2 times your weight).

mind, and spirit does allow for some spectacular displays, such as breaking boards and concrete blocks with a single strike. The explanation lies partly in the repetitive nature of the practice. By drilling the moves over and over, you find that each becomes instinctive, faster than you could manage if you had to stop and think. Another aspect is the harnessing of your inner energy, which is called the life force or *chi*. In Western terms, you use intense focus to bring forth your best abilities, tapping into reserves of strength and stability located in your *center* (what Westerners call the core). The Eastern ideal of this concept is much deeper, and it's the reason that a martial arts master is impossible to budge when his mind is set on staying still. Those concrete blocks don't stand a chance.

Despite all the flying chunks of wood, karate chops, and leaping kicks (and the nasty Samurai in some movies), martial arts are methods of defense, not offense. The culture requires that they be used only in response to an attack. Combat strategy is taught, but the accomplished martial artist will also have learned to remain serene in the face of danger and to walk away whenever possible. Dichotomies such as this one are central to the discipline of martial arts, often referred to with the symbol of yin and yang, which represents the balance of opposite forces.

GEARING UP

Buy nothing before signing up for your first martial arts class. In almost all cases, you will need a uniform, but it is proper etiquette and sometimes required that you buy it from the studio where you will train. If they don't sell uniforms, they will have suggestions about what to buy and where. You may also need some protective sparring gear and weapons, but this equipment should only be purchased after you receive advice from your instructor or the studio owner.

Your first steps, and perhaps the hardest ones, are to select a discipline and a teacher. If you have your heart set on trying your neighbor's class or going to your daughter's *dojo* (the name for a training hall in Japanese forms, also called the *dojang* for Korean styles), you can skip this step—with a caveat: What works for others may not be a good fit for you, so if your enthusiasm wanes, consider researching fresh options before giving up on the sport.

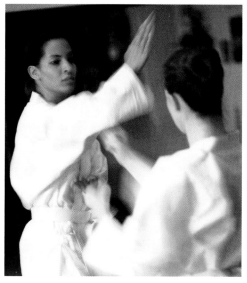

Start with an overview of the different styles. Look in library books to see what the moves are, rent how-to videos, or look online to get a sense of the amount of physical contact. Next, select a few disciplines and look for local schools by checking the phone book, Internet listings, ads in newspapers, or by asking around at local colleges or the parks department to see if they offer classes. Some instructors teach out of their homes as well, and you'll also find clubs you can join that offer sessions. When you've narrowed down the list of schools, check the local chamber of commerce and Better Business Bureau to find out about their reputations.

A sample of the martial arts

Aikido is a Japanese martial art that focuses on harnessing your opponent's power to divert him away from you. The form uses some Jujitsu moves, but emphasizes harmony.

Judo is a Japanese style derived from Jujitsu and is one of two martial arts in the Olympics. The object is to throw the opponent or execute a hold. Punches and kicks are not allowed.

Jujitsu is a Japanese form of grappling. In this art, size is no issue as you use the momentum of your attacker to control and throw him. There are no punches or kicks, but you may use a staff.

Karate comes from Okinawa, off the coast of Japan, and involves striking with bare hands and feet. Karate students learn a variety of stances, blocks, punches, kicks, and take-down techniques. Although the word *karate* is now translated as "empty hand" (it was originally "China hand"), high-degree training may include weapons.

Kendo is a Japanese form of stick fighting in which the sticks stand in for swords. Participants wear protective armor and land blows to the head, chest, or hands.

Kung fu, a Chinese martial art with hundreds of different styles, was made famous by Bruce Lee. Some styles of kung fu focus on kicks, while others emphasize punches; some are fast and explosive, while others are smooth and flowing. Similar to karate, this art includes stances, blocks, kicks, and punches. Kung fu may also include grappling and other close combat.

Muay Thai is a form of kickboxing developed in Thailand. The hands, feet, elbows, shins, and knees are all acceptable weapons in this art, and the competitors now usually wear boxing gloves. Before competing, the boxers complete a ritual dance that also serves as a warm-up.

Qi gong is an ancient Chinese martial art known for flowing movements coordinated with the breath. There is rarely combat in qi gong practice, and it is often taught as a health activity to strengthen, balance, and energize the body.

Tae kwondo is the main Korean martial art and one of two styles in the Olympics. Throwing is not allowed, nor are holds or strikes using the elbows or knees. In combat, kicking predominates. A helmet and protective pads are worn because kicks to the chest and head score points (and can otherwise be fatal).

T'ai chi is the oldest martial art, coming from China. The moves are slow and flowing, looking more like a dance than combat. T'ai chi has been studied for stress reduction, balance, and other health benefits. But t'ai chi is an effective form of self defense.

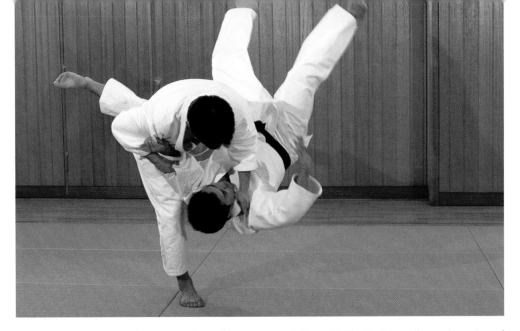

Your next step is to observe a class. Every dojo should allow you to do this before you sign up. Look at how hands-on the teachers are and the amount of contact allowed. Assess if you feel comfortable with the student-teacher ratio and the size of the space for the number of students. Pay close attention to how the teacher treats the students and whether or not they seem proud to be part of the class. If the scene looks promising, stick around after class and ask the students questions, or speak with the teacher and the school's head instructor. You'll want to collect a lot of information, but be aware that you should do your best to show tremendous respect while you're actually grilling the staff. Keep in mind that questioning is considered rude in many Asian cultures and go gently! Ask about the expected level of commitment in terms of class attendance and if students must go to competitions. Find out how long it takes the average student to progress from rank to rank (more than a few months and less than a few years is generally reasonable). And inquire about injuries—there will be some—and steps taken to prevent them. Ask the students about difficulties they face and what they like about the teacher's style. Discuss with the teacher your goals and whether or not he feels he can help you reach them—and expect straightforward questions about your current physical condition and motivation. And be sure to inquire about fees. Most disciplines require promotion tests to move up a rank, and these sessions typically

cost $20 to $100. Find out about the price of the uniform, protective gear, and weapons you'll need as well as the cost of lessons.

Be sure to visit several schools before making your final choice, even if you like the first one. You'll get more out of your training if you mentally commit to more than a few months in class—and you don't want to be half way through the program only to decide you'd prefer a different discipline or instructor. It's common for students to sign up without full investigation and later learn the fit is not a good one. When you've selected your school, ask if you can attend a sample class before committing. Many centers will refrain from the hard sell and welcome your desire to choose well so that you can become a long-term and successful student. This approach follows the tradition and culture that martial-arts masters are expected to give back to the sport. But do be mindful that they must also make a living, which isn't easy when teaching a handful of students.

Be sure to obtain equipment and a uniform before your first session. Buy your uniform as far in advance as you can so you can wash it a few times to soften it a little. In most cases, your uniform should come with a white belt, indicating that you are a beginner, a blank slate. Learn how to tie a square knot in the belt to keep it from falling off. Most martial arts are done barefoot, and you can expect to get blisters from time to time. There are training shoes that are acceptable in some disciplines.

YOUR FIRST TIME

If you have time before your first session, work on areas of weakness in your body, building strength, flexibility, and aerobic conditioning. Even a few sessions in the week prior to class will help. And spend a few minutes organizing your goals for your practice so you can tailor your homework between instruction sessions to maximize your chance for success.

Do your best not to rush to get to your first class. And leave your cell phone home—most dojos forbid them anyway. Prepare your mind by thinking through your expectations and areas of nervousness.

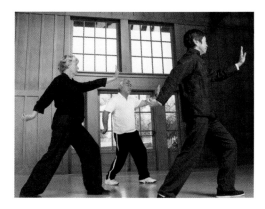

Once inside, put on your uniform (it should be clean and pressed for every class) and find a quiet space to do some light stretching. Expect to be nervous and feel out of place at first. Everything about the experience will seem foreign, from the language to the uniform to the movements. You won't know where to stand, what to say, or when to move until you've had a chance to observe and participate in at least a few sessions. It's even hard to know how to walk through the dojo without getting struck accidentally. To stay safe, consider each martial artist as a skittish horse, giving it wide berth lest it unexpectedly kicks you. If you haven't had a conversation with your instructor about your goals prior to class, it's common to discuss them in the first meeting. The teacher may also tell you more about what is expected, or the first step may be a demonstration of skills. Often, a few instructors or long-term students will display some advanced *forms* (sets of moves) to give you something to aspire toward and show you more of what the discipline entails. The moves are likely to be explosive and accompanied by shouts, used to harness chi energy. These displays may be inspiring and intimidating, but believe it or not, you'll be able to do similar moves if you work at it.

If you're lucky, you'll study alone or start together with other newcomers. But depending on the size of the school and class schedule, you may find yourself in a class with more seasoned students. Instructors and sparring partners should be willing to work at your level as you learn moves, so request changes in intensity or repeated instruction if you need them. If the teacher doesn't break the form down into its parts, ask him or a classmate to do it so you can learn the proper sequence. Repeat them slowly and carefully so that you develop accurate movements. Speed is less important than precision. And hard work is obligatory; you'll be expected to do your best even when you think no one is watching.

While you may be excited to test out your karate chop or learn a spinning kick, expect the first skills and drills to be general conditioning without contact. Jumping right in to flying maneuvers and sparring is a sure way to end up with an injury. Also, it's harder to hit and be hit than you'd expect, so spend some time getting used to the environment before you add this challenge. And remember that students are expected to be humble, so even if you do have the ability to do a few skills, it's best to refrain from showing them off.

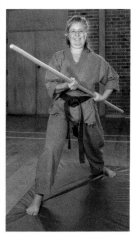

SECRETS TO SUCCESS

Whether you take up the ancient discipline of t'ai chi or a more recent derivation such as aikido, you can have confidence in the path. "These are step-by-step processes of systemized training that has been proven for thousands of years by masters and students," says Sang H. Kim, Ph.D., a tae kwondo champion and retired instructor who has a degree in sports science and has written books on several martial arts. Everything, from the way you stand to the way you breathe, is part of the technique that has been passed down through the centuries, even if it has been modified into a modern system. To maximize the learning, mentally review what you have been taught after each class and practice it, even if the technique seems easy. By visualizing the proper way to do each form, you perfect your comprehension of it, and physical practice will ingrain the movements in your muscles and mind so that you can do them without thought later.

Martial arts masters often teach in a strict manner in which there is one proper way to perform each move. But Kim subscribes to the belief that there is room for personal interpretation. "Learning is a process of copying what is demonstrated by your teacher and then transferring the techniques to yourself," he says. But before you can strike out on your own, you must learn the basics properly so you have a solid foundation on which to build. "The reality of learning is that it's hard work, but the results are definite," says Kim. You can't walk into the studio and try to do what the higher-ranking students are doing. That's a certain path to injury. But if you pace yourself, you'll be rewarded. "The hardship is getting over the physical limitations from age and stiffness," says Kim. "But time and consistent practice work—and you'll be surprised at the easiness of the skills once you learn to do them."

Before each class, be sure to warm up and do some stretching to prepare your body for the challenge of the moves. Try these exercises to get started:

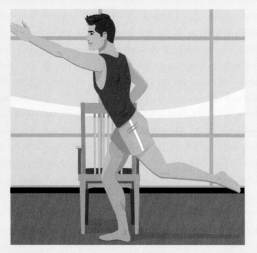

scissor swing

Stand with your right side facing the back of a sturdy chair, your right hand on the chair's back for support. Bend your right knee slightly for a stable base. Lift your left leg forward as high as you comfortably can, pointing the foot. At the same time, swing your left arm straight back. Reverse the swing, bringing your left leg back and left arm forward. Focus on a smooth and relaxed swing more than the maximum height. Do 10 to 12 repetitions, then switch sides and repeat.

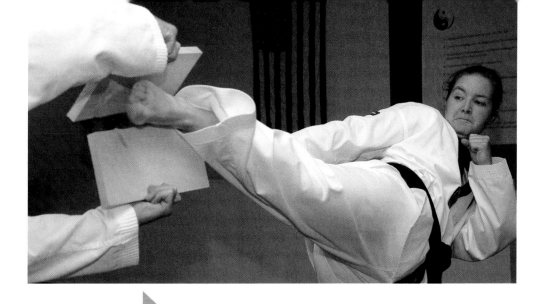

Gary Zarr was a boxer and wrestler in high school. His first experience with Asian martial arts was a type of Japanese karate he tried in his 20s. During his 30s and 40s, he progressed to t'ai chi and, more recently, qi gong. With the classic humility of a student, he says, "By no means do I consider myself a martial artist, but I have been involved over the years and have benefited." And he has learned a lot during that time, much of it beyond the physical maneuvers. An executive at the American Museum of Natural History in New York City, Zarr has an appreciation for learning about different cultures, making his training a natural branch in the ongoing quest. "I became very interested in martial arts in Asia and how the practice is tied into systems of health, philosophy, and art that transcend physical contact," he says. "Martial arts are viewed as part of the cultivation of yourself as a human being; they are instructive when striving to live a balanced and rich life."

Zarr has had a lifelong interest in the spirit of the warrior, reading heroic literature such as the *Odyssey* and explorations of mythology by Joseph Campbell. Studying the heroes of the past, Zarr has learned that in martial arts, the opponent is not the only determining factor in competition. "The ultimate person you compete with is yourself," he says. Whether you win or lose, each time you spar you gain because you learn. And you also gain confidence. A guide—a guru or *sensei*—can help you see the path and stay on it, but to make progress requires pushing your limits physically and emotionally, facing your discomfort and fear. "The degree to which you can get to your own personal edge and explore it is the degree that you grow and evolve," he says. As the great heroes of literature have all discovered, "the light comes after the test."

MARTIAL ARTS

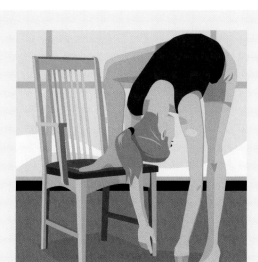

forward bend with branch

Stand with your right leg against the seat of a sturdy chair. Place your right foot on the chair, toes turned out comfortably. Lean forward at the waist, letting your upper body hang toward the floor, your arms and head relaxed, feeling the stretch but no pain. Keep your hips squared to the front. Breathe, keeping your mind focused on relaxing the muscles. Hold the position for at least 15 seconds, working up to 30. Repeat on the other side. Do 2 to 3 repetitions per side.

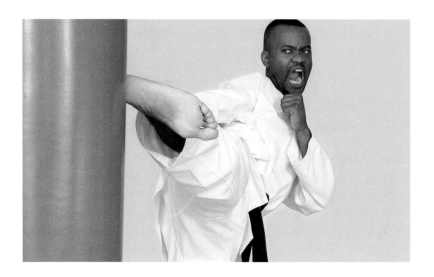

TACKLE THE TRUTH

I'll get hurt in martial arts training

The martial arts are safer than many sports because precautions are taken against injury. As a form of self-defense, the training is designed to help you avoid getting hurt. That's not to say you won't get a bruise or risk twisting an ankle and maybe get knocked down; sparring also brings the risk of someone accidentally knocking the wind out of you by trying to kick in target areas and missing. But as a beginning student, you aren't signing up to get kicked in the head. You may not experience any physical contact until you've mastered quite a few moves, which should allow you a fighting chance to protect yourself.

People who study martial arts are dragon-worshipping fighters

The image of the dragon—or the lion or some other animal—may well be on the door of the dojo. In martial arts, animals and mythical creatures are prized for their strength and prowess. But there's no cult worship involved, even if the practice has a strong spiritual aspect. The focus is on channeling your inner reserves of energy to become the strongest warrior possible. And as a strong warrior, you'll know that you don't need to fight to prove yourself. Unlike their movie images, martial artists tend to be calm pacifists.

It takes years before you can do anything in martial arts

Progress may seem painfully slow at first, but it will come. You should start to develop some skills within the first month, feeling more comfortable and developing a decent understanding of what you will accomplish. If your martial art uses a colored belt system with about six levels, you might get your first colored belt in three to six months. Depending on the discipline, you could achieve black-belt status in as little as three years. That said, you can spend your entire life perfecting your forms and training your mind and spirit. After achieving a black belt in one system, students often go on to learn another one for deeper understanding.

GET MORE FROM YOUR SPORT

Martial arts require stamina and force, plus focus. You can work on stamina and strategy through "court" sports such as basketball. Build strength in the weight room and with yoga or pilates (which also help with focus). Consider taking up other fighting sports, such as fencing, wrestling, and boxing, which are actually martial arts as well. And work on body awareness and balance with gymnastics, skating, and skiing.

To develop your practice, compete. Tournaments offer various categories by rank, age, and/or weight. In competition, you'll have the opportunity to learn from other students, not just the regular pairings at your school. Also, because martial arts are designed to develop your abilities as a warrior, you must go outside your comfort zone and test your skills when you are scared, nervous, or simply in a different location. That's why some systems insist on competition as an element of training. Tournaments are most often held in the late fall and winter and may include three categories: First, you may do forms, or sequences of moves that you select and demonstrate solo, in synchronicity with a team or set to music. The forms will be judged on difficulty, accuracy, power, and confidence—so if you make a mistake, keep going as though nothing were wrong. The second category concerns sparring, which is done in front of judges with a referee. You'll be given points and penalties for various moves. The duration and scoring vary by discipline. Third, in systems that include it, is the breaking contest. You'll be judged on the difficulty of your technique but you'll only score well if you actually break the objects, so choose the toughest moves you can do well.

RESOURCES

→ **www.blackbeltmag.com** is the Web site for the martial arts magazine, covering a variety of techniques and gear, plus a useful link to dojos around the country.

→ **www.fightingarts.com** offers a variety of instruction and information. Click on the "reading room" for articles from beginner mindset to a glossary of the martial arts styles.

→ **www.turtlepress.com** is Sang H. Kim's site, which has a "training tips" section offering a wealth of free information, from history to philosophy, drills to exercises.

→ *Martial Arts after 40* by Sang H. Kim, Ph.D., is a guide to using the martial arts to combat aging, as well as a manual for starting your practice when your body takes a little longer to adapt and heal. The author's strong education in Western sports medicine combines with his training in the martial arts to produce a clear format that will help you reach your goals.

→ *Ultimate Fitness through Martial Arts* by Sang H. Kim, Ph.D., also blends the author's Eastern and Western expertise in exercises that target strength, agility, flexibility, and coordination, plus sections on nutrition and injury prevention. Drills and martial arts moves are described and illustrated, making this book a handy all-round reference.

MARTIAL ARTS

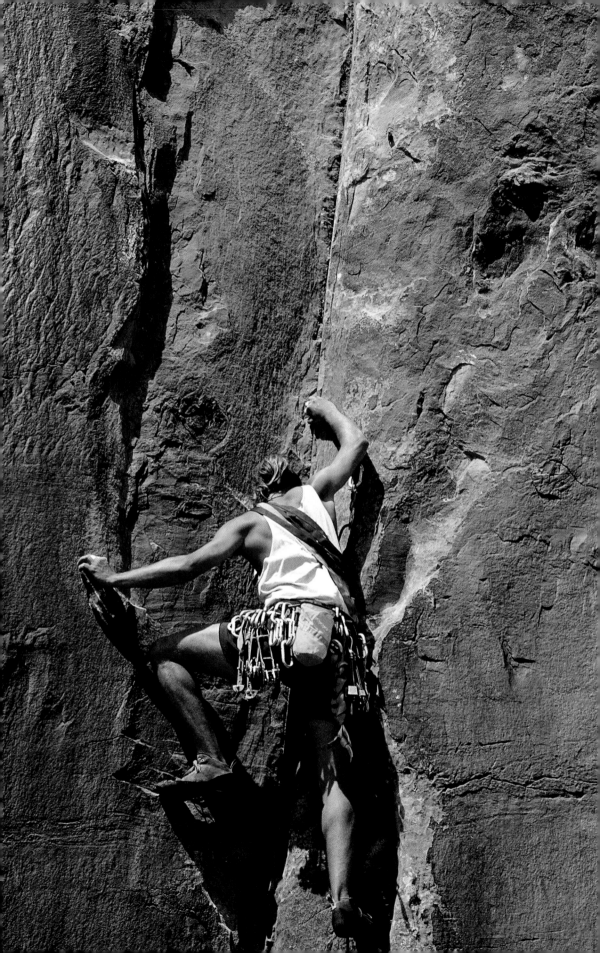

15

ROCK CLIMBING

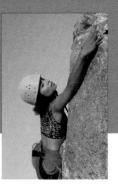

ROCK CLIMBING

YOU'LL LOVE THIS SPORT IF YOU:
- want a sport that challenges your powers of balance, flexibility, and strength all at the same time
- need a mental challenge in addition to a physical one
- enjoy pushing your personal limits
- want to have so much fun you don't realize you're exercising
- enjoy a versatile sport; you can get outdoors in good weather, or practice indoors any time
- love to be out in nature
- like a sport you can do with others
- want something you can do on vacation in some of the most beautiful places in the world

YOU MIGHT NOT LOVE THIS SPORT IF YOU:
- have hand problems, such as arthritis
- are deathly afraid of heights—although this sport could help you work through your fears
- have trust issues; you place your life in the hands of your *belayer*
- dislike the idea of people looking up at your butt while you're hanging in a harness

Climbing is all about challenging yourself. You never stop improving, from the first time you put your foot onto a wall to the elite level, because there's always a harder climb you can aspire to next. And while expert climbers make it look easy, the sport is intense, combining focus, strength, and flexibility. But it's also easier than it may seem to a leery beginner. And many accomplished climbers are so enthusiastic about the sport that they are eager to help a newcomer.

Some climbers first come to the wall because they want a great workout; but they stay because, mentally and physically, the sport is like nothing else. Many people think that they won't like climbing or be able to do it; but you won't know for sure until you try it, because the skills you need are unexpected and untested by most other activities. You'll work your legs and arms to push and pull your body upward. You'll also use your abdominals and back muscles to maneuver for position and try to stay balanced close to the wall. And while novice climbers frequently power-up the climb using strength, more advanced climbers will use finesse, flexibility, and endurance, staying loose and moving in a more fluid manner that conserves energy. The difference is remarkable to watch: an experienced climber may seem to ascend with little effort, using both feet and both hands efficiently, while the novice may struggle for each individual hold. Flexibility is key to extending your reach and being able to twist to find a hold in an awkward position. And you'll develop muscle endurance from climbing.

As much as the physical experience is unexpected, the sport provides even more of a surprise mentally. Climbing is an activity you must truly try to understand, because while clinging to the rock you'll have a visceral reaction that's a combina-

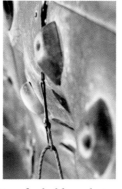

tion of excitement, fear, confusion, and gumption. You must cope with your fear and muscle fatigue while staying engaged enough to plan a route that provides good hand and foot holds all the way to the top of the wall. Other climbers are supportive, offering suggestions for holds and giving encouraging comments, but they can't help your muscles or your intractable mind when either refuses to make another move.

What you do learn over time is that there is a safety net. Your first climbs will be in a style called top-roping, in which a rope runs from your harness up to the top of the rock and then down again to a person called a *belayer*. The belayer reels in the rope as you climb, using a friction belay device to help support your weight securely so you can fall

off the wall without actually falling more than a few inches. Also, the harness and ropes allow you to sit back and rest, if need be. Although resting in the harness would be ruled as cheating in a climbing competition, it is a valid tool for beginners seeking to increase their endurance by taking a short break. When you finish your climb, you'll again sit back in the harness to walk your feet down as the belayer feeds out rope to lower you; this is called *rappelling*.

Rock climbing is sometimes called *technical climbing* or *technical mountaineering* because it involves steep ascents that require equipment such as anchors secured in the rock, sometimes called *hardware* or *protection*. There are a variety of anchor styles to fit different crevices, and there may be bolts permanently fixed in the rock wall on popular routes. Or temporary protection can be inserted by the climber. To prepare a top-rope climb, someone has to get the ropes in place and she may also need to set the anchors.

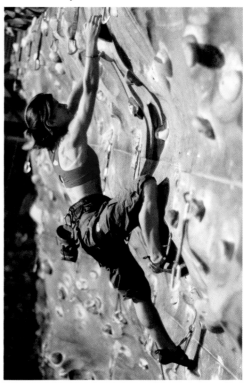

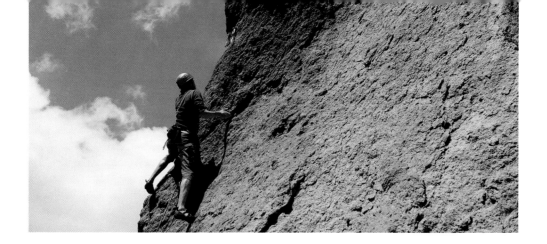

Often, a hiker takes a nontechnical route (a hike) to the top, sets the rope by securing it to anchors or solid natural objects such as a large tree, then hikes or rappels down. When she can't walk to the top, an advanced climber does a *lead climb*, in which the rope is attached to the climber's harness and she secures it to anchors on the ascent. Unfortunately, when a lead climber loses her grip, she will often be above the last anchor and fall a distance before the rope catches, which can mean banging off the rock. And the anchors must be carefully placed so they don't lose purchase with the yank of the rope as she falls, which is one reason this technique is considered advanced.

Historically, rock climbing was not a sport per se but a necessary part of alpine mountaineering. While humans have scaled mountains throughout history for the necessities of hunting or military maneuvers, the birth of alpine mountaineering became an official sport on August 8, 1786, when Dr. Michel-Gabriel Paccard and Jacques Balmat were the first to successfully climb glacier-capped Mont Blanc, the tallest peak in Western Europe, located on the border between France and Italy. The first ascent of the world's tallest peak, Mount Everest, was achieved in 1953 by Sir Edmund Hillary, with Sherpa Tenzing Norgay. It was at this time that notable climbers started to collect "trophy" mountains, with the next feat—the climbing of the tallest peak on each continent—accomplished in 1985 by

SCORE

When rock climbing, a 150-pound person will burn an average of 600 calories per hour climbing up and 420 calories per hour rappelling (or multiply your body weight by 4 and 2.8, respectively).

Dick Bass, followed by Reinhold Messner's scaling of the world's fourteen tallest peaks the following year.

The separation of rock climbing as a sport from the oxygen tanks and frigid conditions of alpine mountaineering began in 1886 when W.P. Hasket-Smith scaled 115 feet up Nape's Needle in the Western Lakes District in England (which he repeated fifty years later at age seventy-four). The next evolution in the sport was rock-climbing competitions. Climbers are judged on how long it takes to get to a certain point or how far they can climb in a set amount of time.

Indoor climbing began as an independent sport during the 1980s. The technique is similar to the outdoor version in that a harness, a rope, and a belay device are used for safety. But climbing walls also have thick mats at the base, rather than ragged rock and hard dirt paths. Also, while the outdoor climber must contend with weather and sometimes wildlife while looking for little ledges, cracks, and knobs in the rock to grasp, indoor climbers have the advantage of temperature-controlled gyms. They don't have to worry about snakes or black flies. In addition, there are easily recognized holds of different shapes and sizes premounted in the wall. The holds are colored to indicate routes, so a climber may try to ascend using only the red holds, for example—although beginners generally use any holds they can reach. The routes are color coded according to level of difficulty, providing plenty of challenge, even though the walls are typically

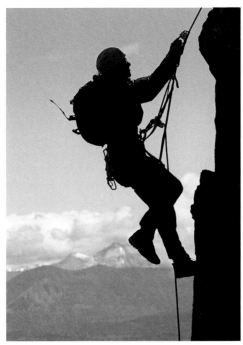

only 30 to 40 feet high. Don't be confused that indoor climbing walls may sometimes be outdoors; the label "indoor wall" implies only that the surface is not natural.

Climbs are rated for technical difficulty. In the U.S., we use the Yosemite Decimal System, which starts at 1.0 for a walk on flat ground and designates scrambling over rock as above 3.0 and below 5.0, depending on the level of difficulty. Rock climbing starts at 5.0 and progresses to 5.15. Climbs below a 5.6 are considered fairly easy. While climbers usually graduate from one rating to the next, some people will find a particular route more or less challenging because of their particular abilities. Part of the rating is based on the steepness of the ascent, but the numerical designation also takes into account the types of holds and ease of selecting a good route. It does not consider any psychological aspects, however, which may make a route seem harder or easier. Also, you may see ratings for the number of anchors in the rock. These are G for good, PG for pretty good, R for *runout* (large spacing in some areas) and X for no anchors at all.

Chances are good you won't choose your first climbs yourself, but it's a nice idea to keep a record of the technical ratings so you can watch your progress and tell guides of your abilities. Start by deciding to climb indoors or out. Then choose a gym for an indoor climb or a guiding company for a natural ascent. Look in the yellow pages, check listings in climbing magazines and Web sites, and ask people who work at local outdoor equipment stores to suggest guide companies. You can also look for learn-to-climb courses created by national organizations such as the Appalachian Mountain Club and Sierra Club.

GEARING UP

For your virgin outing, climb with a school, gym, or group that will rent you all the necessary gear. Wear comfortable clothes appropriate to the weather or temperature conditions, keeping in mind that you will be cooler while standing around (which happens a lot in group climbing situations) and much warmer when working your way up the rock. Remember that natural rock is abrasive on bare skin and can shred fabric. Close-fitting clothes are often a good choice so they won't get snagged as you climb. And trim long fingernails before you go so you don't suffer painful breaks. For sunny days outside, consider sunscreen, sunglasses, and a bandana to wrap around your brow and prevent sweat from dripping in your eyes. Bring water, snacks, and a pack for all of your gear. Bring antiseptic wipes and Band Aids in case of scratches and scrapes. And don't forget the camera to document your accomplishment.

At indoor walls, you can continue to rent the harness and shoes (indoor climbers don't usually wear helmets) for years because it's all conveniently kept on site so you have nothing to bring. When you're sure that you want to keep climbing, you'll want your own harness and shoes (and, when outdoors, a helmet). Go to an outdoor retailer that has a rope hung from the rafters so you can test-drive the fit of harnesses. Tell them your street shoe size, but expect rock climbing shoes to feel too tight—that's how you get a good toe-hold on the wall. They are worn without socks. The helmet must protect your head from falling debris, so make sure it fits snuggly and won't wobble as you climb. Another good purchase is a chalk bag that hangs from your belt. Your hands will sweat, especially when you're nervous. And chalking your hands is part of the mental preparation for the sport as well as a vital factor for improving your grip.

Continue to rely on your guides and instructors (or advanced climber friends) for ropes, anchors, belay devices, and other gear until you have developed the skills to warrant owning your own set.

YOUR FIRST TIME

Whether you sign up to climb indoors or out, do yourself a favor and warm up and stretch before meeting your instructor. Outdoors, you may loosen up with a hike to the wall. Indoors, do some walking or light exercise on

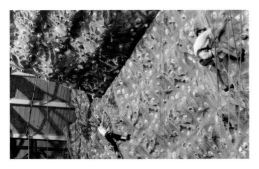

a cardio machine. Don't do so much that your muscles are tired, but try to get limber for the best experience. The first part of your lesson will include how to get into the harness and secure the rope to it with a *figure-eight and follow-through* knot. In most cases, you'll also attach a chalk bag. Next, you'll learn how the belay device works and the responsibilities of the belayer, plus climbing calls. Once the

belayer has checked that the knots, belay device, and ropes are all set, the conversation will go like this:

Climber: On belay
Belayer: On belay—climb when ready
Climber: Climbing
Belayer: Climb on

Prior to this last command, the belayer's full attention may not be on an individual climber. Once "climb on" is said, the climber then heads for the first hold—and the group on the ground is strictly forbidden from distracting the belayer from his task of keeping the climber safe. For beginners, the belayer will generally hold the rope taut to provide a feeling of security as you climb and perhaps some support for your body weight. You can ask for more or less slack as you need it for freedom of motion or added security.

Despite the safety of the rope, many new climbers feel exposed and at risk on the rock. Learning to trust the harness and belayer is harder than it looks. Most novice climbers will immediately adopt a death-like grip that fatigues the hand and forearm muscles. If you can, try to relax your grip, using your arms for balance rather than clinging to the rock. Also, it's common to press up onto tiptoes, which overtires the calves, causing them to shake up and down uncontrollably —amusingly called "sewing machine legs"— because they resemble the needle action. Drop your heels to stretch your calves and the shaking will cease.

Beginners also tend to need long breaks to rest or plan the next move. You'll note that advanced climbers try to keep the action going to use momentum in their favor, but you can't expect to have that ability the first few times out because the sport will feel so unusual and will tax muscles you didn't know you have. Do your best to pace yourself, continuing to move when possible and resting when necessary.

You may make it to the top without falling (but don't be disappointed if you don't). Should you reach the top of the climb, touching the hardware that holds the rope, a clip called a *carabiner*, you'll be ready to rappel. Now comes the hard part: convincing yourself to lean away from the rock and trust that you can safely sit back in your harness out into the air, letting go with your hands. (Note that if you scramble over the top, above the top anchor, you'll have to lower yourself farther, which can be frightening the first time.) Although you can feel the strong pull of the rope from below, your head still insists you will fall if you push away from your safe grasp. Take a deep breath and do it. The relief is instantaneous as your hands and arms relax and your legs and feet rest comfortably on the rock. You should end up sitting, head up, butt down, legs on the wall just slightly lower than your butt. And now you simply walk backwards down to the bottom, which is great fun once you get the hang of it.

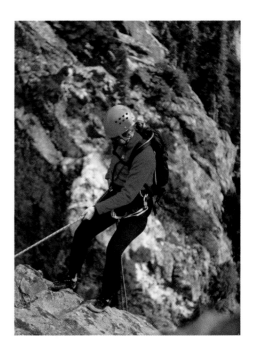

ATHLETE IN ACTION

Eli Katz, 35

"I'm a nice Jewish boy from Brooklyn, a businessman, not a gym rat," says Eli Katz. "But three years ago, I had a gastric bypass operation, and I wanted to stay in shape after the surgery." Katz lost 120 pounds after the stomach stapling procedure and decided to make the gym part of his new life, working out on the elliptical trainer and stair stepper. "If I'm going to lose that weight, I'm not going to get unfit," he decided. But he got too thin, bottoming out at 150 pounds, and needed to build more muscle tone and carefully add a little weight back. He started to lift weights with a trainer, who happened to be an avid rock climber herself. "She'd talk about it and I decided to try it—a new adventure," he says. But he was skeptical. "I hate sports. I'm not the outdoorsy type. I don't rough it. To me, roughing it is staying at a Holiday Inn."

Katz is not the type to judge fitness by how much he can bench press or how far he can run. But he also hates mindless workouts, so he went to the wall as promised. "I didn't expect to want to do it a second time," he recalls. "You see the wall with the notches sticking out and say 'so what?'" But that's because the climbers he saw were experienced and made it look easy. When he climbed on, he discovered the reality. "It worked my whole body; every muscle burned," Katz says, sold on the workout. But more important, he loved the mental aspect. "It was a puzzle to find the next move. You see the route on the wall and try to stick to it—today I'll do the red one—and that's really difficult," he adds.

The climbing is now a part of his workout routine. He bought a harness and shoes. He laughs that he takes off his yarmulke before climbing "because it falls off anyway," he says. And his regular workouts have shifted slightly, adding some moves to improve his climbing ability, such as focusing on forearm strength. "Before the surgery I could not do a pushup or chin up," he says. He's proud of what he has accomplished, but his climbing skills have a long way to go. "I haven't yet been using my whole body and balancing," he says. "I am making the mistake of using my upper body too much, so I burn out too quickly." But his mindset is changing too. Previously, his description of a hike was walking from the car across the parking lot to the mall. Now, he thinks that if the weather were nice, he might try climbing outdoors. "I'm contemplating it, but I'm not there yet," he says.

TACKLE THE TRUTH

My arms aren't strong enough to climb

Before trying it, most people assume that climbing a rock face involves executing a series of pull-ups using your arms alone. But done correctly, you climb by pushing yourself up the wall with your leg and butt muscles as much as possible; your arms are used mostly for balance and some additional pull. Think of it as climbing up a ladder, hand over hand, but with the work largely coming from your legs. You will need a good grip on the rock, often with your arms extended far overhead, which is more taxing than you might predict. But you can climb even if you can't manage a single pull-up, and your grip strength will improve with experience.

I'm afraid of heights and can't climb

Almost everyone has some fear of heights—it's a natural human reaction that keeps us safe. But plenty of people learn to climb despite their fear, or even because of it. If you have any desire to test your mettle and conquer your fear, this is the sport. The ropes will keep you secure, and you can stay fairly low to the ground while building confidence. Try going just a few inches up the rock and then sit back in the harness to see how it catches you. But don't hope to lose the fear completely. A little fear is important to prevent you from taking unnecessary risks. Because you've faced one of your demons, you'll feel a rush from climbing even a small distance up the rock.

I'll get seriously injured climbing

Rock climbing will leave you sore in places you can't name and is likely to produce some scratches and broken fingernails. But if you go with an expert guide on an appropriately rated climb and use the proper gear and precautions, you'll be safe. People just don't fall off a cliff if the harness is secure and the ropes are being used carefully.

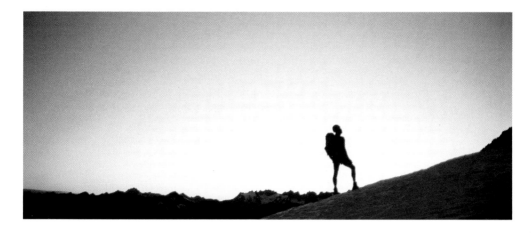

SECRETS TO SUCCESS

Most sports provide a sense of accomplishment in small, irregular doses, but rock climbing can give it to you every single time you go out. Not that you won't have bad days on the wall, but there's always a new technique, a new route, a new height to reach. "You set tangible goals," explains Abby Nelson, a trainer and rock-climbing instructor at the Sport Center at Chelsea Piers, site of one of the largest and most challenging indoor walls in the United States. And as you work toward those goals, you flail and struggle less and start to feel more natural and fluid. "There's a zone that you get into when you feel that you've dialed in the route and you cruise through it," describes Nelson. "It's choreography.

Everything flows from one hold to the next—and you've made that step of accomplishing the climb." And the rush of pride and confidence is infectious.

One great tip for beginners, Nelson says, is that it helps to splay your knees and open up your hips so that you're hugging your body close to the wall. That posture allows you to bring your center of gravity close to the rock, providing a solid platform from which to move to the next hold. Hip-hugging the wall allows you to transfer your weight easily from one foot to the other without slipping or hanging from your arms.

Beginners may also be surprised by how tiring it is to have your hands overhead as you try to grip holds of different

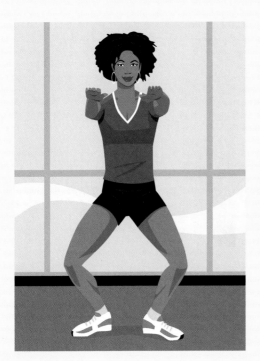

hip-opener plié

Stand with your heels approximately shoulder width apart, feet and knees turned out as far as you comfortably can. Firm your abs, tuck your butt under slightly, shoulders back, head up. Without letting your butt press back at all, bend your knees out toward your toes, lowering your torso straight down a few inches. If you need help balancing, lift your arms in front as you go down. Without resting at the bottom, press through your heels to return to standing. Do 3 sets of 10 reps, building up to 3 sets of 15 reps. As you become more flexible, try to go lower on each dip, taking care not to lose the proper alignment.

shapes and sizes. "Your forearms get hard, which we call 'pumped,' because you're not used to holding on that long, and eventually you just can't hold on any longer," she says. Grip strength is often the limiting factor in beginner climbs. To improve it, hang by your fingertips from a sturdy doorframe for as long as you can, with your legs offering some support from the floor or a stepstool. Also, get a small squishy ball, about the size of a tennis ball, and knead it in one hand at a time.

Even with a weak grip, if you use your legs properly to push rather than trying to pull yourself up the wall, you can conceivably reach the top your first time. "If you can step up stairs, you can probably climb the wall," says Nelson. "Most people have strong legs even when they are deconditioned. We have corporate guys who sit for fourteen hours a day at work, and a good portion of them make it up the wall."

The other limitation is mental. "If I tell you to do a 30-foot bear crawl on the floor, you could probably do it," says Nelson. But when that bear crawl is vertical, people talk themselves out of it. "People have a fear of going up," she says. "Climbing is one third respiration, one third physical and one third mental; tell yourself that you can't make the next move, and it's over." But the opposite is true as well.

Here are two moves to get you primed:

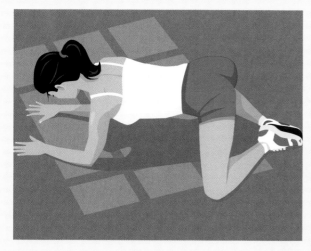

hip-opener stretch

Start on your knees and elbows, with the elbows directly under your shoulders, knees under hips. Walk each knee out to the side for a wider platform and place the soles of your feet together. If you can comfortably go deeper, slowly adjust your elbows forward and knees further out until you feel a stretch in your inner thighs and hips. Don't go too far or you'll pull a groin muscle. Hold just 5 seconds to start. Build up to holding for 20 seconds. Do 1 of these stretches after each set of pliés.

GET MORE FROM YOUR SPORT

Rock climbing is a unique sport, and training in other activities can only bring partial benefits on the rock. But even if you get to climb as much as you would like, and can fully maintain your fitness with this sport alone, it's vital to do some other flexibility training. Yoga and pilates are perfect compliments, because they combine some strength and flexibility with body awareness and balance. Many rock climbers also do trail running, hiking, cross-country skiing, and mountain biking to access new climbs, improve stamina, and help keep body weight low (the less you weigh, the less you have to push up the rock).

Two related sports involve more technical skills. To reach new heights, some climbers embark on multi-day climbs. Called alpine climbing, the sport involves a small team of climbers who carry light camping gear and undertake technical climbs that involve *bivouacs*, or sleeping on slim ledges of rock or a *portaledge platform* fashioned from cords, poles and cloth, and suspended from anchors in the rock. In ice climbing, cold-weather adventurers add *crampons* to their boots, which have metal teeth in the front and under the sole to grip the ice. Climbers kick the front teeth directly into the ice and go straight up. A pair of ice picks is used in addition to anchors because the climbers can't grip the ice as rock climbers can grasp the stone.

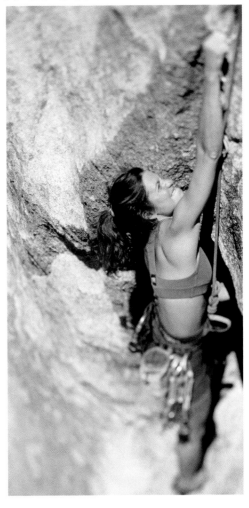

ROCK CLIMBING

RESOURCES

→ **www.abc-of-rockclimbing.com** provides a wealth of information on rock-climbing vacations, climbing techniques, gear, and even common mistakes.

→ **www.indoorclimbing.com** has links to indoor climbing gyms (even indoor ice-climbing walls), directions to popular local boulders, and a comprehensive training guide. This site is one of the more useful ones for beginning climbers.

→ *How to Rock Climb* by John Long, now in its seventh edition, is a classic guide that covers everything from the basics of climbing to ethics and equipment standards.

→ *Knots for Climbers* by Craig Luebben is a compact and concise volume illustrating the basic knots climbers must know, as well as the situations in which to use them.

Take Care of Sports and Fitness Injuries

Research shows that being active is the best long-term strategy for reducing pain—and people who exercise have less arthritis as they age. But every so often, sports participation leads to an injury. Luckily, most aches and pains are minor, and many resolve on their own. The trick is knowing which injuries need medical attention and how to best care for the ones that don't.

Muscle aches and pains Taking up a new sport or learning a new skill in a sport you already play inevitably means new muscle pain. The pain and stiffness is usually worst one to two days after the activity, a phenomenon called *Delayed Onset Muscle Soreness* or DOMS. Try taking the recommended dose of over-the-counter pain relievers, as long as it isn't in conflict with other medical conditions. If you're popping pills often, adjust your activity schedule or talk to your doctor to find other solutions because long-term use of painkillers may cause ulcers and kidney and liver problems. Massage, a warm bath with Epsom salts, and icing the worst points of pain can also help. Topical products such as warming creams do little to promote healing, but if you like how they feel, go ahead and use them. During the healing process, drink extra water, eat healthfully, and get lots of rest.

Skin abrasions and cuts When you injure your skin, the first priority is to stop the bleeding and next is to prevent infection. Wash the area with warm soapy water. For a small cut, try a liquid bandage to seal it. If the cut won't stop bleeding, apply pressure, preferably with a clean cloth, and raise it higher than your heart. Once the bleeding stops, firmly apply a dressing (not so tight that it throbs and swells). You can add insurance against infection by dabbing an antibiotic ointment under the bandage. If the cut won't stop bleeding, seek medical care.

Treat blisters like any skin abrasion. Do not pop them or you risk infection. For rashes and itchy areas, wash them with soap and water, then apply a hydrocortisone cream and a bandage.

Bumps and bruises When you bang a body part, put ice on the spot as soon as you can to reduce swelling and speed healing. A zipper bag with ice or bag of frozen vegetables makes an excellent ice pack. Never put the ice directly on your skin. Always put a towel or other barrier in between. Hold the ice in place for up to twenty minutes, three times a day for the first forty-eight hours after the injury. Later, switch to mild heat to increase circulation to the area.

Sprains and strains The classic cure for a sports injury is RICE: rest, ice, compression, elevation. Try not to put weight on the affected area, treat with ice for the first forty-eight hours, wrap the area firmly (but don't cut off circulation so it throbs or tingles), and prop it up to reduce swelling. When possible, elevate the injury to the same height as your heart to ease circulation.

Again, after forty-eight hours you can switch from ice to mild heat to promote circulation and relaxation in the area. If possible, try not to rely on bracing and wrapping joints for too long because it's preferable to strengthen the area instead of becoming dependent on an external device.

You need medical help if you:
* have a wound that won't stop bleeding
* spike a fever above 101° F
* have difficulty breathing
* are dazed, see stars or other unusual symptoms
* cannot move a part of your body without severe pain
* experience sharp pains
* have an unexplained lump, bump or bruising
* don't start to feel better in two days

INJURIES

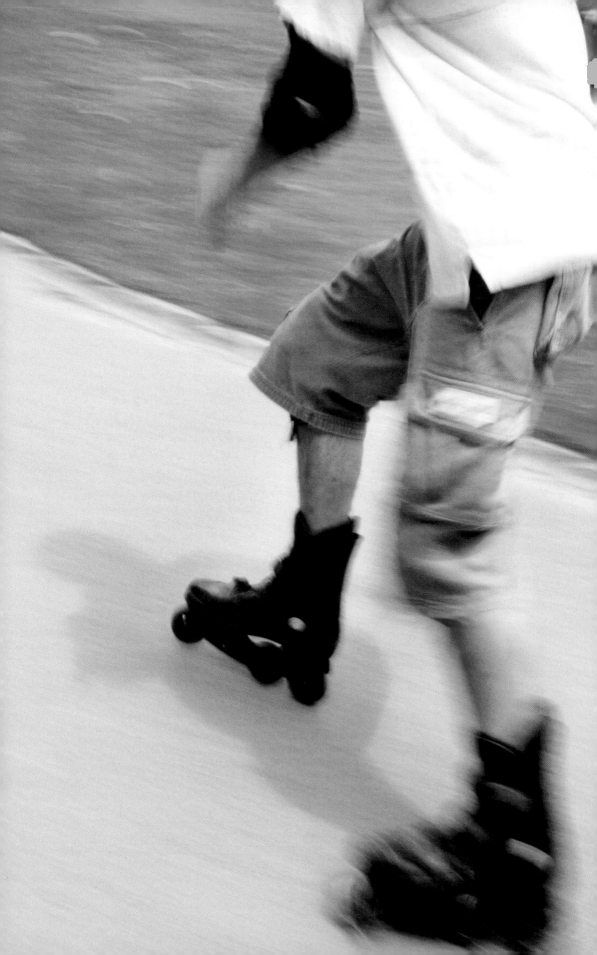

16

SKATING
ICE AND IN-LINE

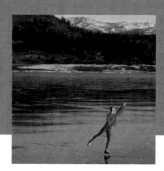

YOU'LL LOVE THESE SPORTS IF YOU:
- want to improve your balance, flexibility, cardiovascular fitness, and strength
- want a lot of fitness benefits from a single activity
- need a mental challenge in addition to a physical one
- thrive on learning new skills and pushing your limits
- enjoy speed and dream of competing
- want to have so much fun you don't realize you're exercising
- enjoy a versatile sport: you can do it outdoors, indoors, or on vacation
- want a sport you can do as a family or with friends
- are interested in playing ice or roller hockey

YOU MIGHT NOT LOVE THESE SPORTS IF YOU:
- have poor balance—although you could use the sport to improve your balance
- are deathly afraid of falling
- don't enjoy going fast
- hate the cold—but you could try forms other than ice skating, or invest in warmer gear

Swoosh! There's nothing quite like the feeling of carving an elegant arc on skates. Skating is fast and fluid, whether you are dancing ballroom-style on the ice or grinding at an in-line skate park. There are too many skating styles to mention, from downhill racing on in-line skates to synchronized skating in a team of eight to twenty-four skaters (which is the fastest growing type of figure skating). And, of course, you can just tool around on your own. No matter what your age and abilities, rest assured that you can find a style that suits your personality. And whichever one you pick, you'll get a great workout that combines cardio, strength, flexibility, and balance in one fun activity. Plus, the feeling of flying over ice or pavement is a thrill that makes the time rush by while you burn calories and get fit.

SKATING

Skating is a rewarding family sport because people at all levels can participate in the same place at the same time. You can start your kids skating as young as three, although some children are not emotionally ready until five, six, or even seven. Before putting a pair of starter skates under the Christmas tree, take your child to watch some skaters in person to gauge his or her enthusiasm, and then try rental skates for the first few outings, or even the entire first season. Rinks rent ice skates and many skate shops rent roller skates. Some outdoor rinks are open for roller skating during warmer weather and also offer rentals.

The skating motion comes largely from the legs and butt, so those muscles get toned the fastest. And don't worry about bulging thighs: Unless you're taking on Bonnie Blair's training regimen, you have nothing to fear. The sport also improves flexibility because you swing your legs quite far as you stroke. Your arms will get a little exercise as well because most of the time you'll be holding them out for balance or pumping them to help you move. Skating will make your abs and back firmer over time, too, because balance comes largely from the core.

Balance is one of the major fitness benefits from any kind of skating. It may sound counter-intuitive to take up a sport that involves falling in order to prevent falls, but skating hones your balance skills, which translates into fewer bad falls in daily life as you get older, when your stability begins to falter. And part of early training on skates should include safety tips such as proper techniques for falling without getting hurt, along with protective gear you should wear (some ice skaters now wear helmets and in-line skaters need a variety of pads). The best way to overcome the fear of falling is to just do it—that is, to fall on purpose. The fear is generally worse than the bump itself. When you're a practiced skater, you'll stay on your feet most of the time, but whenever you're trying to master a new trick, chances are good you'll fall at least once or twice.

From a mental perspective, the fluid grace of skating or the explosive power of speed can be a tremendous release for pent-up energy. Skating can be a moving meditation, with repetition, flow, and physicality combining to provide stress reduction. Struggling to perfect a new skill can require patience, but overall, the sport enhances self-esteem because most people can reach a comfortable level of proficiency.

Another aspect common to all forms of skating is the art of edging. Almost every aspect of the sport relies on finding and holding an edge as you glide or step, no matter which gear is on your feet—blades or

SCORE

If you weigh 150 pounds, you'll burn about 640 calories by doing an hour of vigorous ice skating. (To calculate your hourly burn rate, multiply 4.25 by your weight in pounds.) For in-line skating, you'd burn 850 calories in an hour if you weigh 150 pounds, the same amount as running (or 5.67 multiplied by your weight).

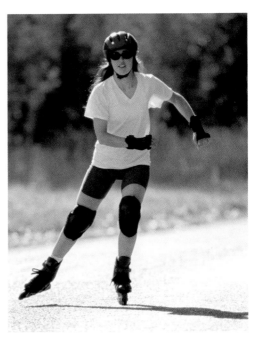

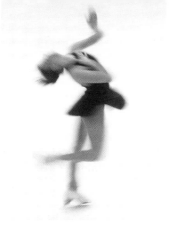

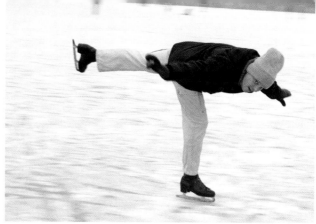

FIGURE SKATING

wheels—or which style of skating you do. To understand edges, think about watching a motorcyclist maneuver through a turn by dipping over to one side of the wheels as the rider's shoulder tips toward the ground. An in-line skater swiveling down a slalom course tips both boots to one side in the same way on each turn. To execute a classic hockey stop, a skater glides sideways on tilted edges with both boots tipped to one side, and then pops straight up, perched vertically and immobile. This maneuver is challenging to learn but very effective for stopping on a dime. Roller skating on four wheels is less about edging, but you still lean your body the way you would riding a motorcycle to help the skates carve around curves.

While it's not necessary to study physics just to learn to skate, being able to visualize the edges while in motion can make the sport easier to master. For example, beginners often falter because they approach skating like walking, trying to stand erect and put one foot in front of the other. The result is stiff, awkward, and ineffective, something like a Frankenstein monster on skates. Instead, to go forward, a skater must keep the torso facing ahead while the legs move to the sides, pushing off the right foot to the right, then the left foot to the left, using the friction of the inside edge of the skate against the ground to propel the body. Ease up your death grip on the person teaching you and give it a try! Trust your feet and glide along. Next, learn to stop. There's plenty of time later for crossovers, backward skating, and spins. Make sure you master the basics before taking on the tricks.

The darling of the winter Olympics, figure skating is not as easy as Michelle Kwan makes it look. But basic skating is not as hard as you might expect, either. Some people step on the ice and immediately have a feel for the sport, while others start by clinging to the boards at the side of the rink, ankles akimbo. However, even the latter group can learn how to glide through a fun workout (and their ankles can be shored up with supportive skates).

As in other sports, it's easiest to learn to skate if you can refrain from analyzing every step and instead just emulate what you see without thinking about it too much. People with dance and yoga backgrounds often take to the sport quickly because they know where their bodies are in space. Kids do well because they're good at mimicry.

It's never too late to take up skating. There are people who began in their teens and went on to become Olympians. Even as an adult, you can aspire to compete in one of the competitions held across the country or internationally and end up standing in the center of the ice holding a bouquet of flowers. And even if you're in it just to learn more and challenge yourself, a recreational skater can take the same U.S. Figure Skating skills tests that are used to rank competitors for their placement in events.

Most skaters who compete join local clubs mainly to get ice time and coaching, but also for help navigating the rules, paperwork, and processes involved in competition. On the positive side, tedious compulsory figures such as the *figure eight* were eliminated from international competition in 1990. The short program, which still includes strict standards for required elements, is more fun to watch, perform, and judge. And after a few tumultuous years with controversial anomalies in judging, a new, precise method of scoring is replacing the classic 6.0 system in hopes of reducing the problems.

Competitive skating is attainable for adult beginners, but the path takes dedicated years of work, even for the most talented novices. On the other hand, learning enough to get a good workout circling the rink won't take long at all. In addition to skating forward, you can expect to master basic skills such as crossovers, backward skating, and maybe a few spins and half jumps—which is plenty for most recreational skaters.

GEARING UP

If you have access to a rink, start with rental skates. They've improved dramatically since you were a kid. Many concessions now offer stiff synthetic or plastic boots that eliminate the weak-ankle problem so long as you lace them securely. One benefit of renting is that the shop will sharpen the blades for you. When you skate on lakes using your own skates, sharpen your blades after twenty to thirty outings. Sharp blades might sound frightening to a beginner, but they actually make it easier to skate. If you've inherited some hand-me-down skates, take them in to be sharpened (yes, they need it). And opt for rentals if the boots don't fit as well as your shoes. Skates that are too small will cause misery; and even with extra socks, skates that are too large will be almost impossible to control properly, which means more falls and less fun.

When you're ready to buy skates, head to a shop that can provide expert advice. If they don't ask about your skating abilities before matching you to a skate, leave. You don't need to spend a fortune, but you do need to be properly fitted. Most major brands serving the pros sell entry-level products for beginning skaters, too. Like sneakers, each com-

pany will have a slightly different shape, so keep trying them on until you find one that's comfortable. Leather skates will take many, many hours to break in, so you want to be able to skate in them while they're still stiff without undue pain, meaning your feet should not feel pinched. To check the fit, make sure you can move your toes, but your heel should be snug. Despite your best efforts, you may find that your skates create sore spots on your feet; if so, ask about having them stretched or buy gel pads that you can insert to ease the pressure.

When you become more advanced, you'll want to invest in a higher-quality skate. Go to a skate shop at a rink so you can test the skates on the ice immediately. Purchase a boot separately from the blades and have the blades mounted to accommodate your body and skating style. Keep an eye out for used skates from elite skaters who purchase new equipment regularly. If you skate at the same rink often, ask the shop manager to watch for an appropriate pair.

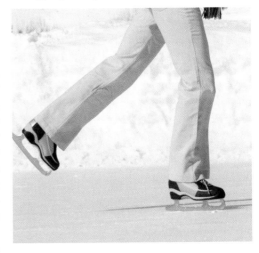

If you own your own skates, don't skip buying blade guards. These plastic covers attach with a spring-loaded strap and serve two purposes when you carry your skates: They protect you from getting stabbed, and they help keep the blades sharp. Wipe your blades clean and let them air dry before put-

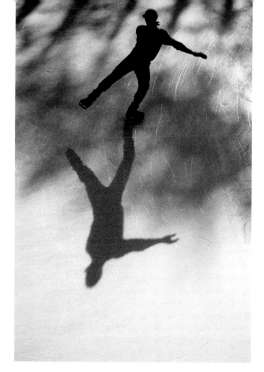

ting the guards on again, or they may rust. If you skate in natural settings, which don't provide rubber mats on the lake's edge, blade guards are especially vital so you can walk to the ice after lacing up your skates. The guards are inexpensive, so purchase a pair when you buy your skates.

Almost any comfortable cold-weather clothing works for skating. Slim profiles are better than baggy outfits because the fabric won't get in your way, but don't wear anything that constricts movement. Dress in layers because you'll be cold when you start, but warm up rapidly once you get going, especially in the legs. Leave the long scarf at home: It could drag on the ice or get dangerously tangled around your neck. Instead, consider purchasing a neck warmer or zip up the collar on your parka. Mittens or gloves are a must for beginners. Skip the knit ones and wear a leather or high-tech water-resistant pair because the ice will be wet when you push up after a fall. Wear thin- to medium-weight socks that come up above your ankles so they are at least as high as the top of the boots. Heavier socks can actually leave your feet colder either by cutting off your circulation or making you sweat (which will turn them damp and chilly when you take a break from the ice). Thick socks can also bunch into painful lumps that lead to blisters.

Many rinks offer lockers. Call ahead to find out if you should bring your own lock; otherwise, you may be forced to buy a new one. Some rinks allow you to leave your shoes and other items near the benches where you'll change into your skates. If so, have adequate pockets to carry keys and money zipped up so they won't fall out onto the ice—and leave pocketbooks and other valuables home.

Skate shops sell a small hook that makes it easier to snug up your laces. These gadgets aren't necessary, but they are convenient—especially if you're trying to get several kids ready in short order. If you're outfitting your kids, helmets are recommended up to age six.

YOUR FIRST TIME

January is National Skating Month, with events at rinks around the country, making it an excellent time to find deals on admission, rentals, and lessons. But you can take up skating anytime—even in the heat of July, you'll find indoor rinks with a clean sheet of ice and not many skaters. If you're going to an open-skate session at a rink for your first foray into the sport, call ahead to find out when they clean the ice: Every few hours, all skaters have to leave the ice to make way for the *Zamboni* to lay down a fresh layer. Try to schedule your arrival during that time so you can boot up while the Zamboni makes its rounds—and hit the rink with a fresh coat of smooth ice. It's actually easier to skate on new ice. And you'll be guaranteed a few hours before having to get off the rink for the next cleaning, which is plenty for a first experience.

It generally takes at least fifteen minutes to prepare to get on the ice. First, lace up your skates: Don't tighten them so much that you cut off circulation to your feet, but do make sure they are snug because floppy boots ruin any chance you have of controlling the skate. For the same reason, don't tuck your pants legs into your skates unless they're slim leggings. If the skates are very stiff, skip one eyelet where the laces turn to go up the boot, which will allow the ankle to flex more easily. Pull your socks up higher than the cuffs of the boot so the tops won't dig in. Check that your clothing is secure and strategic pockets are empty (you don't want to land on your butt and onto your keys!). Next, stand in your skates to get your balance. You're good to go if you can walk comfortably in your skates, but if your ankles roll, your skates are too loose; if your feet cramp, they're too tight. Be careful to walk only on rubber mats or with covers on your blades so you don't ruin the edges.

Now you're ready to take to the ice. The first time you skate, try to stay out of the way of speed demons. You're usually safe if you keep to the outside, near the *boards* (the walls of the rink). The central section is typically used for lessons or figure skaters practicing complex moves. If it's not crowded, it can be a good place for a beginner to try out new skills. The rounded corners of a rink typically provide a quiet place for practice, too, as most skaters gravitate toward the center of the loop on turns. Rinks generally have skaters moving counter-clockwise for the majority of the time, with a switch every so often that's announced and coordinated.

Lessons aren't essential for beginning skaters. You can often grasp the essential elements by watching others, or with a little coaching from friends and family. However, if you're very nervous or had a prior negative experience, sign up for a professional session to improve your odds of success. Rink guards can help if you fall, but don't expect private coaching from them. Finding lessons is easy because there are countless Learn to Skate programs registered with the Ice Skate Institute (www.skateisi.com) and another 800 basic-skills programs registered with U.S. Figure Skating, the same group that sanctions competitions, performances, and exhibitions, and sends skaters to the Olympics. You can find a local center using the zip code search on their Web site, www.usfigureskating.org.

Beginner classes typically are held in groups of about ten, with most skaters at the same skill level. The course will last for six to eight weeks, meeting once a week. Most rinks also offer private lessons, but unless you need intense hand-holding, save these for later when your skills are more advanced. Any time you skate, be sure to stop and go home as soon as you feel fatigued. You're far more likely to fall badly when your muscles and mind are tired. On a lake, be sure you're not the last one skating—you never want to be alone on the ice in case of a problem.

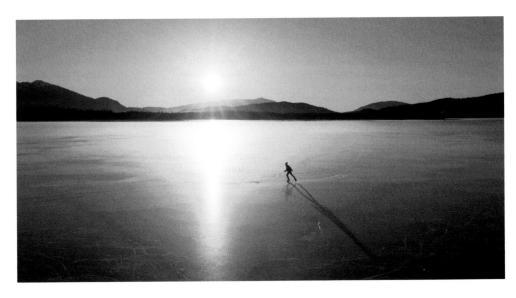

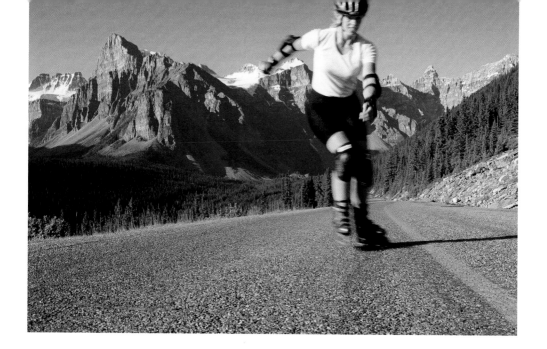

IN-LINE SKATING

The very first roller skates, built in the 1700s, were in-line skates. But they were tough to maneuver and not a popular seller. In 1863, the classic quad skate was invented and the ease of skating made it instantly popular, relegating in-line skates to the sidelines. It wasn't until 1986, when Rollerblades hit the mass market, that in-line skating found its stride. The Rollerblade founders were ice hockey players looking for off-season training skates to mimic the skills of ice hockey skates. The first artistic in-line competitions were held by U.S.A. Roller Skating in 1996, and three years later, the in-line hockey championships were held at the Pan-American Games in Canada. Now considered old fashioned, it's quad skates that you don't see often.

In-line skating is not hard to learn, and many people find it easier than ice skating because the broad "blade" surface is more stable. The physical benefits are largely the same as ice skating—leg strength, core toning, flexibility, and balance. Psychologically, in-line skating affords stress reduction through smooth, fast strokes and elegant gliding, but you can also cover a variety of terrain for sightseeing and escape. There are clubs that take in-line treks on a regular basis. You can find out about them through local outdoor sources or skate shops. The wheeled sport can be done almost any place and any time of year (there are even skates for skating on trails, such as two-wheeled GateSkates), although in-line skating is tougher on wet ground or broken surfaces.

The average recreational skater will buy one pair of in-line skates, most often from the industry leader Rollerblade, and "roll around" the neighborhood, on bike paths, sidewalks, and streets. People of all ages often skate together or skate alongside jogging or cycling friends and family members. Young skaters, who have the advantage of a low center of gravity—and who are often less fearful—are generally the ones who advance to trick skating in skate parks, often referred to as *aggressive* or *extreme* skating. These indoor or outdoor centers have ramps (called *roll-ins*), *half-pipes*, and obstacles such as *spines* (to slide along). Older speed junkies tend to opt for downhill racing. And if flying down a hill at 35 miles per hour doesn't satisfy your inner gonzo, you can try *kiteskating*, hitting speeds up to 60 miles per hour, as you're pulled along behind a performance kite. It's advisable to know at least three different ways to stop that don't involve crashing, before trying any speedy form of skating. At these speeds, it's essential to maintain control.

For those who have a competitive bent, there are downhill races, artistic skating competitions, and an aggressive skating circuit.

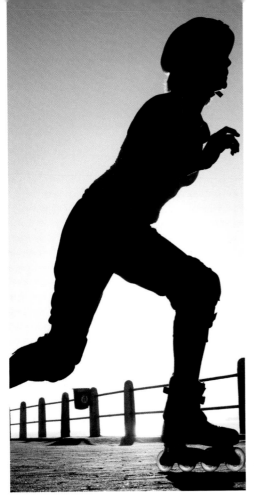

Once you have the skills and the appropriate skates, it's easy to get involved. There are on-line resources to help you find any kind of in-line event.

GEARING UP

To start, rent a pair of skates at a shop or rink. Every Goodwill and Salvation Army store has a bevy of used skates tossed off after one or two tries by people who find they don't like the sport (a reaction often brought on by the feeling of being out of control, because the skater doesn't know how to stop). When you're ready to own your first pair, used skates can be an excellent bargain, provided they are in good shape and fit well. A sloppy fit that lets your foot wiggle a lot inside the shell translates into sloppy skating and that above-mentioned feeling of lacking control. As with ice skates, don't expect to pad out the difference with extra socks or you'll risk blisters and have a mushy ride. In classic recreational skates, look for boots with a strap around the top, which provides added sup-

port. In-line skates typically have four wheels and a heel brake on the right foot. If the skates you're wearing have been used (by you or anyone else), take a look at the wheels and the brake to be sure there's enough rubber to meet the road. If not, buy replacement wheels from a skate shop.

In-line skaters should wear protective pads and a helmet. Knee and elbow pads are popular for preventing road rash and bad bruises from the usual falls as you learn to skate. When you fall forward, it is natural to put out your hands to block the fall, which typically results in a broken bone if you're not wearing wrist guards that have a stiff metal or plastic underside. A helmet is not often seen on adult skaters, but consider this: Head injuries do happen from skating falls—and they can be a lot more serious than a broken wrist. Don't skip this piece of gear. The same helmet you use for cycling is fine for a beginning skater, and they aren't expensive.

Beginners can buy padded shorts that make falling a little less painful. But the garment is bulky and unattractive. If you're balance-challenged or prone to the black-and-blues, go for it. Otherwise, don't bother. Chances are good you won't need this kind of padding for long.

Socks for in-line skating should be thin to medium weight so you can feel your feet connect to the boots for enhanced control. It's generally most comfortable to choose a style that comes up higher than the tops of the boots; although in-line skates are soft inside, hundreds of strides can still leave your calves chafed.

Any comfortable clothing works for in-line skating. Make sure nothing can get caught in the wheels. And as a beginner, don't wear anything you'd prefer doesn't hit the ground (because chances are good you will fall at least a few times). Sunglasses are helpful on bright days, but choose lenses that aren't glass, so there's not the slightest chance of having them break into shards. You'll want your hands free, so bring a backpack or fanny pack to carry keys, water,

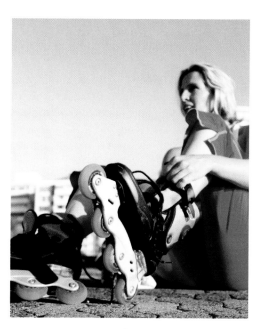

snacks, shoes, and other gear. Leave the iPod and headphones home if you'll be out near cars, bikes, and pedestrians so you can hear them coming.

Hockey, racing, aggressive skating, and other specialty pursuits require specific skates and gear—and some disciplines have traditional garb, as well. If you progress to one of these advanced styles of skating, check for information online or at skate shops.

YOUR FIRST TIME

Before you put on your skates, go someplace with flat terrain and few hazards on the ground such as pebbles and big cracks in the road or sidewalk. A well-maintained parking lot or paved section of playground (such as a basketball court) are good choices. Now

---

ATHLETE IN ACTION

Wade Corbett, 60

"I didn't know about the toe pick; it was a heck of a fall," says Wade Corbett of his first time on the ice when he was in his 30s. "I decided I'd better take lessons after that," because learning as an adult is difficult, he notes. "When I first got out there, I was petrified," he says. "The ice is a different planet, and we weren't born to do this." Despite his fears, Corbett took to the sport right away. "It was beautiful to just fly on the ice."

Back in the '70s, when he started skating, there weren't competitions for adults. Instead, Corbett put years of dance training to use by setting his sites on figure skating shows. "Before long, I was jumping and spinning. I joined the Ice Theater of New York."

By the time he was in his mid-30s, when he had done ice shows, from

California to Brazil, the first adult competitions were getting started. Corbett signed up immediately, and started skating daily and taking lessons again. Between his dancing skills and ice time, Corbett had an edge on many of the other adults in the first competitions and often won. He still does, going to at least one competition a year and often coming out on top in his division, which he calls "50 to death." Corbett loves to travel to the competitions and comments that they are friendly, not like cut-throat elite events. However, he says, "I'm almost never happy with my performance; I always feel I can do better," he says. Now that he's older, he starts his training earlier. "I never know when a competition will be my last." He had major back surgery six years ago that threatened to retire him from the ice, but he finds he's skating better now, albeit with a back brace. And he does admit that the sit spin hurts, but he still polishes off jumps—he just

appreciates the ability more now. "I have arthritis, I have bursitis, and if I fall the wrong way, it's back in for surgery," he says. "So I don't do the axel or double Salchow." Corbett prides himself not on fancy tricks but on clean, elegant skating. "There's nothing like doing the beautiful edges and interesting choreography," he says.

Corbett, who has turned his passion for skating into a career as the head of the skating school at Sky Rink at Chelsea Piers, says that he tries to instill that same appreciation in his students, "not just the love of jumps." He's there six days a week, out on the ice with every class, evaluating every student. He also teaches a few private lessons, directs the hockey prep program, and does choreography for competitors. Despite his personal love for competition, Corbett says the skating school's primary focus is on teaching people how to be proficient on the ice so they can enjoy the sport.

SKATING

you're ready to strap on your pads, secure your helmet, strap on your skates… and stop. It's too easy to gain speed on skates unintentionally, so the first step is to stand up and practice how to stop. The way you slow down and stop on in-line skates isn't difficult, but it's far from intuitive—hence the number of people who drop the sport after one or two tries. Here's one way to learn: Stand up carefully in a flat spot where you can hold on to a chair, bench, banister, wall, or person with your right hand. Place your feet a little wider than shoulder-distance apart, bend your knees slightly, lean forward from your hips, and place your left hand on your left knee. Stay in this position until you feel balanced and stable. Next, put all of your weight on your left foot. Slowly roll your right foot forward without moving the rest of your body. When the foot is as far forward as it can comfortably go, tip up the toes to touch the brake to the ground. Now shift your weight as though squatting and press down through both feet, making the brake press hard into the ground. Hold this position for a few seconds; then return to the starting position. Repeat the process until it feels comfortable; then do it again without holding on. When you can do it on your own, you're ready to roll, so to speak.

You only need a few basic skills to tackle most rinks, parks, and paved bike paths. Avoid sand, gravel, or water because they'll make you slip or trip. And watch other skaters to pick up more handy techniques, including new ways to stop and tricks that are fun.

To learn quickly or progress to new levels, look for lessons. Skate shops are a good resource, as are roller rinks. Local clubs may also offer seminars or skate outings where advanced skaters might be amenable to coaching novices.

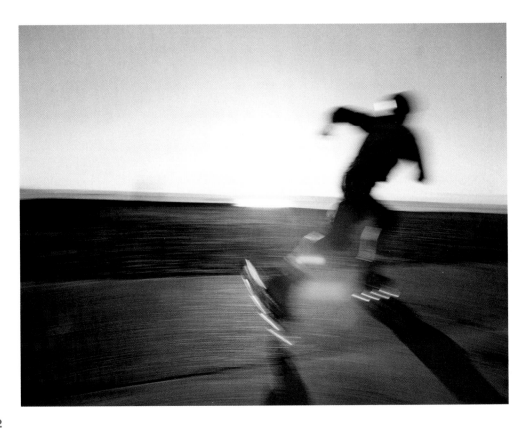

TACKLE THE TRUTH

I have weak ankles, so I can't skate

Look around a rink today and you won't see many people with their ankles tilting out. For the few you do see, take a closer look and you'll notice that their skates are to blame. Appropriately stiff boots will support your ankles so you won't wobble on top. Skating requires a connection through the feet and the skates between your body and the surface. With proper equipment that's worn correctly, weak ankles are not an issue.

If I fall, I'll get seriously hurt

While it's not impossible to get hurt falling, skating isn't riskier than most other sports. You can prevent almost any potential injury by learning the mechanics of a safe landing, wearing appropriate protective gear, and maintaining control. When you fall, keep your body loose and don't resist the motion. Roll or slide if you can. And be sure to tuck in arms and legs rather than extending them, because an outstretched limb is likely to break. The same goes for your head: Tuck it in for safety. Beginning skaters can expect some bumps and bruises from falling, but if you exercise caution there should be no lasting consequences. On the other hand, if you have a physical condition such as back pain or osteoporosis, ask your doctor if it's okay to skate conservatively, as long as you do your best to avoid hard landings.

There's nothing to do but go around in circles

Whether on an ice rink, frozen lake, or on wheels at the local park, you can always add to your skating repertoire. Practice some more complicated moves such as *three turns* (which look like the numeral 3) or take up hockey, which requires precise skating abilities. You can also learn dance steps or join a novice's synchronized skating group. Even simply taking lessons can be a social event with a fitness payoff. On in-line skates, you can participate in local skating tours, skate marathons, and rolling vacations. There are skate parks to explore, or you can learn to figure skate on wheels. And skating is a great sport to take on vacation, whether you're slicing the ice near your chalet in Switzerland or taking an in-line tour through the tulips in Holland.

SECRETS TO SUCCESS

Nobody wants to think about falling, but as a beginner you can be sure you'll do it once or twice at the very least. Therefore, one of the key skills in skating is learning how to get up, says Kenny Moir, executive director of figure skating at Sky Rink at Chelsea Piers. "Don't try to stand up from sitting," he warns. You'll just slip and bounce down again. Instead, get on all fours, bring one foot up onto the skate, place that hand on the knee, then press up to standing. For stability, keep your knees softly bent, hips bent, and hands on your knees, with your feet parallel and hip-distance apart (if you're on a hill on wheels, do this perpendicular to the slope so you don't start downhill before you're ready).

Now that you know how to get up, here are some tips that can make this process less necessary: The first "step"

on skates feels a lot like getting on an escalator—your feet may feel like they are taking off without the rest of your body. In response, people often stiffen up and lean backward, but that posture will put you off balance and frequently causes feet to fly out from underneath as the body goes over backward. Instead, try to keep your weight low and forward for better stability and balance. Try to stay supple, not locking your knees or hips, and glide with your weight on both skates. When that feels comfortable, practice releasing your weight from one foot at a time without lifting the feet off the ice. Next, you're ready to lift a foot and glide on the other. And last, push off with one foot, pushing back and away slowly, pressing down on the inside edge of the skate while standing balanced on the other foot. At the end of the stroke, the push skate is lifted and

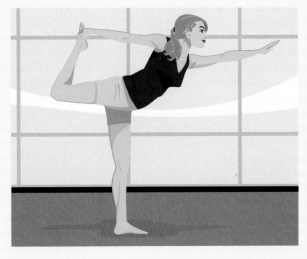

SKATING

royal dancer

Stand with your feet together, knees not locked, abs firm, shoulders back, head erect. Wiggle your toes and visualize planting your feet on the ground. Lift your right foot behind you, tilting forward from the hips, and place the top of your foot into the palm of your right hand, with the hand to the outside of the foot, fingers pointing in. Lift your left hand to shoulder height in front of you. Press your left hand forward, tilt your torso forward from the hips and gently lift your right foot as high as you can. Find a point of balance, keeping your head up. It helps to look at a fixed spot. Hold for as long as you can. Repeat on the other side.

returns to center (it helps to picture a speed skater). You're off!

Once you can move forward, it's easy to learn turns by taking small strokes and placing the skates a little farther in the direction you want to go each time you put down a foot. If your feet hurt inside your boots, check to see if you're clenching your toes out of nervousness. Wiggle your toes and try to relax your feet for relief. The next key skill is the step or the hop. A small step or hop is effective for avoiding a fall when you are confronted with a pebble, crack, or other obstacle. The key is to stay balanced as you avoid the obstacle by picking up your skates with the proper timing. A step is like a regular walking step in which you keep your weight forward enough for momentum but not so far that you fall on your knees. You'll need to step on and off a rink, and you can take a slightly larger step to mount a curb on in-line skates. Hops are easiest to learn when you have both feet squarely under your body and your knees slightly bent.

Before and after a skating session, it helps to stretch, advises Moir. Skating uses a lot of muscles in the legs, butt, and back, which can stiffen up, especially when it's cold. Do some foot and ankle stretches, because carrying a heavy boot on your foot is a lot more work than toting around the weight of a typical shoe. If you have time to work on your balance when you're not skating, try some yoga moves in which you stand on one foot. For example, the following moves can lessen the wobble factor:

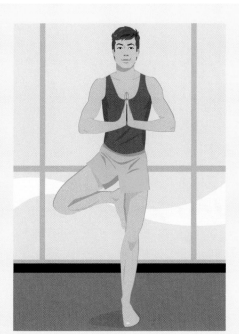

tree pose

Stand with your feet together, knees not locked, abs firm, shoulders back, head erect. Wiggle your toes and visualize planting your feet on the ground. Lift your right foot and place it on the inside of your left leg as high as you can, with the right knee out to the side. Use your hands to help position the foot, then try to let go and place your hands in a prayer position. Find a point of balance, keeping your head up. It helps to look at a fixed spot. Hold for as long as you can. Repeat on the other side.

SKATING

GET MORE FROM YOUR SPORT

If you love skating, consider taking up downhill skiing or snowboarding to put your skills at edging and balance to good use while still providing physical challenge and the rush of speed. Or, if you're a proficient skater, consider trying hockey (roller or ice) to add a new sport to your roster. Hockey can keep you challenged for years because it's hard to simultaneously manage skating, puck handling, and strategy.

Skaters tend to have strong lower bodies, which is a natural advantage for sports such as cycling and running. Pilates, yoga, and dance work well to foster flexibility, balance, and coordination, which are vital for all kinds of skating but especially welcome for artistic and figure skaters. Gymnastics is another activity that will improve your skating and vice versa, especially as you learn more about moving your body in precise patterns.

When you want to combine travel and skating, check out in-line treks or Nordic skating tours (which use a different style of ice skate).

Two good on-line resources are:

➡ www.zephyradventures.com for in-line tours in the U.S. and overseas.
➡ www.Nordicskater.com/tours offers ice-skating treks in the northern U.S. and Canada, plus a few overseas destinations.

For a learning-to-blade vacation, try Camp Rollerblade. You'll fit right in. The average age of students is forty-six, and everyone is a beginner. The camp is all-inclusive, so you don't have to make any arrangements. Kids can come along with adults (www.camprollerblade.com).

Advanced figure skaters can apply to train in a summer camp at Lake Placid, where the program includes top-notch coaching and complementary fitness skills such as trampoline and pilates (www.lakeplacidskating.com). There's also an annual winter adult camp at Ice House in Hackensack, New Jersey (www.icehousenj.com). And check out the adult clinics lead by Olympic coaches and skaters at Ice Works in Aston, Pennsylvania (www.iceworks.net).

RESOURCES

➡ **www.usfigureskating.org** is the official site of United States Figure Skating, where you can find links to local learn-to-skate programs and competitions. The site also has pages describing how to skate.
➡ **www.iceskatingaddict.com** is a site geared specifically toward the adult figure skater or ice dancer.
➡ **www.InlinePlanet.com** is a site packed with info and tips about fitness, racing, gear and getting started on in-line skates.
➡ **www.RollerSports.org** is the site for the International Federation of Roller Sports, the governing body for in-line skating competitions.
➡ *Figure Skating for Dummies* by Kristi Yamaguchi covers topics from buying skates on a budget to judging, passing tests, and selecting choreography.
➡ *Figure Skating School* by Peter Morrissey and James Young provides an overview of classic figure skating moves.
➡ *In-line Skating Basics* by Cam Millar has an overview of every aspect of skating the beginner needs to know.
➡ *Get Rolling: The Beginner's Guide to In-Line Skating* by Liz Miller covers everything you'd expect from the title plus more, including some advanced skills.

SKATING

Staying Warm and Safe in the Cold

You know to wear a hat and dress in layers on frigid days, but sometimes that's not enough to stay comfortable—or alive—when you're out snowshoeing, trail running, or ice skating. Fortunately, thanks to high-tech materials and creative designs, the latest gear leaves little excuse to be housebound when the mercury drops.

Update your layers. You want to play, not change outfits all day. Select gear that's versatile, like a parka with venting zips for sweaty runs that you can close on a chilly lift ride. Purchase a wicking base layer, fleece mid layer, and water-proof breathable outer shell. If there's extra in your budget, try a soft shell as an outer layer on mild days or impenetrable middle layer on brutally cold days.

Add accessories. Try slim glove liners that you can keep on when you take off the big mitts (so your fingers don't freeze while you unfold your trail map). Add a balaclava-style hat, neckwarmer or neoprene face mask that you can pull over your nose, mouth and cheeks; they're great to breathe through when cold air hurts your lungs. Consider battery-operated or instant charcoal hand and foot warmers to prevent frostbite on long days out in the cold.

Don't slip. Unless you have studded tires, skip the cycling when the ground is covered with ice—a Spinning class is safer. But when you do head out to snowshoe or ice skate, take care of how you tread on ice. The most stable step on snow or ice is flat footed with short strides. Keep your weight balanced as evenly as possible on both legs. If you start to slide, try to skate or hop out of it. Proceed down steep terrain sideways to prevent slipping straight down. Choose footwear with deep treads such as Vibram soles. Consider adding a traction device that has studs or teeth to grip the ground.

Learn to fall. The best way to prevent injuries from falling is to learn to fall correctly. Try to stay loose. Stiff body parts are more easily injured than soft, relaxed ones. And learn not to "break" your fall with your hands (a sure way to break your wrist, arm or collar bone). Protect your head, knees, and elbows from direct impact, if you can. Try to land on the padded parts, like your butt.

Learn more. If you trek in the backcountry, you'll need emergency survival skills and avalanche training. Look for listings from adventure schools such as Boulder Outdoor Survival School (www.boss-inc.com) or take a read through *Surviving Cold Weather* by Greg Davenport.

Reminders

* Wear sunscreen, sunglasses or goggles
* Prevent windburn with lip balm and face lotion
* Drink a lot—you won't notice it, but you're sweating
* Bring a friend, a cell phone and maybe a compass if you'll be out of sight of others
* Tell someone where you're going and when you'll be back
* Take off wet layers as soon as you can; they increase your risk of blisters and frostbite
* Eat warm foods because they actually do heat you up from within

Online outdoor outfitters
www.LandsEnd.com
www.LLBean.com
www.REI.com
www.SierraTradingPost.com

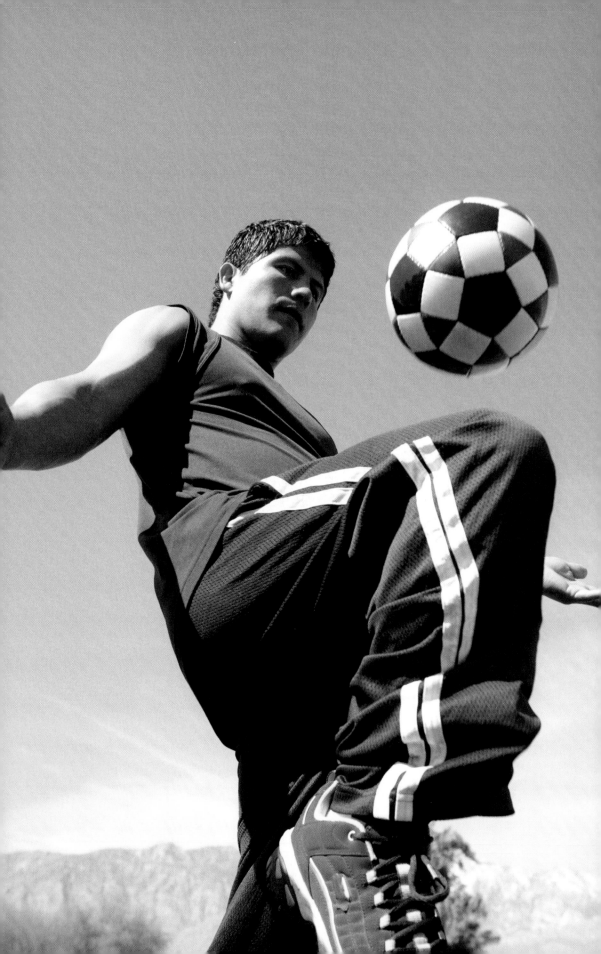

SOCCER

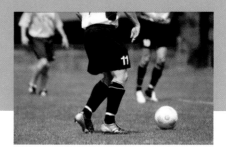

YOU'LL LOVE THIS SPORT IF YOU:
• want to improve your cardiovascular fitness, balance, and agility
• love strategy—need a mental challenge in addition to a physical one
• prefer a sport that's easy to learn, but one you can improve in over the years
• are quick on your feet
• want to be so engaged that you don't know you're exercising
• dream of competing
• enjoy team sports, camaraderie, and social activities
• like to have a set role because you play a specific position on the team
• prefer a sport where it's easy to get together a pick-up game

YOU MIGHT NOT LOVE THIS SPORT IF YOU:
• are completely lacking in speed, coordination, and aim
• have chronic knee pain
• prefer to set your own schedule rather than rely on teammates

Soccer is the most popular sport in the world, although everywhere else it's called football. While it doesn't rank as the national pastime here as it does in many other parts of the globe, participation in the U.S. is on the rise. Part of its appeal is that it's an easy game to learn, with few complex rules, and little required equipment. Young children can master it sufficiently to have a fun time, yet the game can challenge elite athletes when played at its highest level. And everyone gets a good workout from kicking the ball and running up and down the field or dashing around the goal area trying to prevent a score. Another reason soccer appeals to adults is because the rules forbid intentional hitting, kicking, and other painful forms of physical contact.

SOCCER

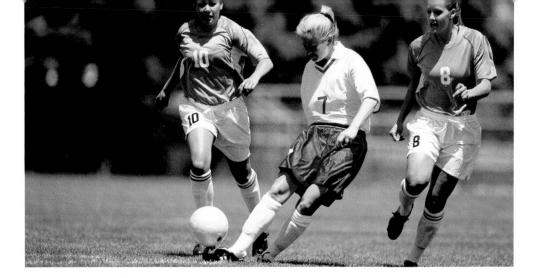

Soccer can provide an intense aerobic workout, although you may spend some time sitting on the bench waiting for a chance to play (teams often have alternates in case of injury or exhaustion and for tactical substitutions). On the field, soccer requires quick footwork, balance, aim, agility, coordination, and strategy. The rules are simple—there are only seventeen of them—but the game itself can be complex. The best players anticipate their opponents' moves and also adjust their plans with split-second analysis of new situations.

Stated simply, the object is to score a goal by moving the ball to the end of the rectangular field using any body parts except the hands and arms. Each team has a *goalkeeper* who strives to keep the other team from scoring. The keeper is allowed to use his hands when the ball is within the goal area, which is outlined on the ground, and he spends most of his time near the net. The laws of the game state that teams may have between seven and eleven players each on the field. Positions other than the keeper—*defenders* who helps protect the goal, *forwards* who try to score, and *midfielders* who switch between the two other roles as needed—are not delineated in the official laws but are fairly universal.

Most of the rules in soccer are straightforward. For example, when the ball goes out of bounds, the last person touching it is deemed to have had control and the other team is given the throw (the one time in the game when touching the ball with the hands is allowed for players other than the keeper) to put it back in play. A referee on the field will make the call on all aspects of play, from goals to penalties, and his word is final.

Early in the history of soccer, which was played at schools throughout England during the 1800s, rules were far more varied. In 1863, when the Football Association met to set the first standardized rules, a split occurred over whether the ball could be carried; opinions differed as well over the practices of kicking, tripping, and holding other players. The groups that disapproved of banning these options split off and formed the rugged sport of rugby.

Almost any flat field can serve as a makeshift *pitch* for a soccer game. Officially, the playing field should be 100 to 130 yards long and 50 to 100 yards wide. Regulation fields have a number of markings, including penalty areas and a halfway line. For a pickup game, the most important designations are the boundaries and goals. The game is played in two halves, traditionally forty-five minutes long, with a halftime lasting no more than fifteen minutes in between.

The most prestigious competition in men's soccer is the World Cup, held once every four years. The Olympics comes next in

SCORE

If you weigh 150 pounds, you'll burn about 360 calories in an hour of soccer—which takes into account that some of that time is not spent in active play but either waiting for the action to come your way or sitting on the bench. (To calculate your hourly burn rate, multiply 2.4 by your weight in pounds.) For competitive play, you'll burn about 540 calories in an hour (or 3.6 times your weight).

importance, its value diminished because of restrictions on the numbers of older players, which may disqualify some of the best professionals. The women's Olympic teams do not suffer the same restrictions.

With leagues for all ages in virtually every corner of the country, soccer is an easy way to join a team and compete at any level. Youth soccer programs have introduced many families to the game, spinning off adult divisions because envious parents also want to get on the field.

GEARING UP

Soccer requires minimal specialized gear. T-shirts and shorts are traditional, along with good sneakers or cleats (which are very helpful to prevent slipping). Soccer players wear high socks to hold shin guards in place underneath them lest the guards slip when kicked. If you don't like the feeling of the guards against your skin, wear a second pair of socks underneath. The laws of soccer forbid the wearing of jewelry on the field because of its potential to cause injury. Hats with brims are also unsafe. If it's very cold, serious soccer players tend to wear a snug base layer under shorts rather than pants that might restrict movement.

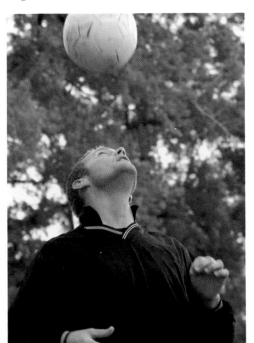

Goalkeepers may opt to invest in padded uniforms to protect themselves when they fall after leaping for the ball. Jerseys come with padding in the sleeves and shorts are padded too. But in introductory play, the keeper isn't likely to launch horizontally to block a shot, so special gear isn't necessary.

If you play in a league, you'll likely need two uniforms (or one reversible uniform) with your number and sometimes your name printed on the jersey. Some teams wear one color for home games and the other for away games. Or they can wear one color most of the time unless it's the same as the opponent's color, in which case the home team must switch to their second option.

Bring plenty of water and snacks to a soccer game—an hour and a half of running around requires restocking the body's stores.

The only required piece of gear is a soccer ball. Traditionally black and white, they now come in a rainbow of colors, but regulation balls are always twenty-seven to twenty-eight inches in diameter. You can purchase lightweight goal posts with nets to set up your own pitch, but games in backyards and parks are often conducted using cones as markers or just a few jackets or caps on the ground.

YOUR FIRST TIME

If you don't know how the game is played, try reading a book or visiting a Web site that explains the seventeen basic rules. Then check out the action at a local match (you'll find one in any park or schoolyard; fast-paced professional games on television are tougher to follow). Next, buy or borrow a ball and try to move it around with your feet. Walk while gently kicking it and then run (called dribbling), kick it with different parts of your foot, tap your foot on top to stop it, then change direction and start moving again. Work with the ball until you have some comfort with how to make it move where you want. Then recruit someone else or find a wall and practice kicking the ball where you want it to go and receiving it when it's coming toward you. These two skills, passing and receiving (also called *controlling*), are more vital than being able to kick a goal. You can also practice *heading*, which is deflecting the incoming ball with your head. However, this skill is somewhat advanced, and you're unlikely to use it on the field in your first few games.

Now you're ready to play. Your training sessions may already have generated requests for a pickup game from friends, family, and neighbors. If not, venture out to the nearest park or playground to see if you can rustle up some interest. If that fails, try posting a notice on a bulletin board or local Web site. And if all of those efforts don't yield results, find a league and jump right in. As long as the team is aware that you're a beginner, you'll do fine. Being part of a team has many benefits for new players: You'll get drills and practice sessions conducted by a coach, plus tips from seasoned players. And you'll get to play regularly, which is the key to success in most sports.

Teams typically hold practice games called *scrimmages*, which don't count for league standings but provide excellent opportunities to try out new skills and get a preview of another team before you play them for points.

When you arrive for a scrimmage or game, do some light activity such as jogging to warm up, then stretch, especially the calves and thigh muscles. You'll have a designated position on the field, playing offense, defense, midfield, or keeper. If you've done your homework, you'll understand your role and know the basics about what to do with the ball.

The game begins with a kickoff from the center and continues until one of three things happens: One team scores a goal, the ball is

TACKLE THE TRUTH

You have to be able to run a marathon to make it through a soccer game

You do run a lot in soccer, but not 26.2 miles. The game involves sprints and stops, and there's generally enough time for recovery in between the intense sections. As part of a team, you'll have ample opportunity to pass the ball to someone else if you need a breather. You'll get fit running up and down the field, and you may be exhausted the first few times you play. But you'll also find some very unfit people out on the soccer field. It's a game that's open to anyone.

You stand around so much in soccer that it's not a good workout

Defense players and keepers may be able to stand still if they want to, but the best players are constantly adjusting position to be ready for the action in case it heads their way. You should be moving up and back, side to side, as the ball moves over the field, on your toes and ready to jump in the fray. Don't exhaust yourself by simply running in circles, but don't stop moving either, unless you need the time to recover your breath.

I can't play a game until I know all the rules

Because it's not overly complex, soccer is a good game to learn on the field. Familiarize yourself with the basic rules just by reading about them, and then pick up the nuances, tactics, and tips while you're out there doing it. There's no better way to learn than right on the field.

kicked out of bounds, or a serious penalty occurs and the ref stops the game (these usually involve intentional physical contact with another player). For minor fouls, the ref may wait until the action stops for another reason before imposing a penalty. After a goal, play will begin again with a kickoff. An out-of-bounds ball is thrown in from the point in which it went out of play. And fouls are handled in various ways, with penalty kicks from different spots and sometimes a caution or eviction from the game for a player. If you've read up on offsides rules as well as proper conduct on the field, you can attempt to play a clean game—but keep in mind that most players cause unintentional fouls, so don't fret if it happens to you. Relax, have fun, and ask for pointers on your performance from your teammates so you can continue to improve.

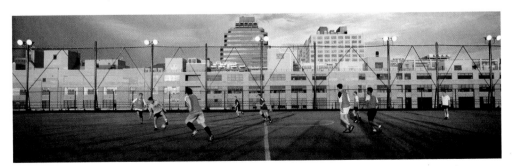

SECRETS TO SUCCESS

Part of what makes soccer so enjoyable, but also a bit challenging, is that adults don't tend to hop on one foot or run backward in most daily activities, says Ron Restrepo, the youth soccer director at Chelsea Piers Field House. These moves are common in the game, and you'll feel like a kid zigzagging all over the grass. But you may also feel sluggish and off kilter. "You need to practice the movements until they become automatic so you can do them at a fast pace," Restrepo advises. "It's not like running track or running in circles—you constantly make quick changes in direction on the field."

The feeling of the varied moves combined with working the ball creates a sensation so foreign that many adults hesitate and get tense. "They start out looking like robots," says Restrepo. To play effectively, you must relax and stay loose. Good soccer players are light on their feet, hovering on their toes, constantly ready to move. They rarely stand stiffly surveying the scene but follow the action with their bodies, anticipating the arrival of the ball at any moment. It's a fluid game, with players acting like a school of fish darting and changing direction in a flash. But gaze off toward the spectators and the ball could whiz by in an instant.

The game moves quickly, so decision-making must keep pace. If you wait until you've got the ball to decide what to do, you'll often be too late to make the best play. Instead, Restrepo teaches soccer

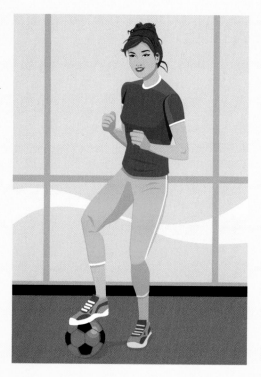

around the world

Stand facing a soccer ball. Rest your right toes on top of the ball, knee bent so your hips stay even. With your left knee slightly bent, hop to the left around the ball, singing or counting out loud to maintain a steady pace. When you've completed a full circle around the ball, keep your right foot on top and hop backward to the start. Repeat the drill with your left foot on the ball. Complete the entire sequence 3 times, building to 10.

students to anticipate receiving the ball and look around before it arrives. Scope out the players on your team and your opponents, and decide a course of action. Then you'll be ready to execute your plan as soon as the ball comes to you. The danger is that you'll be so busy looking around you'll miss the ball, but that's why you practice—to get the timing right. You can work on this skill on your own using some stationary objects as substitutes for players.

Also practice receiving the ball with different parts of your body—anything except your arms and hands—from your hips to your head. Sure, it's easier to "catch" the ball with your feet and lower legs, but the time will come in a game when you can't do it, so it's best to have the skills ready in advance. The same goes for dribbling with your nondominant foot. Everyone has a preferred side, but you can't always have your preference in competition, so be sure you can manage both. And work on looking down the rest of the field as you dribble (instead of down at the ball) so you will be able to watch the other players and scope out where you want to go when you've got possession of the ball. Try these drills to improve your skills:

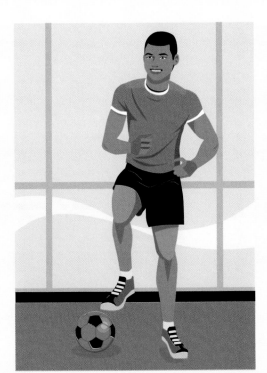

over the world

Stand facing a soccer ball. Leading with your right foot, hop over it. Run in place for 9 steps, then hop backward over the ball, again leading with your right foot. Run in place for 10 steps, then repeat the forward-and-backward pattern leading with your left foot. Repeat the entire sequence 5 times. Next, stand to the left of the ball, hop over it to the right, leading with your right foot, run in place 10 steps, hop over to the left, leading with your left foot and run in place 10 steps to complete the sequence. Repeat the sequence 5 times.

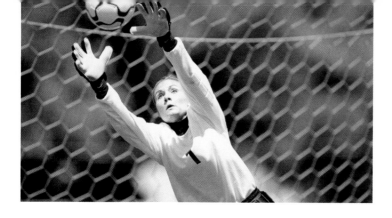

GET MORE FROM YOUR SPORT

When you want to improve your soccer skills, look for a local league so you can play more often, or sign up for lessons. You can also try a camp; while most camps are for kids, there are some for adults. For example, the Soccer Academy in Maryland offers an adult program each summer (www.soccer-academy.com). You can also sign up for the more ubiquitous coaching camps, which will teach you drills and strategies—just call in advance to be sure the instruction suits your level of experience.

If you enjoy soccer and want to extend your season, you can play an indoor version. There's also beach soccer if you want to get a change of venue. To crosstrain while honing your skills, consider taking up volleyball and basketball, both of which enhance your sense of teamwork and awareness on the field. Rugby is another possibility for soccer players looking for variety. American football has less crossover, except when a soccer player who is a great distance kicker becomes a kicker on the team.

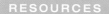

RESOURCES

⇨ **www.ussoccer.com** is the Web presence for the U.S. Soccer Federation, which is the governing body for the American game. The site includes information about players and games. They also have a link to a complete set of soccer rules.

⇨ **www.soccer.org** is the American Youth Soccer Organization's Web site, but they have an excellent short description of the game and rules that apply to any age.

⇨ **www.usasa.com** is the site for the United States Adult Soccer Association. Their listings can help you find the adult leagues in your area.

⇨ ***Step-by-Step Soccer Skills*** by Dave Smith, Pete Edwards, and Adam Ward covers basic ball handling, conditioning drills, and game tactics with a straight-forward writing style.

⇨ ***Complete Conditioning for Soccer*** by Sigi Schmid and Bob Alejo gives workouts and drills to help you prepare physically to take your game to the next level. This guide will also help you use soccer to get into great shape.

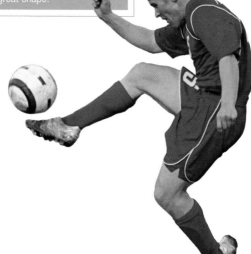

Getting Bargains on Gear

When gear is a necessary part of the game, you don't have to miss out on the fun because of a small budget. Here are some ideas on how to gear up without breaking the bank—from deals on new equipment to the best resources for used items.

Rent and Demo First It seems expensive to pay for one-time use of skis, bicycles, golf clubs, and skates. But it costs a lot more to buy stuff you end up not using. Not only should you test out the sport first—and more than once--but trying a variety of equipment can help you make smarter decisions when you're ready to buy. Demos are not just for skis. For example, the *Golf Digest* site links to retailers offering demo dates.

Get Deals Online Some Web sites offer deep discounts. Try these reputable sites:
* www.Zappos.com for footwear
* www.RoadRunnerSports.com for running stuff
* www.TheFinals.com for swimming items
* www.SierraTradingPost.com for outdoor gear
* www.PerformanceBike.com for cycling
* www.Overstocks.com for any items
* www.Epinions.com for reviews and good prices

Also, search for the name of the sport or the type of gear using the words "discount, bargains, or deals." If you don't know the retailer, check the return policy carefully before purchasing.

Wholesale Clubs The big retailers such as Costco and BJs stock brand-name gear in season, from kayaks to skates. Many clubs have a one-day pass you can use without joining (but beware of fees).

Buy Second-hand Some sports, most notably skiing and ice skating, are known for gear swaps. Ask an instructor or expert athlete for tips on finding them, or check out stores such as golf pro shops and bike shops. While used equipment might appear to be in good shape, make sure it's not so old as to be outdated. Before you purchase pre-owned goods, read a review and

go online to learn the key features and components. For example, shaped skis make it much easier to learn, so don't buy a straighter pair even if they're only $25 and have never been used. In many sports, there's completely different gear for each variant, so you'll need to determine your style, such as classic versus skate for cross-country skiing.

A few items should never be purchased used. Don't buy used sneakers because the materials form to the foot and break down too quickly to fit properly and offer sufficient support. And don't buy used protective gear such as bicycle helmets—it's just not worth the risk that the equipment has a flaw. And damage is not always visible.

Some good sources for used gear include:
* Play It Again Sports (www.playitagainsports.com) is a store where you can buy and sell used athletic equipment (and some new stuff, too). The selection varies by location—the New Hampshire stores have a lot of skis; in New York, there's more skating and golf gear.

* eBay, but only if you know the product well or you find a local seller and can check it out in person. Ask plenty of questions about the age, condition, and return policy before you bid. And double check the shipping costs.

* Your regional Craig's List site and Pennysaver are excellent options for locating sporting goods you can try in person prior to purchase.

* National associations, regional clubs, and local universities. For example, when the local college rowing team updates its fleet, you might get a great deal on a single scull or ergometer.

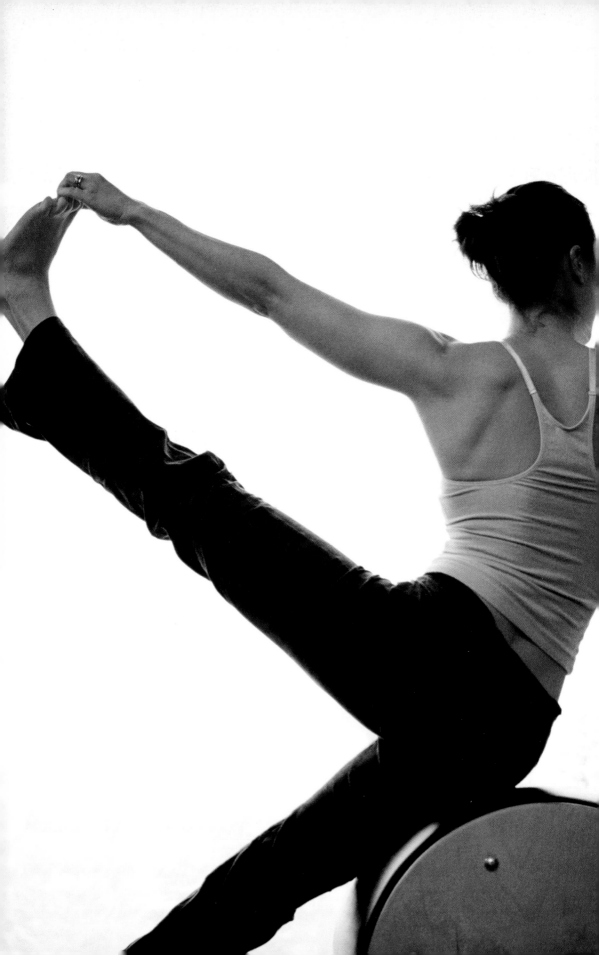

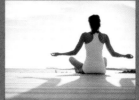

18

STUDIO
YOGA AND PILATES

YOU'LL LOVE THESE SPORTS IF YOU:
- want to build flexible strength, balance, and an injury-resistant body
- crave amazing abs and a full-body workout in one activity
- need a way to reduce stress
- thrive on learning new skills but love quick results, too
- need a sport that challenges the mind as well as the body
- have physical limitations (great for pregnancy and postpartum)
- want an activity you can do for life, alone or in a group, with the kids, anywhere and anytime

YOU MIGHT NOT LOVE THESE SPORTS IF YOU:
- are impatient; these activities require practice and are not easy to master
- don't like hands-on instruction
- are uncomfortable if a teacher delves into spiritual topics
- need social interaction as you practice; classes are often not chatty
- are competitive; yoga and pilates emphasize going at your own pace

Yoga and pilates share a surprising number of similarities, starting with the venue. You can learn each one in a studio, not just in gyms; and you can practice at home if you like. Both activities center on the conscious awareness of body movement, and you can make slight variations on the classic styles that convey your abilities and personality. In each activity, it's vital to have an instructor who can teach you proper form and provide feedback on how your body is positioned. Through coaching and repetition, you learn body awareness as well as how to make the moves flow from one to the next in a beautiful series.

There's a great deal of overlap in the main physical and mental benefits of both pursuits. Yoga and pilates improve your flexibility, agility, coordination, and strength, particularly core strength. Both activities are full-body experiences. Pilates and yoga will enhance your abilities in everything else you do, from golf to carrying groceries, gymnastics to washing the car. You'll be surprised at some of the benefits: Strength in the center of your body improves your sense of balance and positioning, which can greatly improve your skiing, for example. Core strength can also make it easier to give birth. No physical aspect of your life is untouched by these activities. From a mental perspective, these practices are soothing and energizing at the same time. After class, you may feel calm but wide awake at the same time.

Each of these activities has a number of different styles. In yoga, there are forms that emphasize athleticism, meditation, and relaxation or other goals. In pilates, there is a type that concentrates on physical rehabilitation, another that is more athletic. Often, the proponents of one style are well-versed in other types, but in some cases the different camps prefer to keep their distance from one another. Enthusiasts may find that one style is a perfect fit while others may sample many modalities, since they all have slight differences in physical and psychological benefits.

Anyone can do yoga and pilates. The moves are easily adapted for pregnant and postpartum women, who have a lot to gain from improved breathing and core strength. If you have back pain, sign up—before it gets worse—for a targeted yoga or pilates training session. The emphasis on core function and flexibility is just what an ailing back needs—as long as you work with an instructor who is schooled in selecting appropriate poses. If you want to do a little research first, there are plenty of books and videos on the topic of back pain and yoga or pilates practice. (A quick internet search will point you to several good sources.)

Yoga and pilates work well for people at any age. The vast variety of styles means that any person can find a type of yoga or pilates that works well. Mommy-and-me yoga classes are available for parents who need to bring young children along or want to introduce them to the activity. Elderly practitioners are renowned for being in great physical shape while maintaining a high level of mental function.

SCORE

It's difficult to give a set calorie burn for such varied activities. But most beginners tend to do a fairly gentle form of hatha yoga. For that style, which is on the same level of athleticism as stretching, a 150-pound person would burn about 180 calories in an hour (multiply your weight by 1.2 to get your hourly burn). A 150-pound athletic person capable of an energetic style with more sweat (similar to an aerobics class) can burn up to 475 calories (that's 3.2 times your weight).

Like yoga, the calorie burn of pilates will vary greatly depending on the energy level of your practice. A beginner who weighs 150 pounds will generally burn about 215 calories in an hour. (To calculate your hourly burn rate, multiply 1.4 by your weight in pounds.)

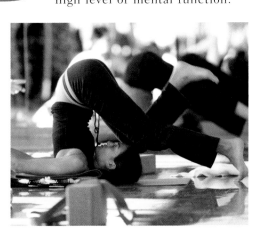

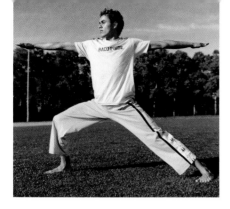

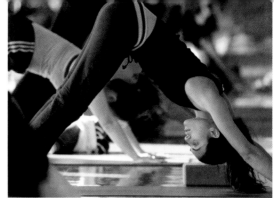

YOGA

Despite its reputation, yoga is not just a bunch of pretzel poses assumed by new-age vegans chanting "Om." You'll find everyone, from executives to professional athletes, in a yoga studio, and the practice can be as gentle or as taxing as you desire, because there are thousands of poses and variations that you do at your own pace. Even a seemingly easy posture such as the *corpse* pose—in which you lie on your back in a comfortable position and breathe—can be a challenge as you attempt to focus your mind and forget the next three things on your to-do list while relaxing the tense muscles all over your body.

There are many reasons people come to yoga—for improved flexibility, to get stronger, for better balance, to slow down and relax, to lose weight, to improve posture, as a spiritual pursuit, or all (or none) of the above. Yoga has so many potential benefits that people who practice it often make seemingly exaggerated claims about how much it does for them. Yet these yoga fans are not wrong. This ancient practice has been shown to provide dozens of benefits for the body and mind, including improved fertility, reduced risk of heart disease, better sleep, happier relationships, and more. Also, yoga practice rarely leads to injuries as long as you select poses that provide appropriate challenges for your body and its quirks. It all adds up to a remarkably useful activity.

The form of yoga first mentioned in history about 3,500 years ago is very different from the types that are popular today. The first detailed description calls yoga a method of breath control, possibly used to enhance the singing abilities of priests. Yoga's history is linked to Hinduism and Buddhism, and early writings call it a path toward enlightenment.

The physical style of mainstream modern yoga evolved from a branch called *hatha* yoga, which relies on poses or *asanas*. It wasn't until the 20th century that anyone began to codify the physical benefits of hatha yoga practice, yet these are the main reasons yoga is popular today.

Many people drawn to yoga for physical gains are pleasantly surprised when they accidentally discover its mental benefits. You don't need to do anything special to reap the rewards. After practicing yoga for a while, it's common to find that it's easier to eat well, sleep deeply, and feel less stressed. Also, studies have found that the discipline and calming effect of yoga can help you focus at work, in school, and in personal pursuits such as stopping smoking or losing weight. Using yoga to still the mind and body to allow for deep spiritual reflection is optional.

While some yoga beginners study one-on-one or travel to an intensive retreat, most begin with a novice's class at a local studio. There are some high-quality teaching videos, from a course in the physical techniques—*Leslie Sansone's You Can Do Yoga*—to a basic session covering the whole mind/body and breathing experience—*Yoga Zone's Introduction to Yoga* (both available at Collage Video, www.collagevideo.com). But save them for after your first few sessions with a teacher in person, because you need someone to give you specific pointers on your form as you learn each pose. One way to begin yoga is to try a few classes at a local gym. Health club classes are typically designed to be less spiritual and more physical. And because their students are often new to the practice, gym instructors are generally good at introducing the moves. However, a yoga studio typically offers more in-depth-study opportunities as well as more styles and more class times from which to choose.

As far back as 800 BC, yoga splintered into different disciplines with different goals, and it is equally diverse today. New forms are developed all the time, whenever a guru develops a variation that's distinct. Some yoga studios teach a variety of styles while others specialize, so call ahead to ask which style of yoga is taught. *Vinyasa*-style yoga is the most popular, with classes of varying intensity focusing on flowing postures and simple breathing. Within Vinyasa, there are specific disciplines, such as the *Iyengar* form, in which you hold poses for longer durations, or athletic *Power Yoga*. Another popular type is *Bikram*, which is sometimes called "hot" yoga because it's practiced in rooms heated to about 105 degrees Fahrenheit. Any class that is simply called *hatha* yoga is usually a mixture of styles incorporating such classic poses as *downward-facing dog* and *plank* in a flowing series called the *Sun Salutation*. In addition to the many forms of yoga, there are also yoga hybrids (such as *yogilates*, which is a yoga/pilates combo) or focused classes (such as yoga for golf players).

Once you've picked a style and studio, you may need to experiment to find a pairing of class and instructor that suits your sensibilities—from relaxing to sweaty, spiritual to drill sergeant. Yoga instructors aren't required to have a set type of training or certification, although reputable studios insist that instructors complete a training program or have a credential such as certification from the Yoga Alliance, which requires at least 200 hours of teaching experience. (Their Web site lists registered instructors and studios; www.yogaalliance.com.) Also, be sure the class you choose first is geared toward beginners—even if you are an accomplished athlete in other sports. More advanced classes will not include the explanations you need to learn the poses. A teacher may use the Sanskrit names for poses, the English equivalents or both. For example, corpse pose is also called *savasana*.

GEARING UP

Yoga is easiest to do barefoot and wearing comfortable clothes. You'll spend some time upside down, so remove jewelry that might flop around. Wear a shirt you can tuck in or one that hugs your body so it won't ride up. Avoid anything that constricts movement, from your waistband to your watch (it's hard to have your hands on the ground in a push-up position with a tight strap on your wrist). Leggings or bike shorts work well, as do yoga pants. Be sure the waistband won't slip down as you move—a drawstring style can be helpful. Overly loose clothing can get in your way and prevent the instructor from easily seeing your body position.

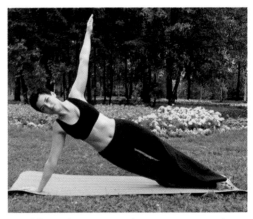

Most classes provide a yoga mat and any props you might need. A yoga mat doesn't cost much, so once you've determined that you enjoy the activity, buy your own to sweat on in class and use at home. The mat used for yoga is called a "sticky" mat because the surface is slightly tacky in order to help hold your hands and feet in place. You can do yoga on a rug at home, but when you're putting your face on the floor, it's nice to have a clean mat. A carrying bag makes it much easier to tote your mat to class. And if you plan to practice at home, you might want to purchase such props as blocks, a bolster, or a strap. You'll learn how to use these items in class so that you can get into and hold a pose correctly until you gain the flexibility to do so without props. You can now buy yoga props at regular sporting goods stores and department stores, and online.

YOUR FIRST TIME

At most studios, you will arrive in an entry hall staffed by an attendant. Here you can check the schedule, pay for your class, and often peruse such offerings as books, yoga bags, and clothing. There may be a changing area in case you come in street clothes. And there is generally a spot designated for shoes, which are left outside the studio.

Inside the yoga room, pick a mat and select a section of floor. If the room is not crowded, leave enough room between you and other classmates to spread out in every direction. It's fine to pick a spot toward the back of the room where you can watch others, but be sure you're able to see and hear the instructor well.

For beginners, the beauty of yoga is that you can work at your own level without falling behind, as you would in an aerobics class. A good instructor will offer modifica-

tions for novices as well as deeper variations for advanced beginners in the same room. (Some people remain beginners at yoga for their entire lives and still get plenty out of the practice.)

Class generally begins with some breathing and light stretches to get the body prepared for more complex moves. The breathing is deep into the lungs and regulated to match movements, or vice versa. When your muscles are warm and your brain is focused, you'll be better able to reach, bend, and hold poses that challenge your balance, flexibility, and strength. Poses typically increase in difficulty over the course of the class. You may find it difficult or impossible to hold the poses for as long as instructed or complete as many repetitions. When this happens, remember that yoga is called a practice because the ability to do it grows with each session and no one is expected to execute every pose perfectly. It's appropriate to come out of a pose and rest at any point during class. The instructor is trying to challenge the most adept yogis in the room, and you should not expect yourself to do everything they do on your first visit. Most yoga classes end with relaxing positions such as the *child's pose* (kneeling, forehead to floor, arms relaxed by your sides, palms up) and the corpse pose. The instructor may end by saying *namaste*, which is a salute to your spirit.

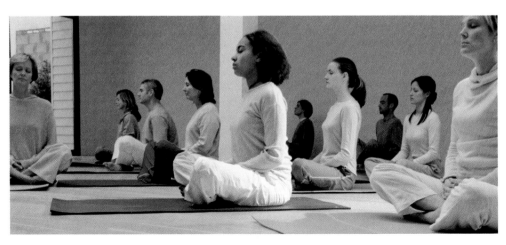

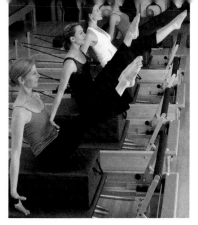

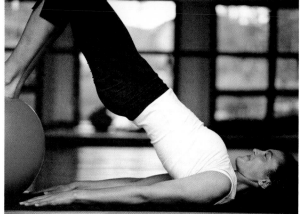

PILATES

For the uninitiated, pilates seems both intimidating and inspiring. The exercises are precise and sometimes rapid. At a studio that offers traditional pilates machines (not just mat work), the equipment resembles a selection of torture devices. The physique of the veteran practitioner is carved and lean, and the muscle control is remarkable. While it's not hard to see the appeal or the benefit that pilates could have on sports or even day-to-day fitness and health, it's daunting to picture getting started. Add a dose of confusion about how and where to start, or even how to pronounce the name (it's *puh-LAH-teeze*), and the feelings of inertia can be overwhelming. Pushing past the fear, however, is well worth the effort. And when you do start, you'll be surprised to find that you've been doing a little pilates all along. The program uses moves similar to the toning and stretching you do on a fitness ball, with a core roller, or using exercise bands (many of which were actually derived from pilates).

Despite those hardbodies you see in the videos and at the studio, pilates is perfect for the not-so-perfect, ailing, or aching body. If you take a lesson using equipment, it supports you as you move, making it easier to accomplish exercises that will improve your abilities. In fact, pilates was developed by German-born Joseph Pilates to overcome his own physical limitations—he was sickly as a child; as a young adult, he studied everything he could to learn how to overcome his body's limitations, including yoga, gymnastics, and human anatomy. He developed a regimen he called *Contrology*. Testing each exercise, he transformed himself into an athlete. Later, as a nurse in British hospitals during World War I, Pilates brought the benefits of exercise to bed-bound patients by using bedsprings to create resistance for their arms and legs. The strange devices he created were the precursors of modern pilates equipment (some of which still resemble a cot with springs). After emigrating to New York, Pilates focused his practice on the large population of dancers who lived there, a natural market for his message of flexible strength and injury resistance. He gained a powerful reputation for rehabilitation and worked with such stage luminaries as Martha Graham and dancers in the New York City Ballet.

The practice of pilates remained a quiet backwater—the domain of dancers and a few other fans—for decades. Not long after Joseph Pilates's death in 1967, however, the method was discovered by Hollywood and soon became the next big fitness trend. Unfortunately, the newfound popularity brought serious squabbles and even court battles over who could claim to teach pilates (or Pilates, or the Pilates Method). Today, factions in the pilates field remain, each claiming to be Joseph Pilates's "real" legacy, with each side supporting a slightly different style.

For a person who simply wants to take up the practice, it's difficult to know whether to begin with "authentic" pilates, reaLPilates, Stott Pilates, Balanced Body, Power Pilates, or some other style. Each technique is a little different, but all are based on the teachings and movements of Joseph Pilates, so each program has value—and some will be a good fit for your personality and abilities while others might not. For example, Power Pilates can be quick and intense, and often appeals to athletes, while Balanced Body is a combination of classically regimented pilates with a blend of rehabilitation for a gentler style more suited to a couch potato or an injured body. The classic styles are more exact in their adherence to the teachings of Pilates, while contemporary forms have added adaptations based on new research or philosophies. If you try one form of pilates and don't enjoy it, consider trying another rather than giving it up.

There are two types of pilates practice: on apparatus and on mat. When you work on the apparatus, you typically have a private lesson with an instructor showing you the

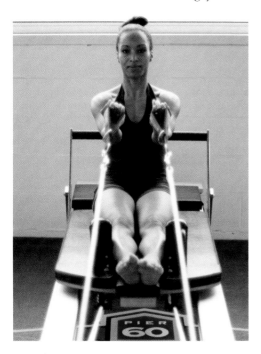

ropes, so to speak. For mat, the typical experience is more like a toning class in a gym, with a group spaced around the room working with one instructor. Pilates mat uses props such as the ball, roller, bands, and a device called the Magic Circle—a metal ring you squeeze for resistance. Mat classes are, naturally, far less expensive than the apparatus lessons, and they are easier to find because any gym can offer them without a

large investment in equipment. Ironically, while the apparatus looks intimidating, the moves are easier because the springs support your body. It's also extremely helpful to have some one-on-one coaching as you begin this activity because the positions can be quite foreign, and there's a lot to remember as you try to execute them.

No matter which style of pilates you choose, your experience will include instruction in use of the breath and talk of the *powerhouse*. Pilates breathing has some similarities to yoga in that it is conscious and deep, but the technique is a little different. Often, in pilates, you breathe in through the nose and out through the mouth, trying to draw the breath into the lower ribs. Breathing is tied to the movements, but the pacing of breath may be rapid or elongated, depending on the exercise you are executing. The powerhouse is sometimes called the core, meaning the abdominals and back. Depending on your instructor, however, it can reach as high up as the heart and as low as mid thigh. Joseph Pilates felt that by focusing on the trunk, you would work the vital organs, thereby improving your health.

The six basic principles of pilates are control, concentration, centering, breathing, precision, and fluidity. In theory, you integrate all six at the same time, but attempting to do so is a challenge that taxes even the most adept athletes. Achieving just one or two is an excellent start. In the process, you build body awareness, which improves your abilities and reduces injuries in other activities.

Finding a pilates class is a little confusing because of the various forms (mat or equipment) and factions. There is no single sanctioning body or instructor certification that you can look to. Some teachers may not have had much training, while others spent years becoming experts in the field. Before you sign up for a lesson or class, ask about the instructor's training and the form of pilates he or she teaches. Get a sense of the techniques and learn the lingo by checking out a

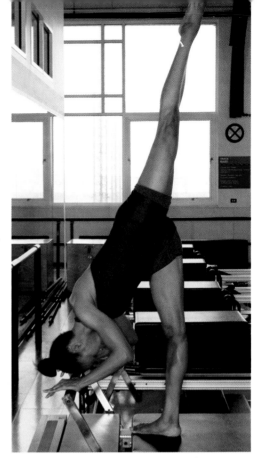

pilates video such as *Winsor Pilates Endless Fitness For Beginners*, which is a perfect introduction to the practice (and includes excellent guidance and modifications for physical limitations as well). *More Than Mat Pilates: Beginner* is a workout based on apparatus moves that have been adapted so they do not require equipment—along with detailed explanations so you fully understand the concepts. And *The Quick and Dirty Guide to Pilates* is a DVD with a unique feature: You can change the camera angle to see more detail of how to perform the move. (All three tapes are available at www.collagevideo.com.) But don't forgo instruction and use only tapes, because you'll definitely need help getting the positions just right while remembering the six principles.

GEARING UP

Pilates is best done barefoot and in comfortable clothes. Because the regimen includes inverted postures, it's desirable to leave jewelry home and wear clothes that won't flop in your face. You can buy pilates shoes or wear socks if you are uncomfortable in bare feet, but neither is necessary nor recommended.

For pilates practice at home, you can use a yoga mat or purchase a specific pilates mat, which is usually thicker for greater protection of the spine. There are a variety of items you can use in your home practice, such as a fitness ball, resistance tubing, balance boards, Magic Circle, and a foam roller. These pieces are available for use at pilates studios and in most gyms as well. To purchase them for home use, look in sporting goods stores or online.

YOUR FIRST TIME

As in yoga, many people find it most comfortable to try pilates first in a familiar setting—as one of the numerous courses offered at your local gym—before heading to a studio. But if your gym is like most and only offers a pilates mat class, you might consider a one-

on-one with an instructor using the apparatus. This approach is especially appropriate if you have physical limitations or have not been exercising. The most famous piece of equipment is called the *reformer*, which looks like a bed with a big bar in place of the footboard and a sliding section of mattress. There are cords attached to springs, each having loops at the end to hold with a hand or foot. Lying on the platform, you will be shown how to do a series of moves called *footwork*, which look like a variety of squats done lying down with your feet in different positions reminiscent of ballet. The supported position protects your back and minimizes the weight you lift. As you get stronger, the apparatus is adjusted to add resistance.

Joseph Pilates developed a full-body workout on each piece of apparatus. Most studios will have the main pieces: The *cadillac* looks like a metal four-poster bed with traction devices and a trapeze. The *chair* is a box with a bar or two on one side to push up and down. The *barrel* is a curved platform about three feet high that looks a little like a gymnastics vault, and it may have a short ladder attached nearby.

The goal of each session is to work the entire body. Often, your instructor will create a circuit, moving from one piece of apparatus to the next rather than completing a workout in one place. Your first session will likely last thirty-five to forty-five minutes and include a few moves on different pieces of equipment and a lot of discussion. The experience will probably feel unnatural at first. When you wake up the next day, your abs will feel sore in a whole new way, and you'll be more aware of your back. Your posture will begin to improve right away.

If you start with a beginner's pilates mat class, you will receive the same instruction on finding and using your "powerhouse," seeking to gain control and concentration, plus improving the flexibility of your spine while strengthening your core. You'll do familiar moves such as the plank and learn new exercises such as the pilates one hundred and leg circles. These are the same moves done on the apparatus, only without the helpful springs and bars. Mat classes can be as physically demanding as yoga, and the instructor must keep everyone in the room challenged. So go at your own pace to avoid injury or excessive muscle soreness. The goal is to progress slowly and properly, especially because mental focus is vital to the practice and is complex to learn.

ATHLETE IN ACTION

Malcolm Bartow, 47

Life as a 40-something has been good to Malcolm Bartow—he has a good job, nice house, a convertible to drive, plenty of dates and friends, plus buddies who like to go catch the local band on Saturday night or tune in to a football game. An engineer in South Carolina who spent time in the army, Bartow has a bit of a tough-guy exterior; he seems far from the type you'd expect to be drawn to yoga. But spend a minute in conversation with him and you quickly learn that he's well-read, funny, warm, and insightful. Perhaps that inner light is why, as he puts it, he was ready and the teacher just "appeared."

A few years ago, Bartow's then-girlfriend got him a book: *Babar's Yoga for Elephants*. The humorous story about how elephants invented yoga was just the thing to entice him into trying the discipline. Because his work requires travel, Bartow found it appealing that practicing yoga doesn't require much equipment or space. He used to

jog, but some trips are to places where even that sport isn't practical—say in a hotel surrounded by highways.

"My girlfriend taught yoga and had a healthy lifestyle, which influenced me," says Bartow. "When she left, I went through the mourning period, all the anger and frustration, and depression—and I needed to exercise for relief." Having already learned the basics from Babar and some pointers his girlfriend had given him, he decided to take up yoga. "It's low impact, and it's one of those things you can do all your life until you drop," he says. "Now I'm at the point when I'm looking at what I'm going to do in retirement in thirteen years."

For Bartow, yoga is an outgrowth of his fascination with meditation, which began in high school during the early '70s. "Then, I used short meditations to relax when my mind was going a mile a minute," he recalls. Interested in trying it again, "I started going to a Zen meditation class at the Unitarian Universalist Church," he says. He tried to sit in the cross-legged lotus position and was too stiff. "That's when I started doing yoga every day." Not only does his practice

make him more flexible, but the yoga itself is similar to meditation. "It's the same focused breathing you do in meditation," Bartow says. "When I've done my fifteen poses, I'm very relaxed." Calm and limber, he then does his meditation. Today, yoga comes up often in Bartow's conversations with friends and colleagues. "It usually starts with, 'Wow, you've lost weight,'" he says. "I've lost twenty pounds over the last four months—it's regular exercise," he adds. (He also notes that he stopped drinking at the same time, which helped quite a bit.) Often, he finds that others are closet yogis. "Yoga has become popular in the last five years," he says. "My friends and I are getting older. People I know are getting knee replacements—I don't want to do that." Yoga is kind to the joints and builds strength, which stabilizes them. He's also found that he has more stamina, wants to eat better, and needs less sleep in order to feel rested. "I don't know if the sleep is because of the meditation, the yoga, getting older, or what," he says. But he's not giving any of them up to find out.

SECRETS TO SUCCESS

"People come expecting a single physical benefit—stress control or relief for an achy back, for example—but once you start, you'll discover that there's much more," says Noll Daniel, who teaches his signature Urban Yoga Workout at the Sports Center at Chelsea Piers and other locations in New York. In addition to strengthening and stretching the entire body, both modalities teach body awareness and focus. "You learn to make the connection between the body and the mind, to focus on each movement in order to obtain the benefits," says Daniel, who worked as a pilates instructor before taking up yoga. This focused movement will bring many beneficial physical effects, from better posture to a more comfortable way of moving in your daily life. And the intense focus of this discipline conveys mental benefits as well that bring calmness and clarity.

One way to maintain that focus is to pay attention to the pattern of your breathing, says Terrence Carey, a wellness and movement coach at The Sports

Center at Chelsea Piers who is certified to teach Balanced Body pilates and has extensive training in the classical method. During yoga or pilates practice, try to visualize breathing into the areas that are working. This concentration is called "mindful" exercise and is integral to both practices. Breathing can be quite a challenge that can make your limbs quiver with exertion, but working muscles need oxygen. Also, each exhalation carries away the toxic chemicals in your cells that result from exercise such as lactic acid, the stuff that makes muscles burn from exertion. As you struggle through a move, it can be calming to imagine the breath cleansing the body.

Awareness of your breathing will also show you where you hold tension in your body, which will aid in reducing stress. You can practice the breathing outside of class, and you may find it a useful tool for calming yourself when you are agitated. Although you can do a short session of yoga or pilates, neither of these practices

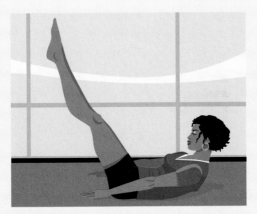

pilates one-hundred

Lie with your back on the ground, arms alongside your body. Lift both legs straight up in the air, thighs pressed together. Lower your legs until you feel a slight tension in your abs; hold them there. Next, lift your head and shoulders into a slight crunch, bringing your arms a few inches off the ground, palms facing down. From the shoulders, pulse both arms up and down 100 times. Don't forget to breathe! Inhale for 5 arm pulses and exhale for the next 5, repeat. Each 100 reps makes a full set.

is effective if done in a rush. When you set time aside for a few moves, prepare yourself as best you can to avoid distractions (e.g., bathroom breaks, ringing telephones, hunger). Spend a little time limbering up and paying attention to your breath before heading into the poses. And leave a few minutes for reflection at the end of your session before you have to dash off to the rest of your day.

Whenever you do yoga or pilates, it's vital that you move at your own level of ability, without comparing yourself to the person on the next mat. It's fine to look at someone more advanced if it inspires or helps you, but try to go at the pace that works for your body. Also, keep in mind that your abilities will vary from day to day. Sometimes you'll be fresh and rested, and other times you might be more distracted or "off your game." Work at the level that feels right at that moment.

Be patient with yourself as you try these new activities. Even if you are very athletic, executing the flowing motions well requires practice. Be prepared to repeat the basics over and over. One day it will click, and you'll experience the graceful intensity of the practice.

If you choose to dedicate some serious time to pilates or yoga, you could become adept and possibly end up teaching others. Your instructors themselves are most likely to be studying on a continuing basis, and some of them may not be much more advanced than you. Sometimes you'll find you get the best instruction from someone close to your level, because he or she will remember exactly how it feels to struggle with the kinds of positions you are finding difficult.

It's challenging to study pilates or yoga if you aren't very flexible or have weak abs or a bad back—but both practices will improve these areas. If you want to prepare for your first experience or progress more quickly, take some time to work on flexibility and torso strength before or between sessions. Here are a few moves to get you started:

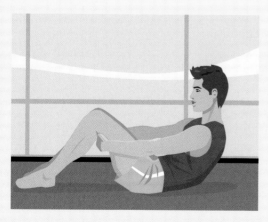

rolldowns

Sit on the ground, knees bent, feet flat on the floor. Hook your fingertips behind your knees. Inhale and elongate your spine, pushing your head as tall as you can. Exhale through pursed lips, slowly rounding your back down until your arms are extended. If you can, continue to round down, letting your fingers slide down along your thighs. Hold at the lowest point you comfortably can. Then, inhaling, roll back up. Start with 1 set of 10 reps and build up to 3 sets of 30 reps.

TACKLE THE TRUTH

Yoga and pilates are cults, not exercise routines

While both activities can include a strong spiritual aspect, neither yoga nor pilates is a cult. Yoga is often practiced for its ability to still the body and mind for introspection and awareness, but no religious doctrine is required. Pilates is founded on some of the concepts of yoga, but while it shares a mental focus, it, too, is not based in any religion.

Fans of yoga and pilates can be highly enthusiastic—and sometimes intimidating—in their expansive spiritual claims for each regimen. And they are likely to do their best to persuade you to give it a try. But you are welcome to take what you like from the practice and discard aspects that don't feel comfortable. There is no religious evangelism in yoga or pilates.

Only thin women do these activities

The tradition of yoga and pilates began with men. Centuries ago in India, only men were permitted to study yoga. It was virtual heresy when women were first taught the asanas or poses. Pilates, for its part, was of course invented by a man, first to condition his own body and then to speed the healing of injured soldiers. The first American pilates studio was run by Joseph Pilates and his wife Clara, working with male and female dancers.

Today, you will find more women than men in yoga and pilates studios, but the disciplines are equally effective for both sexes. Football, hockey, and basketball pros have taken up yoga or pilates to improve their games. So have runners and triathletes.

Any person of any size, shape, or gender can benefit from yoga or pilates. If you have areas of weakness or pain, a carefully designed program can help you recover, make you stronger, and improve your physical abilities. Both programs include modifications to moves so that anyone can do them safely and effectively.

You won't get fit doing yoga or pilates

Wrong. These activities include moves that work the entire body. They can leave you sweaty and sore in places you never knew existed. One thing is guaranteed: A session of yoga or pilates can challenge your body in new ways, making you stronger and more flexible. Joseph Pilates is claimed to have said this about his regimen: "In ten sessions you will feel the difference, in twenty see the difference, and in thirty you'll have a whole new body."

GET MORE FROM YOUR SPORT

Just as pilates and yoga can enhance your experience in other sports, there are many pursuits that can have a positive effect on your practice. Any activity that develops your breathing ability, builds focus, strengthens the core muscles, or improves flexibility or balance will make it easier to do yoga or pilates. Swimming is helpful for enhancing body awareness and breathing skills. Weight lifting builds strength. Perhaps the most closely related sports are gymnastics, skating, and rock climbing, which combine flexibility, balance, agility, and strength. Any form of dance aids in a number of areas, from body movement to breathing to focus. Studying music is helpful for developing rhythm, and singing or playing wind instruments can improve your breathing.

In addition to taking your individual practice wherever you roam, you can find classes in hotels, spas, and studios all over the world—even in the fitness centers on cruise ships. Yoga retreats vary, from bare bones centers with communal quarters and dawn-to-dusk practice to luxury hotels that offer a variety of classes along with massages and gourmet meals. Kripalu is a famous intensive yoga retreat in Lenox, Massachusetts. Unlike yoga, the intensive pilates training camps are typically oriented toward teacher training (www.kripalu.org).

RESOURCES

➡ **www.yogajournal.com** is the robust Web site for the eponymous magazine that provides just about everything you might need to get started. You'll find information and tips about beginning a yoga practice, finding a teacher, practicing poses, as well as a section that helps you select moves that match your abilities and goals.

➡ **www.allaboutpilates.com** is a site that explains the basics, with plenty of common-sense attitude. The site explores the different factions with less bias than most sources.

➡ *Yoga Journal: Yoga Basics* by Mara Carrico and the editors of *Yoga Journal* provides a complete overview of yoga, including history, descriptions of styles, breathing, meditation, and plenty of poses.

➡ *30 Essential Yoga Poses: For Beginning Students and Their Teachers* by physical therapist Judith Lasater, Ph.D., covers the basic poses with detailed photos and pointers. The book also provides information about starting your practice, breathing techniques, and more.

➡ *A Pilates Primer* by Joseph Pilates and William Miller is an explanation of the program and its philosophies by the founder himself.

➡ *Pilates: Bodies in Motion* was written by physical therapist Alycea Ungaro, who was trained in the classic method of pilates and operates a studio in New York called reaLPilates. Her book is a thorough explanation of mat moves that are helpful for beginners, including several photos per exercise, a checklist of alignment pointers, plus photos of common mistakes.

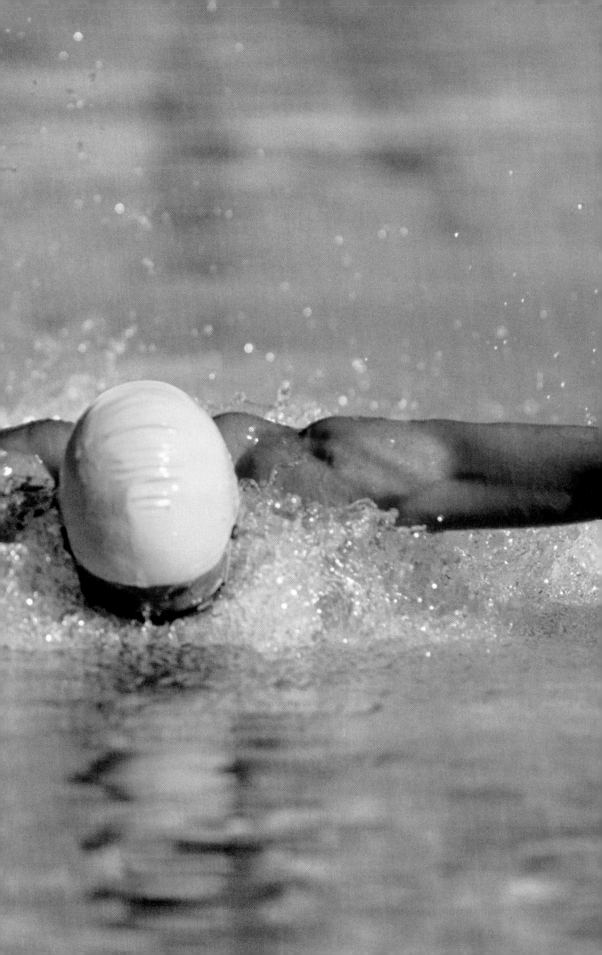

19

SWIMMING

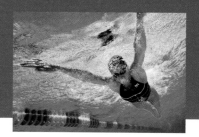

YOU'LL LOVE THIS SPORT IF YOU:
- want a tough cardio and muscular workout from head to toe
- like to learn the basics quickly, then spend years mastering a sport
- enjoy a sense of serenity while you exercise intensively
- like a sport with indoor and outdoor options
- have any kind of injury or disability—almost everyone can learn to swim
- enjoy the camaraderie of a team but prefer to win or lose on your own merits
- prefer a sport that requires almost no gear
- need a sport you can do with your kids in tow

YOU MIGHT NOT LOVE THIS SPORT IF YOU:
- are afraid of the water
- find it difficult to get to the pool, change, shower, and dry your hair after every workout

Water can be called a "great equalizer" because the ability to swim is not solely a factor of fitness. Some elite athletes flail in the pool while unfit folks glide through the water like sleek dolphins. Almost anyone can swim, no matter what shape your body is in or how strong you are. For many people who have physical limitations, swimming is the most appropriate sport, offering a safe way to exercise. The same is true for the rest of us, because water is both buoyant and provides strong resistance, delivering a tough workout with little chance of injury. Swimming is the perfect sport for people who are overweight because a bulky body feels light in the water, not hampered by the extra pounds as it would be on land. But the sport is far from the province of the flabby. Take a look at the physiques of champions and you'll see that swimming is serious exercise. And if you're still in doubt, ask a triathlete which part of the race is the hardest; many will answer that it's the swim.

Swimming is an intense cardio workout—so hard that many people initially can't make it back and forth in the pool for a single lap without stopping. It also works many muscles, requiring major locomotion from the shoulders and arms, the body core and legs. Learning to kick efficiently is one of the skills beginners struggle to master, because the technique is far from intuitive, yet when done well, it provides quite a strong push. It also requires practice to learn how to pull strongly with the arms and develop a comfortable breathing rhythm. And once you've managed a decent stroke, there's plenty more to work on, from flip turns to additional stroke styles.

Mentally, the sport demands focus and discipline because it's tempting to decide you've done enough or slack off on the intensity when swimming lap after lap. Yet it can also be soothing to the mind to be enveloped by the water, and swimming's repetitive motion while performing laps can be meditative.

Lap swimming is a lot different from splashing around in the water. People who work out in the pool put their heads down and go, back and forth, slicing through the water with trained breathing and smooth strokes—at least they aspire to do so. The most common style you'll see in the pool is the classic *forward crawl*, with a breath after every other stroke or less often. The *backstroke* is also popular, and most people find this stroke an easier one to begin with. The *butterfly* and *breaststroke* are far more complex, and relatively few swimmers excel at these strokes today. The breaststroke was the main form of swimming when it first became a competitive sport in the early 1800s. A version of the crawl was introduced in England in the 1870s. The butterfly evolved from the breaststroke in the 1940s.

There are individual events for each stroke in modern swim meets, medley races combining the strokes, and relays with several swimmers completing set distances. And for a completely different challenge, there's also synchronized swimming. Earlier in Olympic history there were also obstacle swims, underwater swims, and a single distance event called the "plunge for distance" that was a dive and a motionless glide. The first few Olympic medal races, in the late 1800s and early 1900s, took place in open water, moving to a pool in 1908. Today, competitors enjoy pools that have wave-reducing gutters and lane markers plus controlled temperatures and electronic timing devices.

Aquatic centers across the country have designated sessions for athletes of different abilities, often with some time reserved for open swimming at any level, family swimming, and water aerobics classes. Water familiarization programs now begin when babies are just a few months old. To those who didn't learn as children, it can seem daunting to face a pool full of splashing kids. Some venues are for adults only, and almost all centers have restricted times when the scene is more mature and calm. Most aquatic centers offer lessons at all levels and ages, as well. And while it may seem as though every American learned

SCORE

Paddling around without swimming laps for an hour burns a whopping 300 calories for a 150-pound person (or your weight times two). Synchronized swimming averages 420 calories in an hour for the same size person (or 2.8 times your weight). When you get into swimming laps with specific strokes, here's a look at how the burn adds up:

Pace	Calories/hour*	Calories/hour/lb
Slow crawl, 50 yards per minute, moderate effort	420	2.8
Backstroke, moderate effort	420	2.8
Breaststroke, moderate effort	540	3.6
Butterfly, moderate effort	600	4
Fast crawl, 75 yards per minute, vigorous effort	600	4

* 150-lb person

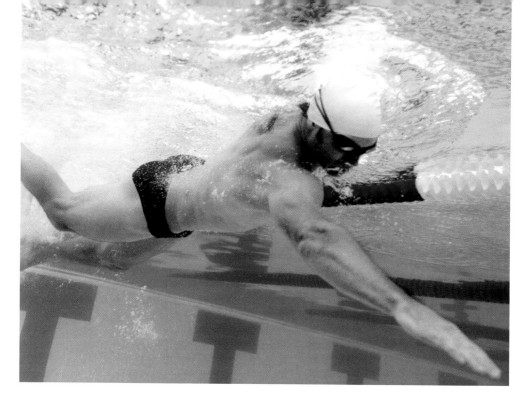

a perfect crawl in childhood, there are many adults who show up for beginner classes in every state, every year.

GEARING UP

While you may already own a bathing suit and even a pair of goggles, choose carefully and consider getting new gear when you're ready to take up swimming as a serious pursuit toward fitness. Bathing suits that chafe and goggles that leak can make you miserable in the pool—sometimes so much so that you never return. To avoid numerous disappointing purchases in the search for goggles that fit your face well, start at the pool. Ask a staffer if there's a collection of abandoned goggles that you can test to find a style that suctions well to your face's shape. You don't need to swim with them; simply press them in place and see if they hold firmly without discomfort. When you find a style that works well, buy your own and test them in the pool. If the lost-and-found bin doesn't produce a pair that fits appropriately, consider asking swimmers for their advice and if you can try on their favorites. You'll find that many avid swimmers are happy to share what they've learned in this often-frustrating quest. High-end sporting goods stores may also have a selection of goggles.

For swimming suits, you don't need expensive competition-quality models, but you also don't want a bad fit. When you try on suits, jump around in the dressing room, bend over, swing your arms, do your best to dislodge it the way the water will. Check carefully for uncomfortable seams, baggy fabric that might bunch in awkward places, and decorative trim that could get in your way. Recreational suits from competition brands are often a good choice. Look in your local sporting goods store rather than in a department store, where advice might be less expert.

While you're shopping, grab a swimmer's towel. These quick-dry and thirsty little cloths will save you loads of laundry. Also, consider a two-pocket gear bag that allows you to keep your wet stuff separate from dry items. Grab a combination lock if your pool has lockers (you don't want to swim with a key dangling off your suit), and flip-flops to wear from the locker room to the pool deck and back (you can pick up athlete's foot from the floor). If you find yourself inadvertently breathing in water through your nose, pick up a nose clip. And if you want to protect your hair, or your pool requires it, buy a swim cap. The classic latex models provide the most protection for hair, but silicone and Lycra versions are softer and more comfortable.

After you learn the basic strokes, you can jumpstart your technique by using "pool tools." They aren't expensive, and you can usually find samples to test at the pool before purchasing your own. Consider using small fins, a kickboard, and webbed gloves or paddles. Pull buoys, snorkels (not the SCUBA kind), stretch cords, and tickers (a metronome that goes in your cap) are also helpful, but save those refinements until you've had a few months in the water at least.

YOUR FIRST TIME

If you don't know how to swim at all, sign up for a session with an instructor. The sport isn't intuitive, and a small investment in learning properly will pay off with your acquiring good technique and making rapid progress. You'll do better than someone who learned as a kid and has to unlearn a bunch of bad habits. If you fall into the category of those who already have some swimming ability, consider a few lessons to improve your form and provide you with skills to work on during your swims.

When you arrive to swim laps, it's expected that you'll rinse off in the shower before getting in the pool. Tie back loose hair so it won't float into your eyes or restrict your arms. Leave a towel, footwear, and water bottle

ATHLETE IN ACTION

Rima Suqi, 40

On a trip to Parrot Cay, a beautiful island in the Turks and Caicos, Rima Suqi got fed up with not knowing how to swim. "They said, 'Just jump in with a snorkel,' and the water was gorgeous. But I couldn't do it," she recalls. Back home in New York, the freelance writer was already a member of Chelsea Piers, which has a huge, sun-splashed pool overlooking the Hudson River. Suqi walked over to the pool, signed up for private instruction, and took the plunge.

That was five years and three instructors ago. Now, when she's not out of town on assignments, she swims four times a week for at least an hour. Even she can't

believe it. Her father is Palestinian and her mom is from Lithuania, so neither grew up in a culture oriented toward water. Suqi was raised in the city by the lake, Chicago, but was never athletic. "My pediatrician told my mom that I had fragile bones, so no sports or ballet for Rima," she says. "I got art and piano lessons."

Suqi took to exercise as an adult, with mixed success. She adored step aerobics in the '80s and '90s, but the pounding took a toll on her knees. "No pain, no gain? That's not me," she says. "I love that nothing hurts when I get out of the pool." Her current coach, who also trains the women's team at New York University, says Suqi is a natural. "She gives me different workouts about once a month," says Suqi, who has mastered all the strokes and swims 2,500 yards per session—that's 100

laps. "The time flies because I have different strokes to do, not just swimming laps," she says. "And there's a sense of accomplishment when you complete the session. I try to push myself for time and to improve." The latest quest is to conquer the flip turn. "I'd never done a somersault in my life until last month. I went to a gymnastics class to learn how to do one on land, hoping it would help in the pool."

Her swimming has also given her confidence and has inspired her toward other physical feats. She has since gone on a week-long camping and kayak trip in Baja, dogsledding in Alaska, and on a trek up Kilimanjaro to mark her 40th birthday. "I never thought I would do those things," she says. "But then, I never thought I would swim, either."

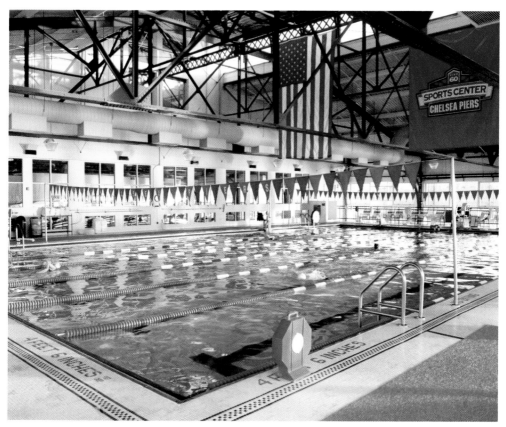

in designated areas—usually there are benches around the perimeter of the room. Stretch your muscles a bit before jumping in, and while you do, peruse the lanes to select the one that's the least crowded or contains swimmers moving at about your speed. Some pools have lanes designated for slow, moderate, and fast swimmers, so inquire on your first visit. Leave the most possible room between you and other swimmers when you jump in. If you're one of two swimmers, you'll be expected to go back and forth in your side of the lane. When there are more swimmers, you'll need to swim in a long clockwise circuit. If you need to pass another swimmer in the loop, tap him on the foot once, then wait until you reach the wall. If he understands the sign, he will stop at the wall and wait for you to pass. Keep this signal in mind in case it's your foot receiving the tap.

Whether you take classes or decide to start swimming on your own, your first challenge will be to build up stamina. Don't expect too much of yourself the first few times out. Have fun, get used to the process of suiting up and moving in the water, and take frequent breathers and water breaks; you do sweat while swimming, even though you don't notice it, so you still need to rehydrate yourself. Try to elongate your body, scoop the water with your hands, and kick effectively. Work on swimming with your face in the water, rotating your torso and head to one side for quick breaths as you stroke. Watch more advanced swimmers who seem to have good form for ideas on body position and technique. Move as slowly as you comfortably can, switching to backstroke if it helps you keep going, so you can add laps and gain stamina.

Coach's Corner

SECRETS TO SUCCESS

Great swimmers make the sport look easy, and the support of the water can at first make it seem that way. But you'll be surprised by the resistance. "One of the biggest surprises in swimming is how easy it is to get to the other end of the pool the first time—and how hard it is to get back," says Glenn Mills, a swimming champ, Olympic team member (in 1980, when the U.S. boycotted the games), and head of Go Swim, a Maryland-based program that provides clinics, classes, and instruction materials such as videos. "Swimming is like running in syrup, and the faster you go, the harder the resistance," he says. Don't expect to complete many laps when you're starting out. In addition to building stamina, it's challenging to get comfortable with the smooth and continuous rhythm of breathing paired with the stroke.

When you can manage more than a few laps without stopping or gasping for breath, look for an experienced swimmer or coach who can give you pointers on form and teach you skills such as flip turns. If you don't know where to find instruction, ask someone on the local swim team for suggestions. When you find a teacher, ask for drills so you can work on different techniques and ideas for using pool tools to improve your abilities. You'll continue to hone your skills for years, learning subtle techniques to move through more water with your hand, how to rotate your hips properly, or how to snap your foot for optimal propulsion.

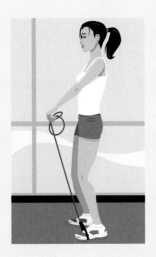
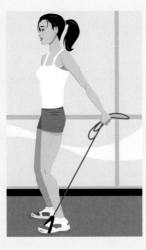

band swims

Stand with your left foot firmly anchoring an exercise band (put your foot through the handle or make a loop so it stays secure). Grasp the other end with your left hand, arm resting by your side so the band has no slack. Stand in a stable position, feet shoulder-width apart, abs firm, head up. Slowly lift your straightened left arm directly in front of you as high as you can without raising your shoulders. Lower the hand to your side and then press it directly back, your arm maintaining a straight position. Lower the band to your side to complete the repetition. Do 10 repetitions, then switch sides and repeat. Work up to 3 sets of 10 reps.

That being said, you can develop a grasp of the basics in just a few good sessions with an instructor. And with diligent practice, adult beginners easily go on to swim in masters competitions (that's the category for anyone over eighteen). The events are further divided into age ranges, making the competition fairer—and easier for those who come late to the sport and are trying to compete against more seasoned athletes. And the meets tend to welcome newcomers. "The events can be as fun—or as serious—as you want to make them; and they are extremely popular," says Mills. There's also an upside to starting later: "You will have the joy of setting personal bests nearly every time you swim," says Mills, "while the long-time swimmer will rarely swim faster than he did in his youth."

An advantage to lessons and competitions is the camaraderie. All that pool time can be lonely, but signing up for sessions or joining a team provides a set of people with whom to practice and swap tips. The other swimmers will also encourage you to perform at your best because someone else is watching.

Here are a few land-based moves to give you an edge in the pool:

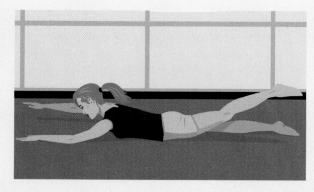

prone swimmers
Lie on the ground, face down. Reach as far as you can with your hands overhead and point your toes, extending your legs as far as possible. Contract your abdominals, inhale, and raise your head and neck slightly off the ground. At the same time, lift your right arm and left leg as high as you comfortably can. While exhaling, lower to the starting position, but keep the muscles engaged. Immediately lift your head, neck, left arm, and right leg with the next inhalation. Exhale and lower to complete 1 repetition. Continue "swimming" for 30 reps. Work up to 3 sets of 50 repetitions.

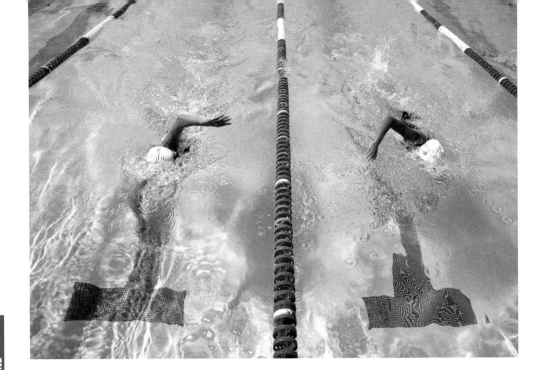

TACKLE THE TRUTH

Swimming laps is boring

Swimming is only boring if you don't progress and learn. Sure, if you slog through lap after lap, you'll feel no more energized than zoning out on the elliptical trainer in front of the television. But swimming is a complex and varied sport, with detailed techniques, a variety of strokes, and enjoyable pool toys to add challenge and improve your abilities. When you swim well, you'll experience a sense of calm euphoria, similar to a runner's high, brought on by rhythmic breathing and energetic movement. If boredom sneaks into your program and you can't afford a lesson to shake it, go online to the many instruction sites, or pick up a book of techniques and look for new ideas to breathe life into your laps.

You can't swim after you eat

This myth has been around for eons, but longevity doesn't make it true. You might not be comfortable completing a tough workout, especially a horizontal one, after a big meal. And flip turns might provoke indigestion on a full stomach. But the dangers of swimming after eating are exaggerated. You won't get cramps from postmeal workouts. Actually, you're more likely to suffer if you are underfed or dehydrated.

You can't learn to swim as an adult— and you're the only person who didn't learn as a kid

Plenty of adults venture into swim class with no idea how to float or stroke. Adult beginner classes are held at pools across the country, which testifies to the fact that you have plenty of company. If you're concerned about your ability to progress or are at all embarrassed, try one or two private lessons when the pool isn't busy to test the waters.

GET MORE FROM YOUR SPORT

Swimming is a full-body activity that accomplishes many fitness goals, but it's important to augment the sport with some land-based activities to develop strong bones and good balance. Make sure your regimen includes walking, bouncing, or some sort of impact activity. Gymnastics and running are great choices for bones, balance, and stamina boosting.

Once you are confident in the water, try snorkeling and SCUBA. There's nothing that makes a long swim more fun than easy breathing and beautiful scenery. You can spend hours getting an amazing workout in the water doing one of these activities. Snorkeling gear is inexpensive and the sport is simple to master once you are comfortable having your face in the water. SCUBA is a little more complicated, but the rewards are worth it. Try a resort course introduction that's shorter than the typical program and includes instructor-led shallow dives (which are plenty deep) to see some of the best underwater venues, such as sunken ships and coral reefs. These classes are offered at some luxury hotels, Club Med locations, and on cruise ships.

Some swimmers get serious about running and cycling in order to compete in triathlons. There are a number of shorter races for training and a variety of triathlon-training clubs and classes across the country.

Swimming clinics and classes are also offered all over the world. Many resorts feature such programs, and there are a variety of destinations if you want to go to swimming camp. For a challenging and memorable trip, consider a swimming-adventure vacation with Swim Trek, which includes swimming from island to island in Greece, Malta, and Croatia as well as island-hopping in other exotic destinations (www.swimtrek.com).

RESOURCES

➧ **www.goswim.tv** is Glenn Mills' site. It has articles, lessons, drills, free video clips, and tips to get you started and keep you moving ahead for months, if not years. He and his team cover conditioning, skills, and general techniques. Mills also contributes articles to the swim pages on the About.com portal, located at www.swimming.about.com.

➧ **www.usms.org** is the site for U.S. Masters Swimming, the group that governs swim events for people old enough to vote. The Web site offers articles about swimming for fitness, plus plenty of training info and links to camps and clubs.

➧ *The Fit Swimmer* by Marianne Brems, a Masters swimming coach in California, provides workouts and tips to turn any lap swim into a challenging and enjoyable training session.

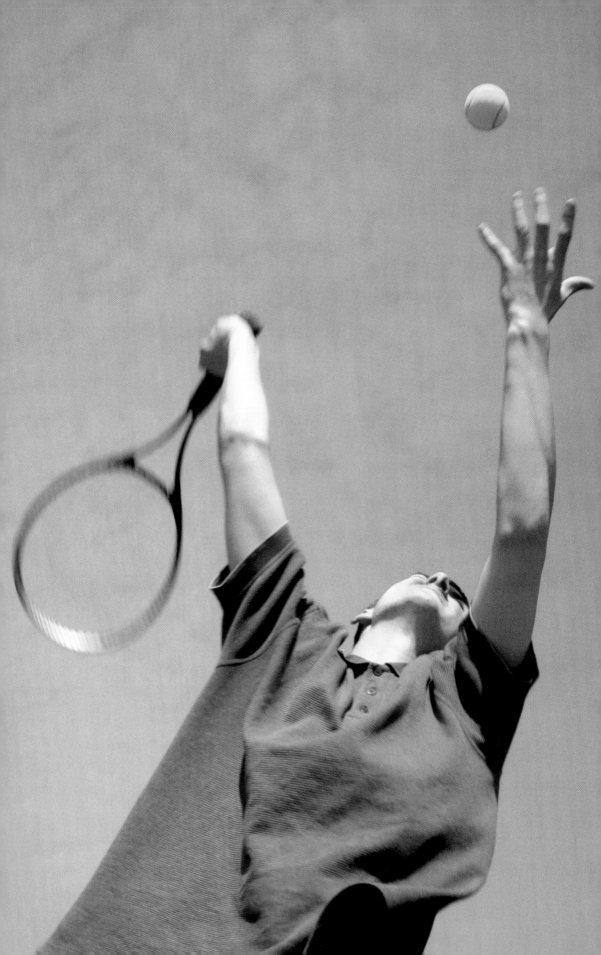

TENNIS

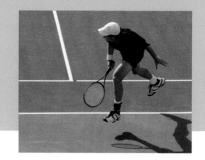

YOU'LL LOVE THIS SPORT IF YOU:
• want a tough cardio workout
• want to develop strong legs and a toned core
• want to improve your balance, speed, and agility
• need a mental challenge in addition to a physical one
• want a sport that you can play—and keep improving at—as you get older
• enjoy playing outdoors
• enjoy the camaraderie of a sport that involves at least one other person
• want a sport that you can play on vacation
• like to take lessons

YOU MIGHT NOT LOVE THIS SPORT IF YOU:
• do not like to move quickly
• prefer solo pursuits
• have a chronic knee or shoulder injury

Once the sport of kings, tennis is now a game played by everyone from pre-school kids to seniors, and across a wide variety of demographics. The aristocratic image still prevails, thanks to numerous private clubs where the rich take private lessons and all-white attire remains the rule. But parks and schoolyards across the country also have courts where competitive —and not so competitive—games are played.

It's easy to get a good workout chasing the ball, and time flies because the sport is so engaging and fun. Watch someone in a serious match and you quickly see that tennis can be a powerful game and a great workout. While the main benefit is cardiovascular fitness, you also develop and utilize muscle strength and gain speed, agility, and coordination. Your legs will get toned running around, and you'll

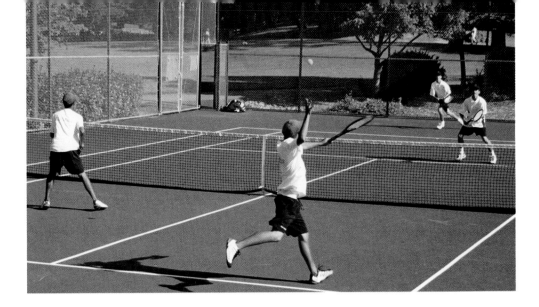

develop a firm core from the stroke, as well as toned shoulders and arms. Tennis can even improve your posture and balance. And, of course, hand-eye coordination is important, as is strategy and quick decision-making. You won't be bored playing tennis. Even if your opponent can easily be trounced, you can still challenge yourself by trying to perfect your ball placement.

In addition to the mental and physical challenges of the game, tennis provides an easy way to exercise outdoors in nice weather or indoors anytime. You can hit against a wall alone to practice skills, take a lesson, or find camaraderie on the court, whether with a single opponent, a doubles teammate, or an entire league of players. Many people play an intensely competitive game, but you'll find plenty of players who prefer to knock the ball around the court, work up a sweat, and not even keep score.

As a form of physical and mental exercise, hitting a ball back and forth on a court has been a pastime for about a thousand years. The earliest precursor of modern tennis was a game of handball played by monks in 11th century France over a string stretched across the monastery courtyard. They also used the walls and roofs of the surrounding buildings to ricochet the shots, like racquetball and squash games do today. The hard ball was tough on the hands, and later players wore gloves and then webbed gloves, which evolved into the use of paddles, then racquets. As early as 1528, Henry VIII played a game called tennis that used a wooden racquet strung with sheep gut to hit a solid ball over a net; however, each serve had to bounce off a sloping roof. That game, called *court tennis* by Americans, is still played at Hampton Court Palace outside London and in a handful of places around the world.

During the 1900s, lawn tennis became popular, often played on croquet lawns; a kit with a temporary net and all the other necessary gear transformed the pitch into a tennis court. Around that time, Wimbledon was founded as the first *lawn tennis* tournament. Eventually, lawn tennis overtook croquet as the amusement of choice for the upper crust. (Early tournaments had no prize money because you had to be wealthy to play.) To earn a living at the game meant a tough schedule of touring as a professional, or teaching at a club. Pro players were banned from competitions until 1968, when Open tournaments were first played. Eventually, the game became available to the middle class and even minorities, changing the lily-white history (white players, white balls, white togs) into the dynamic sport now played at the U.S. Open and on courts all over the country.

SCORE

If you weigh 150 pounds, you'll burn about 300 calories in an hour of doubles tennis. (To calculate your hourly burn rate, multiply your weight in pounds by two.) Singles tennis burns about 420 calories in an hour for a 150-pound person (or 2.8 times your weight).

TENNIS

Scoring in tennis is a throwback to historic French terminology. The points are love, fifteen, thirty, forty, deuce, advantage, and the win. *Love* is zero, which some experts say originated with the null score being called an egg or, in French, *l'oeuf* (pronounced "luff"). The points used to be in intervals of fifteen, but the final number was reduced to forty (perhaps some lazy players got tired of saying the "five" when everyone knew what they meant with the shorthand "forty").

Up until forty, if both players have the same number of points, the score is called as "fifteen all" or "thirty all." Once the score reaches forty, the next player who is ahead by two points wins. At that point, a tied score is called *deuce* (a term thought to have evolved from another French term: *à deux le jeu*, which means "of two the game"—or roughly, "both in the game"). When a player scores after forty, that player is said to have the *advantage*, because he could win on the next point. Advantage in, or "ad in" is when the server could win. "Ad out" is when the advantage is on the receiver's side.

One player will serve for an entire game, then the other for the next game. Games are played in a group called a set, which is won when one player takes six games and has won two more games than the opponent. When both players win six games each, there may be a tiebreaker, rather than continuing to play until there's a two-game lead (for evenly matched players, that could take all day). Three or five sets equals a match. In a three-set match, the first player to win two sets wins the match. A five-set match is won by the first player taking three sets.

Tennis is now played on three surfaces: grass, clay, and hard courts, with grass the least common. *Hard courts* are the easiest to find. They can be made of concrete, asphalt, Astroturf, or other materials. On grass and hard courts, the ball bounces quickly, and *rallies* (hitting back and forth until someone scores) tend to be short and intense. *Clay courts* are softer and slower, with a higher bounce to the ball. The court has a fine coating of dust-like gravel on the surface that can be tough on asthma and contact lenses. But these courts slow the game sufficiently to help beginners learn the strokes, and the ball leaves a mark on the surface, making it easy to tell if the shot has gone out of bounds. If you have a clay court available, try it to feel the difference.

The fancy history, long matches, odd method of scoring, and high-tech racquets might make the game seem inaccessible. But the basics of tennis are easy to learn, and beginners can enjoy the sport right away without spending much on gear. You need only learn a few rules and skills to play a decent novice game. And if you prefer, you can hit the ball around without even that much prep work.

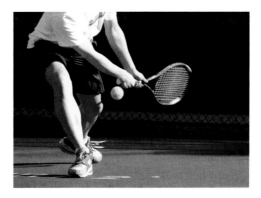

GEARING UP

If the game of tennis seems faster and more power-packed than it used to, you can blame part of it on weight-lifting, which produces stronger strokes and athleticism on the court, and the rest on high-tech racquets. Beginning in the 1970s, the classic wood frames were replaced first by metal, and then by the lightweight but strong graphite composites such as graphite-titanium. While wooden racquets would warp if they were made larger, the new materials allowed for larger heads and longer strings, delivering more power, fewer missed shots, and a larger sweet spot. The gear improvements translate into 150 mile per hour serves at the U.S. Open—but also an easier time for you learning the game.

When you buy your first racquet, look for one that's fairly large (an oversize head of 100 square inches or more), light enough for you to manage with ease (about 10 ounces), and that has a thick frame (25 mm or more) to deliver more power. Many racquets now come an inch longer than standard (28 rather than 27), which adds power to your swing; but they are a tad harder to control. Unless you are petite or have weak arms, you'll probably do fine with the longer model. For your first racquet, look for one that is balanced in the head weight and handle weight, not head-heavy or head-light.

The best plan is to borrow racquets to try out different styles so that you can learn what you like. When that's not an option, get solid sales help at a specialty store or high-end sporting goods store. Swing the racquet in various patterns to see if it feels comfortable. Make sure the grip fits your hand size. When you're ready to buy, you can get a pre-strung racquet for under $100 that will be perfect until your skills advance quite a bit.

Next, you need tennis balls. It's proper tennis etiquette to bring an unopened can of balls with you every time you play, even if you don't use them. For court play, you can pick up a can of three balls from any sporting goods store or online. Advanced players will open a fresh can at least once a week because the balls go flat quickly. Mildly flat balls don't bounce as far, which can be an advantage as you try to learn because the game will be slower. But a flat ball can also mean you need to run farther to get to the shot. Try old and new balls to see which you prefer. And keep in mind that other players often prefer fresh, faster balls.

To make learning easier, consider a foam ball. These balls have the same weight and bounce like a regular tennis ball, but the Nerf-like foam slows them down so you have more time to set up your next shot. Large sporting goods stores and online retailers have them, under names such as foam warm-up balls or transition balls or sponge speed balls.

Spare yourself some discomfort and pick up a pair of decent tennis sneakers. Playing tennis in running shoes or fashion sneakers can lead to damage to your feet, painful shin splints, or a twisted ankle. Your tennis shoes need a combination of cushioning and support for the leaps, lunges, quick stops, and side-to-side moves of a court sport, without so much weight that you feel sluggish. You don't need to spend a lot to get a quality shoe, but you do need to hop around the store in them to be sure you aren't jamming a toe or slipping sideways as you lunge for a shot.

Most players don't wear sunglasses on the court because they can limit the field of vision, but a hat or visor will help shade your eyes from glaring rays. Look for a soft band at the brow to soak up sweat so it doesn't drip into your eyes and sting them.

You don't need fancy tennis clothes to play, but large pockets are nice for holding extra balls so you can free your hands as you rally. Be sure you can move freely in the outfit you select, including overhead swinging of the arms and deep crouches with your legs. You'll warm up quickly as you play, so if the temperature is cool, wear a light jacket that you can remove.

Bring a bottle of water to the court and wear sunscreen if you play outdoors. A bag and a racquet cover are generally welcome additions to your gear list.

YOUR FIRST TIME

Start out with a knowledgeable friend or tennis professional showing you how to grip the racquet properly and the right way to execute a *forehand*, a *backhand* shot and a basic *serve*. Those few skills will allow you to play your first game, but they can take an entire lesson (or more) to learn because seemingly simple techniques such as the forehand swing start with your stance and involve more than just how you move your arm. Once you understand the basics, practice the swing with just the racquet until it feels comfortable. Then practice your shots by hitting a ball against a wall.

When you are ready to play, arrange a game with an opponent or coach. Leave enough time to stretch a little before your scheduled court time. Do some gentle moving stretches, such as walking with long strides to loosen the hips and swinging your torso from side to side to warm up the abdominal and back

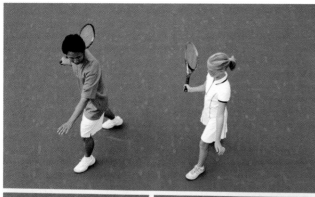

muscles. When you arrive at the court, remember that it's impolite to walk near players in the middle of a point. If you need to cross behind another court to get to yours, wait until the rally is over.

The winner of a coin toss or spin of the racquet will determine who gets to serve first or on which end of the court you begin. The server stands behind the *baseline* (the end line, furthest from the net), to one side of the center line (to the right for the first serve, switching sides for each point). Before serving, the player calls the score, putting his score first, then tosses the ball up, hitting it before it

bounces. The serve must pass over the net into the box diagonal from the server's position. If the serve hits the top of the net, it is repeated. When the serve falls outside the box, it is called a *fault* and the server gets a second chance. Two faults equal a point scored for the receiving player, and hence the second serve is usually a more conservative shot than the first.

For novice singles games, the receiving player generally stands forward of the baseline on the side of the court to which the serve is directed, letting it bounce once inside the box before returning it. After the serve, the players can move about freely on the court. The ball must make it over the net (it can touch en route) and can bounce only once inside the lines of the court. If a ball is out of bounds, do not return it; if you do, it is still in play and you don't get the point. A shot that lands on the line is in bounds. The rally continues until one player misses the ball, it bounces twice, or a shot goes out of bounds. No matter who served, the last player to hit the ball in bounds gets the point. A player who touches the net or drops his racquet while hitting the ball loses the point. The point may be replayed if there is a disagreement about whether or not it was in bounds or if there was a distraction such as the ball from an adjacent game landing on your court.

At the end of the game, the second player takes over the serve for the next game. After the second game, the players switch sides of the court, and the serve returns to the first server, and so on. At the end of play, opponents shake hands at the net.

During the game, it's important to pick up missed balls that lie within the court and close surroundings. It's easy to lose track of them if you leave them lying about, and you could land on one while running for a shot, causing a twisted ankle or nasty fall. If a ball has crossed into another court, do not retrieve it until after the players have paused between points. And if someone else's ball rolls into your court, you can wait until your point is done before returning it. If it's convenient, it's polite to toss it back yourself rather than wait for them to come get it.

Players who like to stay near the back of the court are called baseliners. Some like to rush up and play near the net for a faster, more aggressive game with fewer bounces. This position can intimidate your opponent, but a well-placed lob shot over your head will send you rushing back to return the ball.

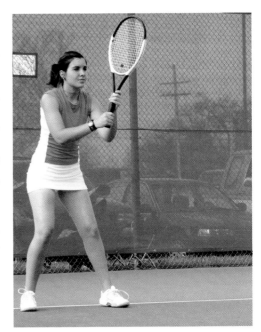

ATHLETE IN ACTION

Barbara DiSchino, 53

Growing up as a tomboy in Texas, Barbara DiSchino loved keeping pace with her two brothers. Though naturally athletic and drawn to tennis, she ruled out the sport while in school because she couldn't master the scoring. She was incredulous when her physical education teacher suggested she try out for the high school tennis team anyway. "I figured I shouldn't play a game I couldn't keep score in!"

At 30, DiSchino finally indulged her interest by signing up for lessons from the parks and recreation department where she lives in Medfield, Massachusetts. Thirteen years later, when her family gave her tennis lessons as a Mother's Day gift, the pro encouraged her to take tennis more seriously. DiSchino joined a local club. "I was in way over my head," DiSchino remembers. In fact, another pro she met, a Tennis Hall of Fame inductee, even told her, "You'll never be a tennis player." Competitive by nature, his com-

ment only spurred her on. "He's gonna eat those words!" DiSchino decided. DiSchino joined a doubles team, although "it was hard to find a partner who would take me on with no experience."

Eventually, she paired up with a patient older woman who helped her learn the scoring and the finer points of the game. But after two years, they had won only four of their thirty-six matches. DiSchino needed more wins.

She joined the U.S. Tennis Association and started playing competitively. "I also begged my way on to a weekend team as a sub for practices or matches or anything," she says. With four kids, an ailing parent and a part-time job, DiSchino worked hard to squeeze her new passion into her schedule. She played weekends and evenings and credits her husband ("my biggest cheerleader") for clearing time on the calendar. The sport helped her lose the post-baby weight she was still carrying around and provided a needed break from stress. When her ill father came to watch her compete, DiSchino was thrilled to win for him. After he died, she says, "Tennis time and cama-

raderie kept me going." The exercise and support of teammates boosted her spirits because she could focus on the ball instead of on her problems. "Tennis is a sport that you have to concentrate on while you are playing, and it is a good 'get-away.' It helped me through a lot," she recalls.

In addition to having supportive teammates, DiSchino matched up with a new partner four years ago, which brought the wins she craved. Clare Donahue keeps a cool head on the court, which is the perfect complement to DiSchino's fierce competitiveness. They make a formidable pair, and in 2004 they won the New England doubles title for their rating (3.5) and received their trophy at the Tennis Hall of Fame. Last year, DiSchino's team earned a spot to compete in the national championship and tied for fifth place.

Not surprisingly, DiSchino isn't content to rest on her laurels. "Because we played at Nationals, we have to move up a level. We are almost halfway through the season, and a first place tie is one point away!"

TACKLE THE TRUTH

You need to take months of pricey lessons to be good at tennis

If you can hit the ball over the net and inside the lines, you're playing tennis. There are plenty of pros who teach tennis and can help your game progress, even with just one session's worth of pointers —and lessons aren't always expensive. You can look for good deals with your local parks department, for example. But you don't need a single lesson to get out on the court and have fun, plus get a great workout. The rules are easy to learn, too. If you're nervous, augment your knowledge with a basic book or get information online.

To play tennis, you have to be very coordinated

The key to a great game of tennis is being in the right place. If you can anticipate the action, which you'll learn with practice, you can get into position to return shots easily. In the right spot, you'll have a choice of a forehand or backhand swing, a smash down the center line or a lob over your opponent's head. But if you're late getting to the ball, you will only be able to get your racquet on it for whatever type of shot is easiest in that position. Rather than focusing on coordination, spend your time learning the game, watching your opponent's strategies, and improving your speed on the court with foot-speed drills (you can find them in any tennis book, magazine, or on Web sites).

I'll get tennis elbow and end up in horrible pain

It's possible to get tennis elbow from playing tennis—and from using tools, vacuuming, playing baseball, and other actions. The condition is more common in beginners than advanced players, because it happens from poor stroke mechanics and off-kilter shots that send strong vibrations up the arm. The ache and pain of tennis elbow, or lateral epicondylitis, is caused by an inflamed tendon—the one that attaches the top of the forearm muscle to the upper arm bone. The condition is a repetitive strain injury, usually because you move your wrist during backhand shots. If your elbow feels sore during or after a game, try a lighter racquet with a bigger head, which allows less of the vibration into your arm and fewer thunks from almost-missed returns. If you have trouble, you can attach a small dampening device (about $5) to your racquet strings or wear a strap ($10 to $20) just below the elbow to halt the vibration's travel. Treat the ache with ice, rest, and an over-the-counter painkiller such as ibuprofen. But don't return to the game doing the same thing or you'll have repeated problems. Request instruction on your stroke mechanics to avoid future flare-ups. You can also strengthen the muscles above and below the elbow to help prevent the problem.

TENNIS

SECRETS TO SUCCESS

When you want to play a game of tennis, it helps to be able to describe your abilities to possible opponents. It's easy when you can say, "I've only played once," but after your skills have progressed a little, it can be harder to describe your level in words. And just because another player has been practicing and playing for years, doesn't mean he's better than you are. To solve the problem, there's a rating system. Player ratings start at 1.0 for someone who hasn't played before and go up to 7.0 for a world champion. At 2.0, you know the basic rules and make some good shots but need to work on your strokes and get more practice, and at 2.5 you can keep a short, easy rally going. A good match is any player within half a point of your rating. "If you're not sure of your level, sign up for a program and the instructor will place you into a level-appropriate group," suggests Bill Mountford, director of tennis for the United States Tennis Association (USTA) National Tennis Center in New York, which is the home of the U.S. Open. You can get rated with a single lesson, as well.

When you're learning and practicing, it's easy to get stymied by everything you're trying to master. Don't be. "Sometimes, it helps just to try to hit the ball over the net and not worry about every detail of stroke mechanics," advises Mountford. To improve, you need a combination of skills plus practice, not simply an overwhelming influx of instruction. On the court, you want to stay light on your feet and ready to move at all times.

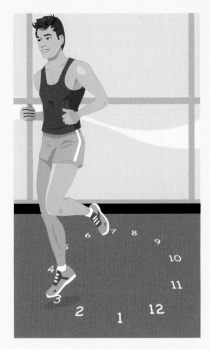

clock drill

Take a piece of chalk and sit on a flat, hard surface, such as a sidewalk or driveway. Without leaning, mark the ground as far as you can reach to the side with each hand. Get up and use the two marks to draw a circle, as if they were 3 and 9 o'clock on a clock face. Mark all the hours around the circle. (If you can't get to an appropriate outdoor location, picture an imaginary clock.) Stand at 6, facing 12. Hop with your left foot to 12. Then hop backwards to 6 with your right foot. Next, hop with your left foot to 10, then back to 6. Hop to 2 with your left foot, then back to 6. Continue to 4 and 8 to finish the circle's even numbers. Again starting at 6, repeat the drill but this time hop forward with the right foot and back with the left. Once you've learned the pattern, pick up the speed. Continue, as fast as you can safely go, for 2 minutes. Build up to 5 minutes.

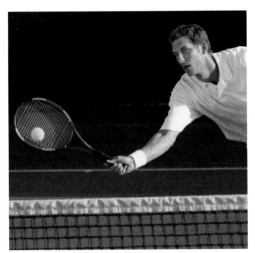

Many shots are missed because the player was stuck in place. To avoid this problem, stay up on the forward half of your feet, knees slightly bent, racquet out and ready to hit. Staying on the front of your feet will absorb the impact of the movement and protect your knees, hips, and back from strain.

Also consider some off-the-court drills. "All the champion players skip rope for fast feet," says Mountford. And they work out with weights, plus do stamina sessions. The game is full of stops and starts, so you want to do some cardio intervals to build your capacity for sprints. And the rapid change of direction that's part of play gets easier if you do leg-strengthening exercises. To get used to the feel of the stroke and build strength, swing your racquet with the cover on or hold two racquets and swing them together. During play, your racquet will feel light in comparison.

Try these drills to improve your game:

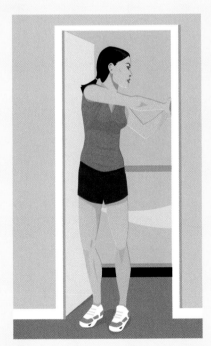

trunk twists

Stand in a standard doorway (roughly 3 feet wide). Step forward about 12 inches. Reach back to the left to touch both hands to the door frame, keeping your feet in position, moving your head to see where you are touching. Return to center. Reach to the right and return to center. Repeat 30 times (stop if you get dizzy). Do 3 sets.

GET MORE FROM YOUR SPORT

Running around on the court after errant shots provides plenty of aerobic exercise. But if you find your game is more stop, retrieve the ball, try again—and your heart rate isn't elevated enough to feel like a good workout—consider trying Cardio Tennis (www.cardiotennis.com). The program incorporates fast-paced drills and skills with up to eight players and one coach on the court and music playing to keep you moving. It was developed by the USTA to provide a tennis-based aerobics class that's fun, sweaty, and can help improve your game. It's offered at parks and clubs across the country, and the format can accommodate players of all levels.

Tennis players tend to enjoy the footwork, hand-eye coordination, and strategic component of fencing, boxing, and martial arts. These sports also incorporate full-body strength, control, and excellent aim. If you want to work mainly on developing fast, strong legs, try step aerobics, cycling, running, or dancing. To improve your balance and core strength, turn to skating, gymnastics, pilates, and yoga.

It's commonly believed that playing racquetball or squash will ruin your tennis game. But these sports are fast and fun, and you shouldn't rule them out unless you personally find they hurt your tennis stroke. And you might just find you prefer one of the other sports. Handball and jai alai are also great options if you can find a game.

Amateurs can play in leagues all over the country that have local competitions. You can also progress to play in national tournaments. But one of the most enjoyable aspects of the game is finding courts in beautiful destinations for play at any level. Many major hotels and resorts offer court time and lessons. For a luxury vacation with some serious tennis coaching, try Topnotch Resort at Stowe, in Vermont (www.topnotchresort.com) or the spa and tennis combination at the Vic Braden Tennis College held at Green Valley Spa Resort in Utah (www.vicbradentennis.com). Braden also offers family camps and a three-day course, which focus on tennis without the spa treatments and hikes.

RESOURCES

➡ **www.usta.com** is the site for the U.S. Tennis Association, where you'll find links to players, courts, and leagues in your area, tips on the game, the rule book and more.

➡ **www.tennis.com** is the website of *Tennis* magazine. It offers a comprehensive guide to buying racquets and shoes, as well as weekly tennis tips.

➡ **www.tennis4you.com** houses a huge archive of articles on shot-making, conditioning and mental preparation. This site is a must-read for both tennis beginners and more experienced players.

➡ *Tennis for Dummies* by Patrick McEnroe with Peter Bodo is one of the better guides in the series. The book covers everything from strokes and scoring to injury prevention and conditioning.

➡ *Visual Tennis* by John Yardell works on the assumption that a picture is worth a thousand words. The popular book is packed with photographs of proper stroke execution, along with descriptions of the finer points of technique.

TENNIS

Staying Hydrated When It's Hot

Sweat much? Good for you. Perspiration, the body's mechanism for cooling down, becomes more efficient when you're more fit. When you play in warm places, your body is "practicing" using its sweat system and getting better at it each time, a process called acclimatization. No matter what your sport, breaking into a sweat sooner than you used to and sweating more indicates that you've made gains in health and performance.

On the other hand, perspiration only counts toward your fitness goals if it's the result of exertion. You won't get fitter from sweating because you've piled on too many clothes. Heat does loosen up your muscles and improve circulation, which is why stepping into a sauna or steam room can relieve aches and muscle fatigue. The same principles apply to your pre-sports warm-up. If you want to wear extra gear until you're warm, go for it. But once you start to sweat, lose the layers.

It's tempting to bundle up because the scale registers lighter at the end of a serious sweat session, but you're not cooking off pounds. In an hour of exercising, you'll lose about 2 pounds (1 liter) of water; a tough game of basketball or beach volleyball under a scorching sun can double that number. But as soon as you have a drink, the weight returns. The body hordes water to replenish its supply because being dehydrated has serious negative consequences—more than you probably realize. If your core body temperature rises too much you can actually fry your brain, causing irreparable damage. Dehydration also causes confusion, fatigue, and headaches. It can lead to constipation, kidney ailments and other medical problems.

You'll need to drink before you get thirsty because the body doesn't sense dehydration early enough. It doesn't take long to sweat yourself into mild dehydration. About two hours before heading out to play, prep your body by downing 2 cups of water. When you're active, drink a cup every twenty minutes at least. And if you'll be at it for an hour or more, switch to a sports drink. These beverages contain salts your body loses in sweat and also are formulated so you absorb them quickly for maximal hydration.

> ★ **FACT:**
> When you're thirsty, you may mistake the signal as hunger. Try drinking a glass of water before sitting down for a snack.

In addition to the dangers of extreme dehydration, keep in mind that even mild dehydration makes your workout less productive; you won't be able to push your body as hard as you can when you stay fully hydrated. The dip in performance is partly caused by your heart: When you're dehydrated, the heart has to beat harder to move blood around your body, making you more winded and tired. Also, a properly cooled body burns fat for energy, while an overheated one switches to using sugar—and that's detrimental to endurance and, some experts argue, could reduce weight loss. And mild dehydration can reduce your mental ability enough to make you play poorly.

For the best results, keep your body well-hydrated all day long rather than trying to pound down all the water you need only around your workout. Start with a full glass every morning before you brush your teeth, keep a bottle of a beverage on your desk and in your car so you can sip all day, and fill up at meals (plus, you'll eat less and may lose weight). Just be sure you're choosing water or sports drinks—not sodas and lots of juices—because the calories do add up.

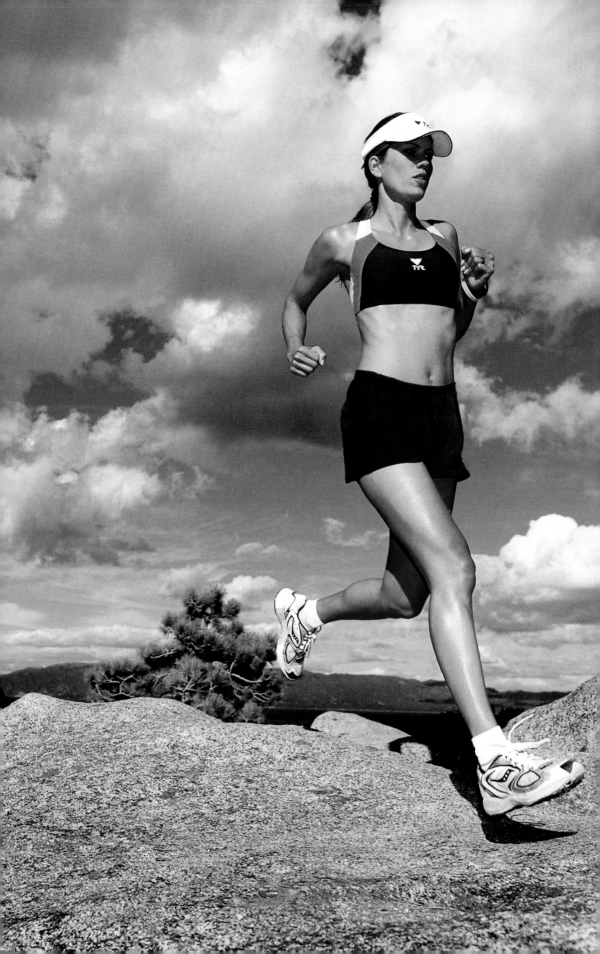

21

TRAIL RUNNING
AND CROSS-COUNTRY SKIING

YOU'LL LOVE THESE SPORTS IF YOU:
- desire an intense cardio challenge
- love a sport that feels good but burns lots of calories
- want a core- and leg-toning workout
- love beautiful scenery
- want to play outdoors any time of year
- appreciate a sport that's so distracting you'll forget you're exercising
- enjoy sport vacations and weekend getaways
- prefer a sport that can be solitary or, depending on your mood, packed with people

YOU MIGHT NOT LOVE THESE SPORTS IF YOU:
- need instant success—these sports involve learning some skills before you're proficient
- never want to fall; these sports don't always involve falls, but they do happen
- fear being out in the woods
- hate being cold, wet, or other seasonal or weather-related discomforts
- have a terrible sense of direction

Give your lungs and heart the best possible workout while enjoying gorgeous scenery and peaceful surroundings. Those are a few of the benefits from trail running and cross-country skiing. Compared to running on pavement, these sports can be far gentler on your joints and provide a better all-around workout. Trail running can involve some paved bike paths or hard-packed fire roads, which are not so different from jogging down the street, but more often you'll run on hiking trails and mountain-bike paths. These softer surfaces, from dirt to sand to grass, are better shock absorbers for your feet, knees, and back. Also, your movements are not limited to plodding forward, one foot after the next. Trail runners sidestep, walk up hills, scramble up rocks, and generally engage in a much more varied set of movements than street joggers. Cross-country skiing is even gentler on the joints, except when you fall. A skier's body moves in a graceful extended line, using all the body's muscles for an unparalleled workout. Athletes who compete in these sports are some of the fittest in the world. If you aspire to compete, there are plenty of options open to people at all levels, with many adult beginners managing respectable results before long. But many more people simply pursue these activities recreationally to get into great shape.

Both sports are incredibly enjoyable. Doing them outdoors is nothing like the treadmill or ski machine in a gym. You get away from congestion and smog, heading off into the woods, but still maintain an intense level of activity that quickly translates into a meditative calm that's energetic yet soothing for a dose of runner's high. Either sport will take you to remote, pristine places some of which may be too far to access at the slower pace of a hike or snowshoe trek. Plus, there's nothing quite like coming in after a brisk workout in the snow to a cup of cocoa or hot soup. Plan your outings around a good lunch destination for the ultimate pleasure; a fireplace is a bonus.

Some trail runners and cross-country skiers are solitary types who enjoy the sports because of the lack of crowds (although it's never really smart to go off into the woods alone, so stick to somewhat traveled trails or bring a friend along). Others seek out clubs and events for the camaraderie. Many athletes use these sports as part of a crosstraining program to complement other woodsy activities, from bird walks to snowshoeing. And families can easily participate as a group; you'll find toddler events at some trail-running races and youth divisions in cross-country ski events.

SCORE

If you weigh 150 pounds, you'll burn about 480 calories in an hour of cross-country running (or 3.2 times your weight in pounds). This number is the closest estimate to trail running, but if you're competing at an intense level, you'll burn more. For cross-country skiing, there is more data available from exercise physiology labs testing the relationship between pace and calorie burn. Check the chart for your burn rate.

Miles/hour	Effort	Calories/hour*	Calories/hour/lb
2.5	Slow, walking pace	360	2.4
4–4.9	Moderate, leisurely	420	2.8
5–7.9	Brisk, vigorous	480	3.2
> 8	Racing	780	5.2
Uphill	Maximal exertion	930	6.2

* 150-lb person

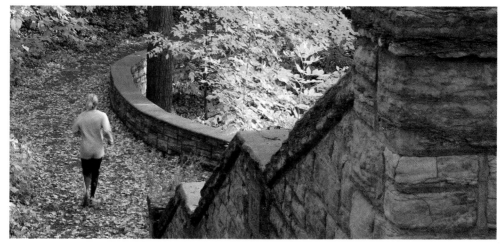

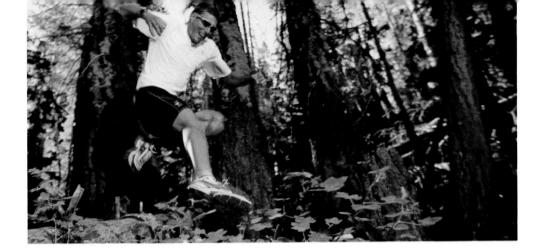

TRAIL RUNNING

Like hiking, trail running has been around for as long as man has walked on two feet. During the early 1800s, a team race called the Paper Chase (or Hare and Hounds) was held as a school competition in England. In these races, one team would dash off, leaving a paper trail over a jagged route, and the second team would try to follow the trail and catch them. The chase was imported to the U.S. in 1888 and shortly afterward morphed into the still-popular college sport, cross-country running, in which points are awarded based on the finishing order for each team member and tallied for the final score.

Trail running is the next evolution, an individual sport with far fewer participants for some events, so runners may be alone on portions of the trail. In competition, the course is marked and longer runs have stations with food, water, and first-aid supplies. There may be checkpoints at which the runner must record his name to prove he has completed the proper course. Trail-running races can be as short as 3 kilometers (about 2 miles), but many are marathons and ultramarathons, with some of the most famous covering 100 miles or more.

On a trail run, you can expect to climb over rocks and tree stumps, scramble up steep ascents (sometimes using a rope for assistance), run through streams, squish in mud, cross deserts, traverse snow-capped peaks, and even run through tunnels and caves. Many of the prestigious races take place at high altitudes, which adds to the challenge. And runners will proceed much more slowly off-road than on a paved course, because of the obstacles, so even for elite athletes, the winning times may seems slow. Of course, a recreational runner can simply head for the local park and do a little running on hiking or bridle paths. Any length of run can easily be translated into an off-road jaunt, but short distances in well-traveled areas are the easiest because they don't require any extra planning or gear. A longer run or more isolated destination necessitates preparations such as getting a trail map and toting along food and water, maybe even a compass or *global positioning system* (GPS).

GEARING UP

The one indispensable item of gear for trail running is, of course, footwear. While some people use off-road sandals or light hiking boots, most runners opt for regular running shoes or trail running shoes. The latter are lower to the ground, often stiffer, and wider for more stability. They also tend to have more pronounced tread for better traction that's spaced wider so as not to get caked with mud. If you are shopping for a true trail shoe, watch out for shoes that have trail-running cosmetics—mainly darker colors—but lack these other adaptations for off-road running. You can buy water-resistant shoes, but since runs could involve plunging knee deep in a stream or up to your ankles in mud, a coating on the shoe won't keep the wet from seeping in over the top, and it may make the shoe stay soggy longer. A better bet: footwear that will dry quickly made of thinner mesh, paired with wool or synthetic socks that won't cause blisters when wet.

Any jogging clothes will work for trail running, but competitors tend to select ultra-lightweight options that are close-fitting so they won't snag on branches or brush.

Fabrics that wick away moisture and dry quickly are recommended for long, sweaty runs. Wearing layers and a hat is vital, because conditions will change from glaring sun to shaded woods. And the usual precau-

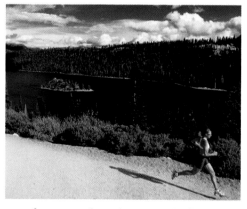

tions for seasonal conditions apply, from sunscreen to bug spray. Also, hydration is an important consideration in trail running. Many runners opt for water pouches with sip tubes in backpacks or lumbar packs, or tucked inside specially designed vests that also provide a pocket or two for some snacks and a map. Some runners carry hand bottles or wear waist packs designed to hold regular water bottles and food. Endurance runners who will be out for more than four hours may rely on calorie-dense foods in small packages, such as energy bars and gels. And they often use salt tablets to replenish electrolytes lost in sweat.

YOUR FIRST TIME

It's easy to start trail running—simply identify a safe, well-marked trail and take your regular run off-road. Or pick up the pace on your hike until you're running some or all of it. Enjoy the scenery and the silence, but keep an eye on the terrain and the time. Running on a trail will take far longer than

you might expect, and overestimating how far you can go while getting back before dark is one of the most common beginner's mistakes. Test out your pace with a short initial outing so you can plan properly. Also, bring more water and snacks than you would for a hike or road run, because you'll be burning more fuel and sweating more.

Don't be surprised if you have to walk on your trail run. Sometimes the footing is too tricky or the ascent too steep to keep running. Even the top competitors slow down for safety or to take a breather. For downhill sections, you'll want to choose your foot placement carefully, which often necessitates a slower pace.

Bumps and scrapes can be part of the territory when the terrain is technically challenging. And beginners sometimes suffer an ankle roll, but top competitors rarely do. The more you run off-road, the stronger your ankle-stabilizing muscles will become. Your technique for avoiding a twisted ankle will also improve, such as learning to correct your footing as soon as you sense the beginning of a roll-over. And you'll learn to better judge the terrain, too. While you're learning, keep your pace slow enough to avoid these minor injuries.

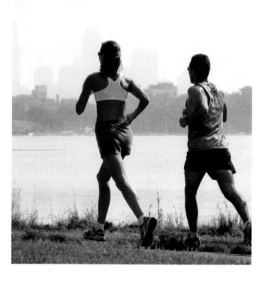

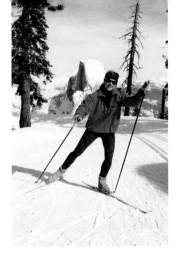
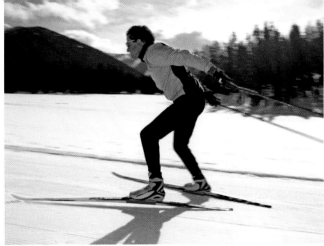

CROSS-COUNTRY SKIING

About five thousand years ago, the natives of Norway invented cross-country skiing as a method of transportation, and the sport is often called "Nordic skiing" (although purists point out that the Nordic category also includes ski jumping). The first recordings of recreational skiing were races in Iceland in 1000 AD. The activity is a traditional sport in Scandinavia, and some of the world's fastest skiers come from these countries—as did the first men credited for bringing the sport to the U.S. Today, cross-country skiing is one of the fastest growing sports in America, according to the National Sporting Goods Association.

There are three styles of cross-country skiing. *Classic technique* involves keeping both skis in a parallel position. Nordic centers that groom trails with a double track are popular places to go for classic cross-country skiing, and some races are designated for classic skiers only. This technique is often recommended for nervous beginners and non-athletes because you start by simply shuffling along on two skis, like walking. It will feel awkward at first as it takes a while to get the proper rhythm of the kick and glide and arm movements. *Skate skiing* is faster and involves alternating pushing one ski out in a V pattern, like ice or in-line skating. This type of skiing is only suited to smooth snow such as is found on groomed trails (without the double track). The motions are harder to learn (unless you're an accomplished skater), often taking a handful of lessons to learn with any proficiency. Wannabe racers often start with this style of skiing because it is faster and used in more races. For competitions

designated "free," skiers may choose to skate ski or use classic style, and most choose to skate. Some races are called double pursuit and require competitors to complete one portion using classic technique while the other is free. The third category, *Telemark* skiing, is named after the Norwegian town where it originated. Although it's officially a type of cross-country skiing because the heel of the boot is not attached to the ski, Telemark technique is designed for going downhill and uses fatter skis with metal edges, more like downhill skis. Many Telemarkers use ski-resort lifts to go up, unlike classic and skate skiers who ski whether the terrain is uphill, flat, or downhill. Classic and skate skiers may borrow the Telemark technique for skiing downhill, although it's more challenging on skinnier skis.

In addition to Nordic centers, you can cross-country ski almost anywhere there's snow cover. After a good snowstorm, you'll find Nordic skiers on the street, on hiking trails, bike and bridle paths, and golf courses.

GEARING UP

Cross-country skiing is sometimes referred to as "free-heeling" because the back of the boot is not attached to the ski. Novices often begin with rentals to test whether they like the sport, to decide whether they prefer classic or skate skiing, and to get a feel for the gear before making the investment. If you choose the classic style and want to cruise local parks and golf courses, you can get a decent set of equipment (skis, poles, boots)

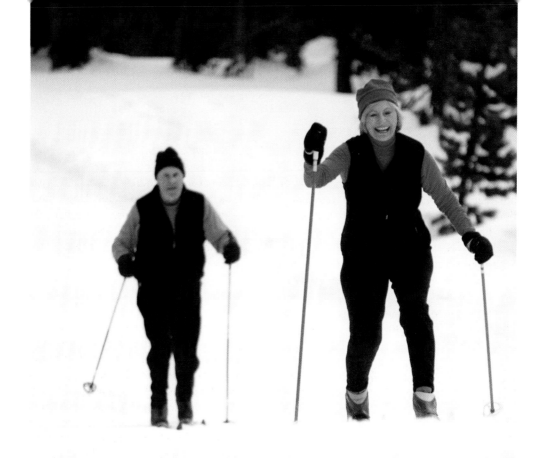

from any ski shop or outdoor retailer. If you aspire to race, consider signing up for a rental/lesson combo at a Nordic center before investing in your own gear so you know more about equipment subtleties before making a purchase.

With classic skis, when you step down on one ski, the center flattens to make contact with the snow, and it must grip to provide traction for the push that propels you forward. When you unweight the ski, the center (called the *kick zone*) comes off the snow and the tip and tail glide. The skis are designed to grip or glide either through the application of different waxes to the different zones, or, if the skis are *waxless*, a pattern is carved in the kick zone that acts as a tread to generate grip. ("Waxless" is a bit of a misnomer because these skis still require a wax coating for maintenance and glide, but they are considerably lower-maintenance than waxed skis.) The waxless style of ski is popular these days for its convenience, but serious skiers may prefer to wax their skis for improved performance, because the etched pattern in the kick zone limits gliding. Waxes are designed to work

with specific snow conditions, based on temperature and whether the snow is fresh-fallen or old. As a beginner, consider renting waxless skis so you can enjoy the sport with less prep time. The reduced gliding may actually be a benefit while you're learning.

Skating skis have more of an edge on their insides to help skiers carve clean lines for forward propulsion. The skis are generally shorter than the classic variety and weigh less because skating is designed for speed.

In addition to skis, you'll need boots and poles. These items are part of the rental package, or you can bring your own. Poles are longer than downhill versions, but similar in that they have a point and a basket at the bottom, a grip and wrist strap at the top. Skating poles are longer and stiffer than the classic style. They are made from a variety of materials, with lighter poles being more expensive and having design improvements to enhance performance, but they are also easier to break.

The boots look like sleek hiking shoes with an extended front to secure into the bindings. Classic style boots are the softest, with "combi" boots falling in between, and skating boots feeling stiffer. But all the boots are light and more comfortable than downhill ski boots, and modern versions may offer breathable insulation and water resistance. Boots and bindings come in different styles that must be matched to work together.

In powder conditions, you'll also want gaiters, water-resistant covers worn over the pant leg from the knee down. Gaiters have elastic at the top and secure under the boot to stay in place, so you don't get wet from the snow, and they offer additional warmth and wind resistance.

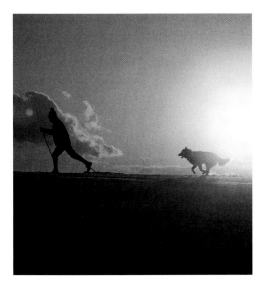

Nordic skiing apparel is designed for winter conditions but is not bulky or heavily insulated, because you generate a lot of heat working this hard. Wicking layers are *de rigueur*. Be careful not to overdress, especially when it comes to gloves and hats, which must be thinner to allow heat to escape so you don't get sweaty and soggy (and then freeze when you stop to catch your breath). The gloves should have palms that allow you to grip the poles securely. A tube-shaped neck-warmer is helpful so you can open your jacket for ventilation without allowing your throat to get cold. You can also pull it up over your face to breathe through to temper air that's frigid and hurts your lungs.

Pack plenty of water. You may not realize you're sweating because of the cold, but you'll probably be working as hard doing light skiing as you would if you were taking a moderate-paced jog over the same terrain. Snacks are helpful, too. Keep the water and food where they won't freeze solid; inside coat pockets work well.

YOUR FIRST TIME

Cross-country skiing is an easy-access sport. You grab your gear, amble over to a good starting location, click in, and you're off. As with any trail sport, you should check your trail map and let someone know your plans before leaving civilization. A rank beginner should take a lesson or get a knowledgeable friend to show you how to ski. It looks easy, but you'll find a steep learning curve in either classic or skate style.

For classic technique, you'll start with a shuffling walk: The arms work in counterpoint, the left pole pushing down into the snow and back as the right foot moves back. At the same time, the left foot slides forward and the right hand comes up front in preparation for the switch. When you are comfortable with the technique, called *diagonal stride*, you can start to lean forward, kicking your heels out at the end of each stroke, gliding on the front ski to cover more distance.

For a change of pace, you can also try *double poling*, which means placing the skis parallel, planting both poles in the snow, and pushing. This technique probably will feel more natural, but it can be quite tiring. On gradual descents or flats, advanced skiers merge the two styles, double poling with a single kick afterwards.

When you find a hill that's too steep to slide straight up, one technique for ascent is called a *herringbone*. Turn your skis out in a V, alternate stepping forward, lifting the whole ski over and up, and make sure the tails don't hit. Hold the poles behind you to arrest a fall or press them into the snow behind the skis to help push your body upwards. If you slide backwards using the herringbone, consider turning perpendicular to the slope and sidestepping up. Both of these techniques seem slow and awkward, but advanced skiers can do them at a run. You'll get the hang of it with practice.

To skate ski, start on flat ground, without the poles (hold them in case you need to avert a fall). Turn the skis out in a slight V. Push down, out, and back with your right ski just as you would with an ice skate or in-line skate. Glide forward on the left diagonal with your weight centered on the left ski. Now reverse the action, pushing off with the left ski and gliding on the right. The trick is to stay balanced on the skinny ski and commit all your weight on the one foot. When you're ready to add the arms, start by using both poles together (double poling) for every other

stroke. Add poles to every stroke if you need more propulsion, such as when going uphill. There are a variety of other poling techniques, but this one will get you started.

Going down a slope free-heeling is less controlled than when you're on downhill skis, so it can be frightening—but it's also exhilarating when you accomplish it without falling. There are several options to choose, depending on the terrain: For a very slight slope, you might manage to point your skis down and glide like a downhill skier. Use your inner thigh muscles to stay stable over the skis, trying to keep them flat so your heels don't roll off. A second option is to *snowplow*, pressing the heels of the skis out, tips together to dig in the edges and execute a controlled slide. When you are more advanced at controlling the skis, you can attempt the deep-kneed Telemark

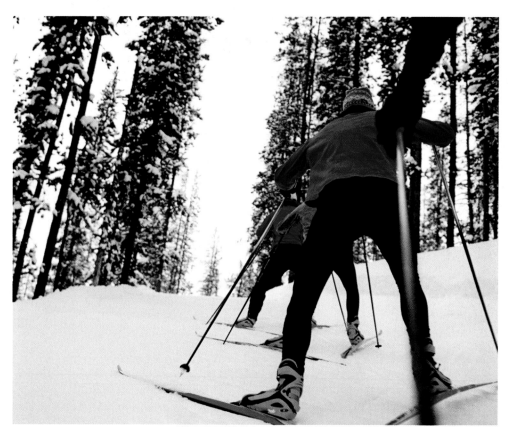

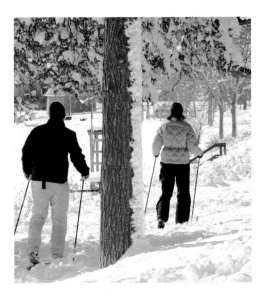

turn. And you can always sidestep down if the hill is intimidating.

The movements are certainly awkward at first, so go slowly and be patient. But don't skip the sport just because it takes longer to master the basic skills—it's intensely good exercise no matter what your skill level, and feels fluid and graceful when the technique clicks. If you're truly struggling, ask for some pointers while you're on the gym's Nordic ski machine to get a feeling for the rhythm and body position of classic style skiing, or try a lesson on snow. Nordic centers, which are often located near downhill ski resorts, typically have teaching professionals who can show you the basic techniques in one or two lessons.

ATHLETE IN ACTION

Paul Spencer, 39

An avid runner who competed in many marathons, Paul Spencer was sidelined three years ago with a herniated disc in his back that required surgery. Back on his feet after the operation, he discovered that long training runs made his back pain flare up. "I was very upset since running was a huge part of my life," he says. But around the same time, he and his wife moved to Bend, Oregon, and Spencer saw skate skiers racing at the local Nordic center. "The technique looked so cool, and I love being outdoors, so I decided to try it," he says. That winter he ventured out a few times and fell in love with the sport—"fell" being the operative word. He signed up for a ski clinic and says: "I was a total klutz and did more falling than any of the 60-year-olds in my class. On flat sections, I'd teeter over sideways. Down hills, I'd take head-first

dives or slide on my butt." But Spencer kept showing up. "One icy day, after I'd fallen about twenty times in an hour, the instructor kept asking if I wanted to head back." He'd probably never seen anyone fall quite so much, but Spencer was a seasoned athlete who went right into skate skiing in order to compete—and even for this kind of skiing, he pushed hard. "Most people don't fall as much learning to skate ski. My wife never fell. She takes hills slowly. I was trying to emulate advanced skiers before I developed the balance," he says. "At the end of the lessons, I was usually sorer in my hips and shoulders from falling down than from my new form of exercise."

Undeterred, Spencer stayed close to the Nordic center lodge, skiing around and around a small oval track, trying to perfect his technique, resting every five to ten minutes. "I was too clumsy to venture out on real trails," he recalls. After about ten lessons, he had a breakthrough in balance and was

able to leave the oval and head for the woods, still falling occasionally, but now managing long stretches upright. He continued training all summer by roller skiing, which uses 2-foot long metal planks with wheels at either end "and no brakes!" he says.

By the next winter, his form had improved, and he joined a race training group. Over the next three months, Spencer completed six races. "I've had good results for someone with my level of experience," he says. "I usually finish somewhere in the first half."

"I've learned that this sport takes a long time to master," he says. "I will have to give it several years before I can expect to do really well." But in the meantime, he's had a revelation: "I cringe when I think I could still be running every day and never have discovered cross-country skiing," he says. "Back then, I couldn't imagine life without marathons, but now I hope I will be skiing for the rest of my life."

TRAILS

SECRETS TO SUCCESS

Much of the culture of recreational trail running and cross-country skiing involves back-to-nature ethics. "It's about getting away from the urban environment, which includes technology," says Adam Chase, president of the All American Trail Running Association, an avid Nordic skier and adventure racer. Even competitors may eschew gadgets such as GPS tracking devices and heart-rate monitors in a combined effort to keep it simple and lightweight. Plus, out on the trail, standard measures don't apply. "Even a good GPS system can't measure distance accurately under the forest canopy, when you're running switchbacks and going up and down, not straight," explains Chase. Event organizers will often map the trail using a measuring wheel or a mountain bike with an odometer. But the events are all about time—and your recreational and training outings are best measured that way as well. Use the RPE scale to set your intensity (see chapter 2 for instructions), especially if you travel to altitude, a factor that will independently increase your heart rate.

The varied conditions experienced during a day in the wilderness and the need to be well-prepared run counter to the desire to carry very little weight. While leaving the gizmos home, cross-country skiers and trail runners may be the first to experiment with high-tech fabrics and innovative clothing designs so they can tote a few ounces less while bringing along necessary gear for safety and comfort such as a jacket or sports drink.

These athletes pride themselves on being rugged outdoors folks, not deterred

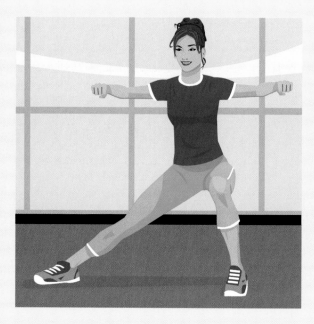

lateral lunges

Stand with your feet shoulder-width apart, abs firm, shoulders back, head up, arms bent at your sides so your elbows are tucked close, fists forward, parallel to the ground. Keeping your torso erect, take a large step to the left with your left foot, bending both knees to lower your butt as far as you can. At the same time, keeping your arms bent, lift your elbows to shoulder height. Press through your left heel and squeeze your glutes as you step back to the start. Repeat to the right to complete 1 repetition. Do 3 sets of 10 reps, building to 3 sets of 30.

by a few bumps and bruises or a little precipitation. So if you're signing up for a group outing, make sure you know the pace and comfort-level the group has in mind. If you're looking for a sedate circuit around the lake, be certain you're not joining in a competitive training loop.

While progress uphill may seem the most taxing in these sports, it's the downhill sections that require the most skill. Look ahead, not at your feet, and slow down. Try to stay light on your feet (or skis); picture yourself floating down the slope. The temptation is to lean back to move more slowly, but you're most likely to fall if your weight is in your heels. In trail running, take small steps to reduce the impact of landings on your body.

"These sports are a serious challenge for the muscles and cardiovascular system," notes Louis Dzierzak, executive editor of *Cross Country Skier* magazine. If you want to get your body ready or do some gym training on the side, focus on intense cardio, full-body strength, and plenty of balance work. "Do some cycling on a mountain bike or road bike, skating or hiking to work your legs," Dzierzak says. If you own a balance board or similar device, use it. "The variety of movements used on the trail will require more core stability than road running," says Chase. You'll also use your inner and outer thighs to stay upright and in control. Focus on these two areas when you do strength work. And try these moves:

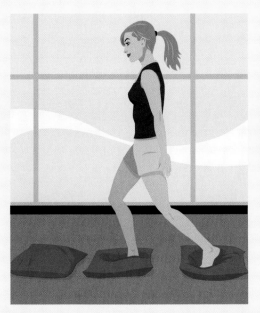

wobble work

If you don't own a wobble board, use this drill to work on your balance. Place 3 regular bed pillows or large throw pillows on the ground and step forward and back as quickly as you can safely with good form. Swing your arms forcefully to add to the challenge, moving them in different directions to test your stability. Keep going for at least 5 minutes because your balance will falter more as you get tired.

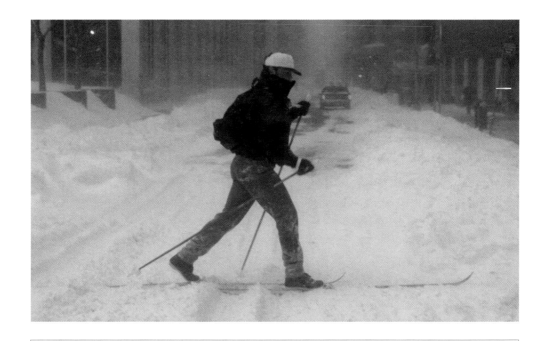

TACKLE THE TRUTH

You have to be a gonzo athlete to trail run or cross-country ski

Not true. You will find fabulously fit athletes participating and competing in these sports, and they often go on to do triathlons, adventure races and other extreme events. And elite athletes from other realms often use these sports for crosstraining because they generate huge gains in fitness and performance while staving off boredom. But for the average person, both sports are easy to scale to your ability simply by selecting easy terrain and shorter distances or by taking frequent rest breaks. And these activities are remarkably good exercise that can whip you into shape quickly, especially because they are so enjoyable you may want to keep going for hours.

You need to live in the country to have access to trails

You don't need to live near the wilderness to enjoy these sports. You can trail run and cross-country ski anywhere there's appropriate terrain. For example, you'll find runners on the bridle paths in New York City's Central Park and cross-country skiers on the gentle hills of golf courses around the country.

The pace is so much slower than on the road that I won't get a good workout

When you're in the woods, all bets are off on speed. The terrain is challenging, and you shouldn't expect to go fast. But that doesn't mean you're getting less of a workout—you're actually getting more because you use more muscles. These sports don't just tone your legs and butt. You'll use your entire body for almost every stroke in cross-country skiing, and often work your arms and torso in trail running, too.

GET MORE FROM YOUR SPORT

People who like to work out in the woods often enjoy other forms of off-road sports, including hiking, snowshoeing, rock climbing, and mountain biking. Swimming, rowing, and gymnastics provide excellent options for full-body, stamina-enhancing workouts to swap in and out with trail running and cross-country skiing. To improve your balance, take up skating, fencing, and martial arts. Nordic skiers often do their off-season training by Nordic walking, which is basically hiking with poles with a focus on maintaining the same rhythmic stride of a skier. There are also roller skis, which look like extremely long in-line skates with wheels at the ends, and also involve the use of poles just like skiing. Skiers and runners often augment their upper-body strength by kayaking and lifting weights.

It's easy to get involved in off-road racing, even as a beginner. And there are trail-running and cross-country ski competitions for kids. In the Leatherman's Loop 10K, in Cross River, New York, there's a category for children as young as one (at three-quarter mile, that's probably too tough for most one-year-olds, who may not even be walking yet!). One joy of racing is the travel. Cross-country ski and trail-running races are held in some of the most beautiful places in the world as well as some of the most inaccessible rugged destinations. There are trail-running competitions in the Sahara Desert, South Africa, and New Zealand, for example. And while Nordic ski racing is an excellent excuse to travel in Scandinavia, you'll also find events from China to the Czech Republic.

The sport of orienteering is popular with trail runners and cross-country skiers. These events require navigation skills as well as physical ability. Each competitor is given a map at the start of the race that shows the location of "control markers"—orange and white flags and a punch that proves you found it. You can get from point A to point B in any way you want, on trails or off, walking, running, skiing, snowshoeing, whatever you choose. You must collect all the punches to complete the race, but there's no specific order required.

If you like to travel, you can go to training camps for either cross-country skiing or trail running. Many ski resorts offer Nordic programs, and Craftsbury Outdoor Center in Vermont is a well-known destination for cross-country skiers who want to improve their skills (www.craftsbury.com). If you want to train seriously in trail running, try Beyond Running, a camp run by physical therapist and ultramarathoner Scott Jurek (www.beyond-running.com).

RESOURCES

➡ www.trailrunner.com is the home of the All American Trail Running Association, with links to races, gear companies, and clubs.

➡ www.trailrunnermag.com, the site for *Trail Runner* magazine, offers articles about gear and technique plus a race calendar.

➡ www.xcskiworld.com has different sections for recreational skiers versus competitors, each packed with detailed information about training, gear, and events plus places to go.

➡ www.xcski.org, the site for the Cross Country Ski Areas Association, has information about getting started, finding trips, and Nordic ski areas.

➡ *The Ultimate Guide to Trail Running* by Adam Chase and Nancy Hobbs is available on the AATRA website, www.trailrunner.com. The book covers all the basics, plus nutrition, first aid, planning for weather, tactics, and more.

➡ *Cross Country Skiing: Building Skills for Fun and Fitness* by instructor Steve Hindman has clear photographs of each technique as well as help choosing a style, selecting gear, getting kids involved, picking destinations and instructors, and starting to race.

TRAILS

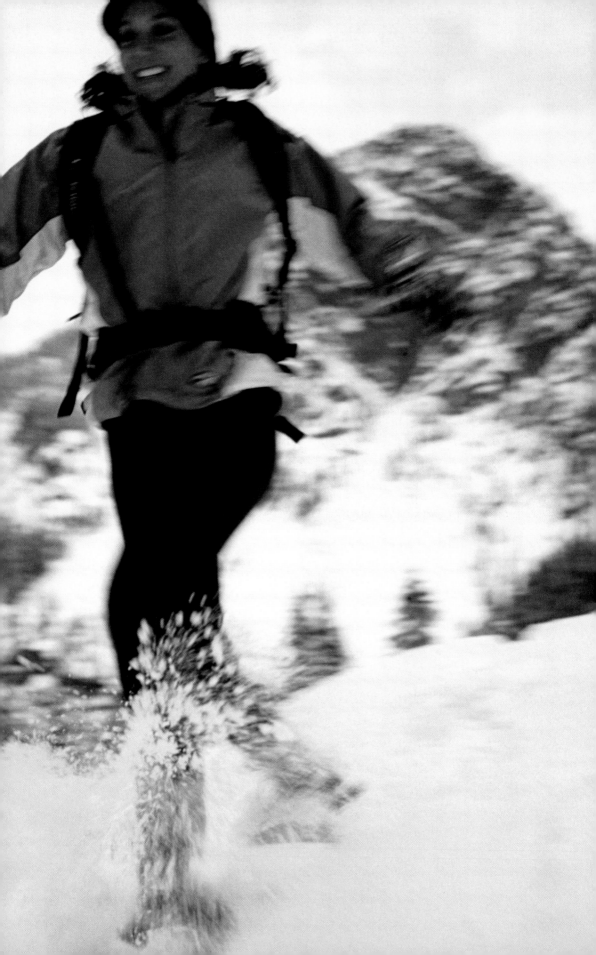

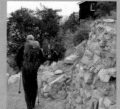

22

TREKKING
HIKING AND SNOWSHOEING

YOU'LL LOVE THESE SPORTS IF YOU:
• want to focus on cardio benefits with a thigh-and-butt-toning workout
• like to play at your own level; you can go for a stroll in a valley or head straight up a mountain
• love beautiful scenery
• prefer to play outdoors
• appreciate a sport that's so enjoyable you forget you're exercising
• enjoy taking sport vacations and exploring new places
• prefer a sport you can do alone or with people (or with your dog) depending on your mood

YOU MIGHT NOT LOVE THESE SPORTS IF YOU:
• have fears about wildlife, woods or solitude
• get lost very easily
• have chronic foot pain
• never want to get caught in the rain or snow
• never like to lose cell-phone reception

Here are two of the easiest and most accessible sports. If you can walk, you can hike or snowshoe with no additional training and not much gear. Locations abound—you can even spend a day hiking in a city or taking a snowshoe trek on the local golf course. You don't need to stray far from home for interesting sightings of flora and fauna, rock formations (or buildings), and perhaps even waterfalls and sweeping views. Or you can undertake a bigger excursion with a multiday getaway in, say, the Alps. You can saunter or speed along, tackle tough terrain or literally go for a walk in the park. The options are endless.

People have been trekking along trails for as long as humans have been walking upright. The earliest outings were utilitarian, including hunting forays, nomads searching for new homes, pilgrimages, and military maneuvers. Some of the most noteworthy historical references to hiking and snowshoeing can be found in the journals of explorers such as Lewis and Clark, who chronicled their journey from Illinois to the West Coast between 1804 and 1806, and in reports of Sir Ernest Shackleton's expeditions to Antarctica a century later.

Even if you never set foot in Antarctica or on Everest, don't underestimate the physical demands of hiking and snowshoeing. Both are serious workouts that provide significant cardiovascular benefits and can improve your health, help you lose weight, and give you more energy. You'll build leg strength and get a toned butt from hill climbs. You get all the benefits of the StairMaster without the monotony. Also, tricky footing will improve your balance and agility. And long outings are great for stamina and burning calories, especially if you carry a backpack.

As rich as these sports are in physical benefits, the psychological gains can be even greater. Every trek, no matter how short, is a mental getaway, a breath of fresh air for your brain that's akin to a mini vacation. If you feel stressed or depressed, this type of exercise has been shown by a number of scientific studies to be as curative as medication but without the side effects. Getting out into a natural setting, stepping one foot in front of the other, and filling your lungs full of air puts you into a relaxed state that reduces the level of stress hormones, lowers blood pressure, and helps you sleep better. And if you take just a few wise precautions against problems such as blisters, exposure to heat and cold, and getting lost, there are no downsides.

SCORE

If you weigh 150 pounds, you'll burn about 300 calories in an hour of hiking—at an average, not-very-strenuous pace. (To calculate your hourly burn rate, multiply your weight in pounds by two). Carrying a pack adds another 60 calories (or .4 times your weight). For snowshoeing or mountain climbing, the average calorie burn is 420 an hour (or 2.8 times your weight). The harder you huff and puff, the more calories you burn—up to twice the usual amount if you're heading uphill at a quick clip.

First, select a trail and research local wildlife and weather. Find out how long it takes the average person to complete the route, then adjust the estimate for your level of fitness. A beginner can expect to cover only about two miles in an hour, or four to five miles in a half day. If you want to bring kids or a dog along, be sure you have reserves of energy to cope with their needs in the woods. If there's a ranger station, be sure to check in before you hit the trail so they know you're in the area and can warn you about unusual conditions.

On any trip, no matter how brief, bring along a trail map, Band-Aids, snacks, and water—about a cup per hour per person. If you'll be out for a few hours, pack a small first-aid kit. For full-day excursions, put together a survival kit with a pocket knife, duct tape, matches, candles, a flashlight, extra batteries, alcohol-based hand sanitizer, rubber bands, a needle and thread, toilet paper, and bug repellent. Pack it all in a plastic zipper bag and bring a few extra bags, too. Bring more water and food than you think you'll consume (never drink water in the wild unless you treat it first or are truly about to die from dehydration). Add extra socks to your kit in case you get yours wet.

Pack everything in a comfortable backpack and consider leaving room to store any layers you shed. For a short trip, try a waist pack with a bottle holder. Take special care with your car keys, securing them in a zipped or Velcro-closed pocket that you won't open on the trail. Tuck in some money and identification, just in case.

Many snowshoers and hikers use poles to aid in balance on challenging terrain. Poles also give the upper body a workout, which burns more calories because you're using more muscles.

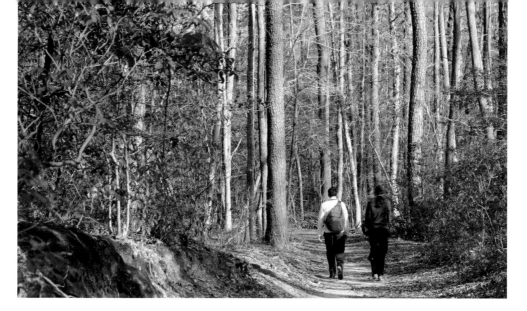

HIKING

The average stroll down a dirt path can be an adventure in itself as you discover animal tracks and enjoy the sights and sounds of nature. But hiking can be much more than checking out the hills and views, fields and flowers. If a walk down a trail doesn't seem sufficient to engage your interest, plan a trek with a purpose: Work up to steeper inclines as you train for an adventure vacation climbing Kilimanjaro or build up your distance until you can do overnight backpacking trips and walk the 2,160 miles of Appalachian Trail that runs from Georgia to Maine. You can also combine conservation work with hiking, helping to maintain trails for groups such as the Sierra Club. Another excellent way to get involved in hiking is to join your local chapter of the National Audubon Society (www.Audubon.org), a conservation group that organizes bird walks. Their treks tend to be more moderate in distance and, often, in terrain. And you can check out events at chapters all across the country for variety.

Hiking might seem as simple as a stroll in the woods, but there are skills you can learn to enhance your experience and improve your safety. One area that rewards attention: the Leave No Trace concept, which in a nutshell means you should carry out your garbage (including toilet paper!), resist the urge to collect rocks and flowers, and leave nothing behind but your footprints—even taking care where you put those so you don't damage natural habitats. It's hard to imagine that a step

or two to the side of the trail could make a difference, but the effect is cumulative. The damage became an increasing problem when Americans took up hiking in droves during the '60s, with the National Parks Service noting a jump from 33 million visitors in 1950 to 172 million in 1970. And the number keeps going up. Each outdoor enthusiast has a small impact that, when multiplied by the millions, ends up taking a large toll.

To add to your hiking skills, consider a learning vacation with the Appalachian Mountain Club or other outdoor-education groups. You can sign on for classes in map and compass reading, wilderness first aid, or how to *Leave No Trace*. Or take guided treks that include lessons in nature photography or tree and flower identification. The trips are inexpensive, the guides are experienced, and the fees help preserve and maintain the trails. Clubs such as these have sessions that are open to all, and some outings for adults, singles, families, teens, and other groups.

GEARING UP

For hiking, the most important item of gear is boots. Keeping your feet comfortable for hours on the trail takes a little more planning than you need for walking around town. First, you'll need to match the type of footwear with the excursion. For short hikes of less than three hours, a sturdy pair of sneakers can work (some hikers even wear off-road sandals). If you decide you like hiking, buy a pair of dayhikers. These reasonably priced boots offer slightly more support than sneakers and should feel comfortable right out of the box. For wet or muddy climates, step up to a light backpacking boot with a little more support and a waterproof liner. They cost a little more but are well worth the price when you have dry, comfortable feet. For serious hiking, such as long trips for which you'll carry a heavy pack, upgrade to stiffer leather backpacking boots for more support and protection. These boots cost more and should be broken in by your wearing them around town for at least a few days before you embark on your trip. If the terrain is rugged or you're going on a multiday trek, you'll be glad to have the bigger boots—but they'll be too hot and heavy for an afternoon in the local hills. Pick the lightest boots that work for the conditions your feet will face.

Make sure your footwear fits properly. When you try on boots, they should feel snug in the heel. Lightweight boots will fit closely in the toe, almost like sneakers. Stiffer boots

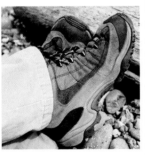

have more room up front on the assumption that you'll be going down steep hills with a heavy pack pushing your body forward—and the extra space keeps your toes from getting jammed. Try several brands to find the best fit, because each one is shaped slightly differently.

Test any new pair of boots on several short outings before wearing them on a hike of three hours or more. If they chafe, they will bother you a lot more when you're walking all day—and they could do some damage to your feet. When you're ready for your first trip to the woods, pad any sections that rub your foot (called hot spots) by attaching a product called moleskin, which you can buy at a drugstore.

The right socks are as important as the boots. Cotton socks will get soggy from sweat and cause blisters. Breathable synthetic and wool-blend materials will stay dry and comfortable. Wear a thin liner sock and then a slightly thicker sock for padding. You don't want huge amounts of cushioning, because the sock will bunch up and cause blisters. But socks that are too small can cut off your circulation. Try seamless styles because seams will rub your feet and cause blisters after a few thousand steps.

For a short trip, wear any clothing that's comfortable. On longer hikes, stay away from cotton clothing because it lacks the vital safety performance of breathable and wicking materials. Wear layers, an insulation item or two if it's cold, and an outer shell such as a waterproof, breathable jacket or parka. Always bring along one more layer than you think you'll need because it's often cooler under the trees than it seems while you're standing next to your car with the sun beating down. A lightweight windbreaker is easy to tote and serves the purpose well. Put on a hat with a brim and sunscreen, plus bug spray. If you're hiking in an area with ticks, wear long sleeves and long pants; tuck the bottoms of your trousers into your socks to provide a barrier. Light-colored clothing makes it easier to spot a tick and stays cool while providing some sun protection. You'll get dirtier faster than wearing black, but you'll be a lot more comfortable.

YOUR FIRST TIME

When you're ready to try hiking, make the first foray a short one. Look for a trail at a local nature preserve that has an easy rating, or sign up for a beginner's outing with a club. Use this excursion to get a feel for the gear and see how you like the sport. If you take on too hard a hike the first time, you'll end up

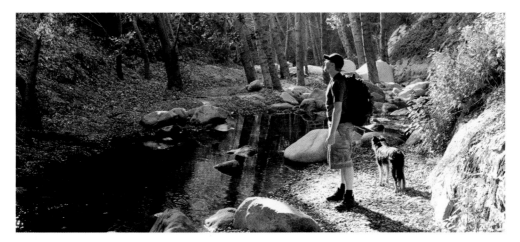

sore and miserable and unlikely to return for a second one. Even if you are very fit and physically ready for a complex route, your outdoors skills are not up to snuff until you've gotten some experience. Plus, a gentle beginning will give you a chance to enjoy the wildlife and the woods. Even if you're with a group, get a copy of the trail map the first time you go to test your navigation skills. If

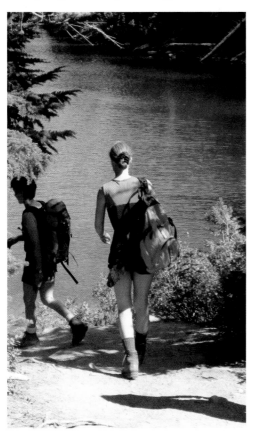

you're hiking at your own pace, check how long it takes you to complete the route compared to your estimate in the guidebook, so you can use it to evaluate future plans.

Hiking is just a "walk in the woods," as the saying goes, but there are a few form pointers that can make it more pleasant. Stand upright, shoulders back and abs firm (although not as rigid as a soldier at attention). Swing your arms or poles comfortably. Lean forward slightly from the ankles and keep your knees soft, not locked out. Instead of looking down at your feet on easy terrain, watch the trail a few feet ahead of you for obstacles. (When the footing is tricky, you'll have to look down to pick a solid spot to step.) Loose material such as sand and pebbles may shift underfoot. If you see sturdy roots or well embedded rocks, these spots tend to make sure footing—especially when you're going downhill, because they will stop you from slipping. Before transferring your weight, however, put your foot down gingerly to make sure the selected root or rock doesn't move. Whether you are going uphill or down, resist the urge to take large steps. Smaller ones conserve energy, allow for firmer footholds, and are gentler on your joints.

If you're wearing a pack, cinch it firmly around your shoulders so that it's snug to your back, and use the waist straps to prevent bouncing. Keep your water handy and sip often as you go. Don't postpone bodily functions—start looking for a good spot as soon as you notice nature's call. And most important, don't forget to look around to enjoy the scenery.

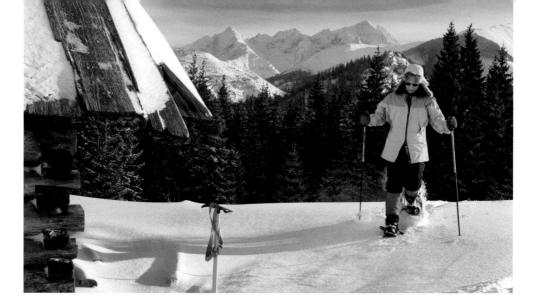

SNOWSHOEING

As far as winter sports are concerned, it doesn't get easier than snowshoeing. Kids can do it from a young age, as can older folks. It's low-impact for knees and other achy joints and can burn major numbers of calories when done at an intense pace. The sport even comes with a fashionable history. In cold regions of the U.S. and Canada, recreational snowshoe clubs were formed during the middle to late 1800s. The clubs had wealthy members who wore attractive uniforms on outings. But back then, enthusiasts had to deal with equipment issues: The old wood and rawhide snowshoes were much larger and heavier than versions we use today, and walking in them was more difficult.

Modern snowshoes are much smaller and lighter, so you can almost walk with your natural stride instead of the bow-legged duck walk necessitated by older models. Today, snowshoes are usually made of metal frames spread with plastic or high-tech fabric decks. Underneath, most models have metal teeth called crampons that grab the ground so you won't slip. Most snowshoes now have bindings that allow you to lift your heel free of the deck for a more natural stride.

GEARING UP

For your first outing, it's a good idea to rent snowshoes, which you can do at some outdoor stores and ski resorts, as well as parks, nature centers, and hiking clubs. Once you've decided that you like the sport, pick up your own pair—they aren't expensive and you can even get used ones. (Renting is also a nice option if you don't want to pack your own pair in your luggage).

Snowshoes come in different styles and sizes, which you choose, depending on your weight, speed, and terrain. Large snowshoes are heavier and less maneuverable, so it's best to use the smallest size to keep you from sinking into the snow. If you're lucky enough to hike in deep powder conditions rather than hard-packed snow, you'll need more loft.

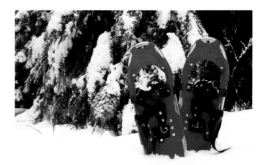

There are sizes for children, specific styles for women, and large sizes for heavier people. Beginners will do well with an inexpensive recreational snowshoe; an oval shape that tapers in the back is easiest to walk in. Buy snowshoes that have a good set of crampons. Bindings should be comfortable, secure, and easy to operate.

When you progress beyond a basic romp in the woods, you might want to upgrade to a

TREKKING

style specific to your plans. For example, backcountry snowshoes are extra durable and have more complex, rigid bindings that grasp your foot securely for long, arduous trips. Running styles are designed not to hit into each other as you move. They often have an asymmetrical tail.

Next up, you'll need boots. Some snowshoe runners wear trail sneakers, but don't try that for a snowshoe hike. On short outings, you can wear regular snow boots or light hiking boots. For longer trips or messy conditions, get a waterproof insulated hiking boot that offers more substantial protection from the wet and cold. Snowboarding boots work well, too.

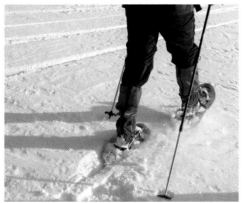

Wear two layers of socks—a thin, breathable inner one and a slightly more padded outer one. The layers move against each other so there's no friction on your feet. As with regular hiking, be sure to pick socks that fit well and won't bunch up and cause blisters. Wear a hat, gloves, or mittens and sunglasses or ski goggles to protect your eyes from wind and glare off the snow. Dress in at least three warm layers: long underwear (base layer), a breathable insulation layer, and a water-and-wind-proof outer shell. Consider using a neck warmer so that you can open your jacket for ventilation without exposing your throat to the cold. And if frigid air is harsh on your lungs, you can warm it slightly by pulling the neck warmer up over your mouth and nose and breathing through

it. In deep snow, wear gaiters, water-resistant covers that attach over your boots and come up mid-calf to keep the powder out of your boots.

When you pack your gear in your backpack, consider which items should not get frozen (water and snacks, for example) and pack these closest to your back, where they will benefit from your body heat. If it's well below zero, put them inside your coat. In addition to the regular safety items you need for hiking, add a snowshoe-repair kit and chemical hand and foot warmers. Also, consult an outdoor retailer to find an appropriate insulation layer in case you need it; your choices include a tarp, sleeping-bag liner, or a medium-weight jacket. Consider bringing warm drinks in a thermos and possibly a pad that's waterproof and insulated to sit on.

YOUR FIRST TIME

Before your first outing, be sure to check the weather report and snow depth, in case a storm might be heading in that would leave you blinded in the woods or needing to dig out your car when you return. If your snowshoes have crampons, make sure there are at least six inches of snow on the ground so they don't get banged up on dirt and rocks.

Adjust your bindings indoors, where you can sit warm and dry. Then hike to the snow before strapping your boots into your snowshoes. Walk around a bit on flat ground to get the feel for stepping with the contraptions on your feet. Snug up your bindings if they feel wobbly—but don't make them too tight or they'll cut off your circulation, leaving your feet sore and cold.

Next, try a slight incline. There are several easy techniques for climbing: The most stable way to go is straight up. With each step, dig in the crampons before shifting your weight onto the foot. If you find you're slipping too much because the path is icy or steep, turn your toes out 45 degrees, step forward with your right foot, then step farther with the left, making sure the tail of the left snowshoe clears the tail of the right one. If you're using poles, plant them behind each foot so you can't slip backward. This somewhat awkward technique is called a *herringbone* because of the pattern it leaves in the snow. It gets easier over time, and advanced snowshoers can actually run uphill doing it. If you still slip backward with the herringbone, try turning your entire body perpendicular to the ascent and sidestepping uphill or zigzagging back and forth across the incline, if there's room.

Once you've gone up, you'll need to learn to come down. In a wide-open space with a gentle slope and plenty of powder, it's fun to bound downhill with big leaps. Only do this if you're sure there's a solid base underneath, such as on a ski trail. For most descents, you'll walk right down, again making sure the crampons have a firm grip before shifting your weight onto your foot. It may feel good to lean back slightly, but don't do it. You're actually safer leaning slightly forward so the crampons can dig in and you're less likely to fall back and hit your head. Keep your poles up in front, not trailing behind you, so that you can plant them ahead if you start to slip. If the slope is steep, consider walking side to side across the hill for a gentle descent or sidestepping down. You can also put your snowshoes side by side facing downhill, sit on the tails, curl your toes, and ride downhill—a technique called *glissade*.

As you go, check your posture to be sure you aren't hunching forward. As in hiking, you want to stand upright but not stiffly, swing your arms and look ahead whenever possible. Looking down and rounding your

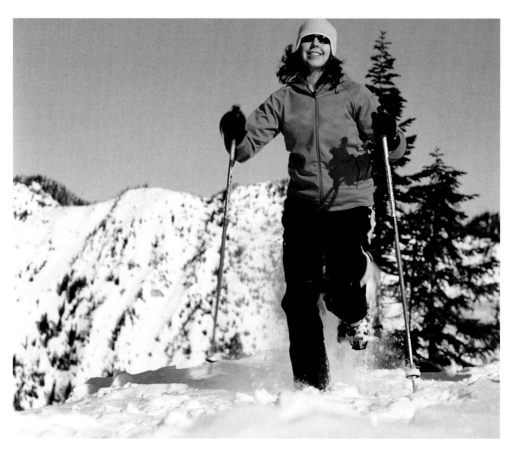

TREKKING

shoulders collapses your chest and won't allow you to breathe as deeply as you can with your shoulders back and chest open.

Make your first outing fairly brief. Consider it a test of your gear. Were you warm enough? Did you sweat a lot? If so, lighten the layers of your clothing for your next outing, because cooling down when wet is a risk for hypothermia. Did your bindings hold well? Were your feet warm and dry? Did you bring enough water? Make any necessary adjustments so you can plan a longer outing next time.

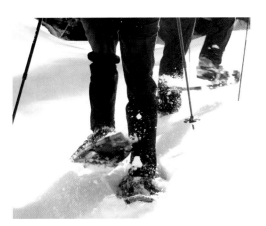

ATHLETE IN ACTION

Jerome Berman, 84

"My best friend started hiking with the Sierra Club and invited me to go along," recalls Jerome Berman of his first trek twenty-six years ago. Not yet 60, in good shape, and a fan of the outdoors, Berman was happy to try it. "We added two other good friends, found it was enjoyable and it became a regular event," he says. The group got their start close to home. "There are hundreds of trails within an hour and a half of where we live," says the Bronxville, New York resident. In 1984, a trek to Israel began a tradition of one overseas hike a year. "We had to watch out for signs of land mines and expended ammunition, and we did a good climb," Berman recalls. "It was a memorable trip, especially because I had never been to Israel before."

Before hiking for the first time, Berman read up a bit about navigation with a compass and a few safety pointers, but he learned almost everything else while on the trail. He's a steadfast fan of waterproof boots and hiking poles as well as synthetic breathable clothing, and he always carries a flashlight. It's

easy for the group to pack properly because prior to any trip, one member thoroughly researches the weather and trails, local dangers, and places for overnight stays. The eldest of their merry band, now 96, no longer comes along, but the other three are still at it and have made few changes in the way they hike. One notable exception: In younger days, they did more camping, but now they prefer taking day trips of seven hours or so before returning to a comfortable bed, with maybe one night spent sleeping under the stars.

Over the years, Berman and his friends have collected thousands of photographs and many more memories. In Poland, the group came across an area where the trail had been wiped out by an avalanche, a surprise that hadn't turned up in their pretrip research. "There was a heavy chain for 50 yards with nothing underneath but a 300 foot drop. You had to go hand over hand." Berman recalls that it seemed fine to make the treacherous crossing at the time, but looking back, he says "Nobody in their right mind would have done that."

An Arizona hike brought another experience he hopes never to repeat. The foursome had picked a spot to set up camp for the night. Popping behind a

tree to relieve himself, Berman looked up to find a 5½-foot rattlesnake lazing in the late afternoon sun a few feet away. "You feel very vulnerable when you're exposed," he says. He scooted away quietly, but brought his friends to a safe distance to take pictures of the creature before moving on to a new campsite.

Most hikes don't have such harrowing tales, but still foster rich memories of sights and adventures. Berman speaks enthusiastically of the unfathomable history and beauty of the Grand Canyon. And he remembers meeting a man in Italy who took time off from work to spend two hours guiding Berman and his friends to an old Roman road. He once took a trek in Sterling Forest, about an hour from home, where the cold winds were blowing 40 miles per hour and the spot for lunch was overlooking a frozen waterfall. Wherever they go, Berman most revels in the "three great joys" of hiking, as he calls them: The physical accomplishment, the beauty of nature, and the camaraderie. "You can unburden your soul on a hike, it comes naturally, and whatever is said never leaves the woods," he explains.

TREKKING

Coach's Corner

SECRETS TO SUCCESS

It's so easy to start hiking and snowshoe-ing that people often underestimate these sports and get in over their heads. "Get some sort of contact with the sport before you sign up for a big goal," says Ben Hendrickson, a personal trainer at The Sports Center at Chelsea Piers. That advice sounds logical, but he's amazed at how often it's skipped. "On a trip I took to Kilimanjaro, there were people who had very limited outdoors experience," he recalls. Knowledgeable hikers, like Berman and his friends, start with local trails and work up to far-flung destina-tions. It's smart to get your early experi-ence in places where, in case you encounter trouble, you know the sur-rounding area and might even be able to call home for a little help from a friend.

Before you head out, come to an agreement with your companions on the type of outing you want—a workout, a slow-and-steady pace, or many stops to smell the flowers. On the trail, stop at least every half hour to assess your posi-tion, drink some water, and have a little snack. The first time you hike any new trail, watch for changes in markings. If you are going to follow the same path back, "look back every five to ten minutes, especially at junctures," says Hendrickson. The trail will look quite dif-ferent when you are traveling in the oppo-site direction—and it can be impossible to determine which way to go if the mark-ings are unclear. Wear a watch so you can keep an eye on the time. When you reach a fork in the trail, check your map and plot your pace against your expecta-tions so you can speed up or change your route to ensure you're back to civi-lization well before dark.

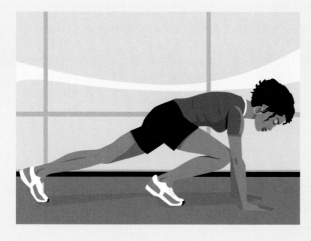

mountain climbers

From hands and knees, extend the legs, place the toes on the ground; form a straight line from the top of your head to your heels. Your hands should be directly under your shoulders, elbows slightly bent. Abs should be taut. Allow your butt to rise as you bring your right knee toward your chest, placing the ball of the foot on the ground. This is the starting position. Spring up off of both feet and switch position, landing with your left foot forward, right foot back. Repeat to return to the start and complete 1 repetition. Do 10 repetitions. Build up to 3 sets of 20 reps.

Increase the length and difficulty of your treks slowly. Flat terrain and short trips don't require much endurance or leg muscle strength, but as soon as you add a few steep inclines, unsteady footing, a heavy pack, or a significant distance, the physical challenge increases quickly. It's much more fun—and safer—if you build up each factor a little at a time. For the average trip, leave yourself a 20 percent safety buffer in terms of time and stamina. Be aware that extreme weather or high altitudes can leave you more fatigued in short order, and build in a larger buffer in these conditions. If you have kids along, plan a hike that ensures you'll have extra reserves of energy in case they need assistance.

As you go, check your posture and technique regularly. It's easy to get sloppy as you settle into the trek or start to get tired. With each step, try to roll through the entire foot, from heel to toe (it's tempting to go uphill on just your toes). A flat foot, slightly bent knee, and firm abs provide the most stable stance to prevent falls. When you go up a steep hill, don't be afraid to use your hands to grip the ground and assist your ascent. If you grasp rocks or vegetation, give a small pull first to ensure your chosen anchor is secure—but try not to do damage by pulling hard and dislodging vegetation or ground cover. Be aware of others who are downhill from you, staggering your position in case you might inadvertently send down a shower of snow, rocks, or dirt in their direction.

If you have time for some off-trail training, try these moves:

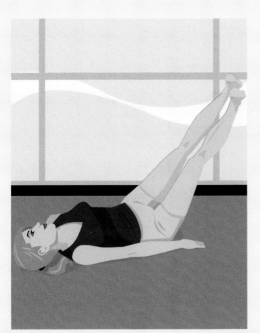

hip crossover

Lie on the ground on your back, hands by your sides, palms down. (If you find you need extra support during this move, pick a spot where you can place your arms overhead and grasp a stable object such as the bottom of a couch). Lift both legs so the feet are directly above your hips, feet pressed together. Using your abdominal muscles, lower both legs to the right as far as you can. Lift your legs back to center in a controlled manner (don't swing) and then lower them to the left. Return to center to complete 1 repetition. Do 10 reps. Build up to 3 sets of 10 reps. Note: If you have back problems, skip this move and do a different abs strengthener.

TACKLE THE TRUTH

You'll get lost and die of exposure

Every so often, there's a much-publicized case of someone lost in the woods because of a freak accident or bad weather. To stay out of the headlines, take these safety steps: Never stray far from civilization by yourself. Better yet, take two friends so one can stay in the woods with an injured companion while the other goes for help. Learn to read a compass and don't count on your cell phone because reception is spotty in remote places—which is exactly where you're going to get lost. Tell someone where you're going and how long you'll be gone so they'll look for you before days pass. Stay on marked trails to increase the likelihood that help will cross your path. For overnight trips, study survival skills. There are plenty of simple steps that can keep you safe, but they aren't intuitive.

You'll get attacked by wild animals

Most wild animals are frightened of humans and will more likely run away than attack you. Notable exceptions are animals that feel threatened (especially mothers guarding their young) or those that have learned that humans carry food in their backpacks. The bigger risks to you in the woods are deer-hunting humans and fast-moving mountain bikers, so be sure to dress in bright colors or choose trails that are off limits to hunting or biking. While animal attacks are rare, you can't just assume you'll be safe on the trail. Learn about the local wildlife and how best to avoid trouble from guidebooks and rangers who can warn of trouble-spots such as nesting areas. Know what to watch for, how to react if approached, and how to stash your pack if you're staying overnight. If your fear of animals keeps you out of the woods, consider snowshoeing. In winter, most wildlife is hibernating, but you'll still see beautiful birds and breathtaking views.

Hiking and snowshoeing are only for granola-crunching tree-hugging types

You'll find a lot of people who love nature out on the trails. But these sports are now so popular that you'll find a fair representation of just about every demographic out there, from Boy Scouts to bird watchers to urbanites. Guaranteed, there is someone just like you who goes hiking or snowshoeing. And most people you encounter on the trails are friendly and helpful.

GET MORE FROM YOUR SPORT

The average person can prep to climb Kilimanjaro, an arduous trip, in about a year of trekking. And there are plenty of exciting places to visit along the way. Almost every adventure outfitter offers spectacular trips at every level, and on trails all over the world. There are offerings that involve camping and cooking out, cabin stays, or even luxurious lodges. You can trek the Great Wall of China or walk on a network of ladders in Ghana suspended high in the trees in the African rain forest. Any place you can hike turns into a snowshoe destination once the white stuff blankets the area. Some of the most memorable snow excursions are in the U.S. National Parks such as Yosemite, Arcadia in Maine, or Denali in Alaska, where a dogsled team is likely to pass you on the trail.

If you want to increase the challenge of your hiking or snowshoeing, there are plenty of sports to try. Orienteering adds an element of navigation and competition as you race to find set locations using a marked map, almost like a treasure hunt. Backpacking with overnight camping gives you extended opportunities to hike and introduces a new set of skills and gear. Mountaineering takes hiking to a new level of technical challenge with more difficult terrain. And trail running adds speed to increase the cardiovascular benefits, calorie burn, and distance you can cover. For snowshoers, there are overnight excursions, races, and club outings. The U.S. Snowshoe Association lists events on their Web site (www.snowshoeracing.com), including races for kids.

If you love these activities because you enjoy getting out in nature and testing your abilities, consider trying other outdoor sports such as kayaking, rock or ice climbing, and downhill or cross-country skiing. Many people who love hiking and snowshoeing also enjoy the body awareness, strength, and introspection you get from yoga, pilates, or even martial arts. Swimming and running are excellent crosstraining activities for outdoor sports because they increase your stamina and help you pace your breathing.

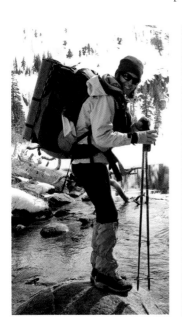

RESOURCES

www.americanhiking.org is the site of the American Hiking Society, and their site can help you find local hiking clubs or trails.

www.abc-of-hiking.com is a good resource for learning about all aspects of hiking, from gear to destinations.

www.wintertrails.org has an excellent section about snowshoeing, including information about getting started.

www.snowshoemag.com provides gear reviews and information about events, plus a state-by-state listing of Nordic centers that are great destinations.

Snowshoeing: From Novice to Master by Gene Prater and Dave Felkey covers all the ground you might need—from history to gear to getting better traction. There are also chapters about snowshoe camping and racing.

The Complete Walker IV by Colin Fletcher and Chip Rawlins stands out above other hiking books for thoroughness (at 864 pages, they cover it all!) and clarity. The authors have been there and done that; they give it to you straight and have fun while doing so.

TREKKING

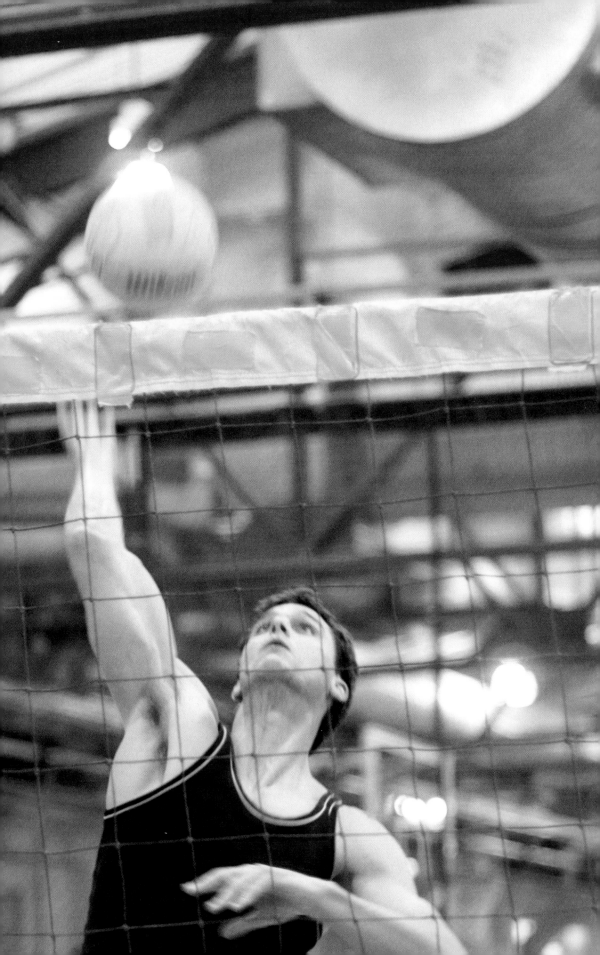

VOLLEYBALL

It's rare to grow up in the United States and never set foot on a volleyball court, since the sport is a classic choice in school physical-education classes. Not everyone has a good experience in P.E.—but if that includes you, don't let it stop you from trying volleyball as an adult. It's not unusual to find that your abilities and interest in the game improve with age.

Volleyball, the second most popular sport in the world (behind soccer), was invented in the United States. A YMCA instructor named William G. Morgan came up with the idea to blend basketball, handball, baseball, and tennis to create a noncontact recreational sport that men could play after work. The game evolved over the next three decades, and in 1928, the U.S. Volleyball Association was created to codify the rules and establish tournaments open to players

VOLLEYBALL

outside YMCAs. Beach volleyball started in Hawaii in 1915, and then became streamlined to a two-man game in 1930. Volleyball joined the Olympic roster in 1964, but the Americans didn't win their first medals until 1984. A player named Karch Kiraly was on that team and went on to win the first gold medal in beach volleyball when the sand game became an Olympic sport in 1996. Perhaps more inspiring for older players, Kiraly and his partner won the Association of Volleyball Professionals' tournament in 2003 just a few months before Kiraly's forty-third birthday, pushing him over $3 million in prize earnings—almost twenty years after his first Olympic gold medal. If he can keep winning international tournaments in his forties, chances are good that you can hold your own at the local gymnasium.

SCORE

If you weigh 150 pounds, you'll burn about 120 calories in an hour of recreational indoor volleyball (or 0.8 times your weight), 180 calories in an hour of competitive indoor volleyball (1.2 times your weight) and 420 calories in an hour of vigorous beach volleyball (or 2.8 times your weight).

Adult volleyball, from recreational to competitive, is one of the easiest team sports to find and join because the game is relatively simple to learn, requires almost no gear to purchase yourself, and is commonly played indoors, outdoors, and on the beach. There are also disabled leagues, including a sitting version for people in wheelchairs. Parks, schools, and YMCAs have nets set up permanently for practice, pickup games, and scheduled play, and many offer adult leagues as well.

Another welcoming aspect of the game is that you don't need to gather a big group; you can play with as few as two on a side or as many as six (or more if it's just for fun). And even though skills may vary from person to person, a team can remain strong as a whole because the positions on the court are more fluid than in most other sports, allowing players to move around quite a bit to play to their strengths. There's even a little-known position that doesn't require serving, a defensive player called the *libero*.

Volleyball can be one intense exercise session. It's a cardio fest that tones the legs and butt from jumping, diving, and running—with added intensity if you play on a shifting surface of sand. Your arms, shoulders, and upper back get strong and lean from hitting and serving. And twisting and blocking motions target the body's core.

Volleyball requires decent aim, but the hand positions used for striking the ball are unlike those used in daily activities and therefore are often learned on the court. You will improve your balance, coordination, and agility. The jumping and running, as well as impact with the ball, make volleyball excellent for maintaining bone strength. And your juxtaposition with others on the court will improve your peripheral awareness, which is useful for activities such as driving.

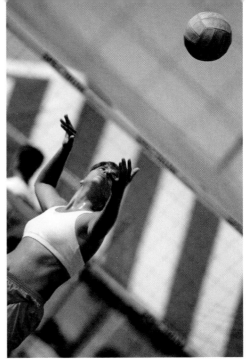

Mentally, the game is challenging. Teammates must work together to set up effective plays, and strategy involves learning the strengths and weaknesses of the opposing players. The action is fast, calling for split-second decision making plus a keen awareness of the positions and abilities of your teammates. And because your position rotates every time your team wins control of the serve, you are constantly adjusting your play.

The volleyball court is a rectangle that varies in size depending on where it is played—indoors, outdoors, or on the beach. The net is similar to tennis' net but set higher than your head, with specific heights for different age ranges and a lower setting for women. Games are played to fifteen or thirty points, with a two-point spread required to win. International rules for indoor games (called *sets*) require a team to win three sets in order to win a match—or, if the teams are tied two sets apiece, the fifth set is a tie-breaker played for fifteen instead of thirty points.

GEARING UP

To play volleyball, you'll need a ball and a net, but unless you want to buy a setup for your yard, it's common to make use of the court and equipment at a gym, beach, or YMCA. It's nice to have a ball to practice with, and they are not expensive.

Many people wear bathing suits to play beach volleyball, but shorts and a shirt are

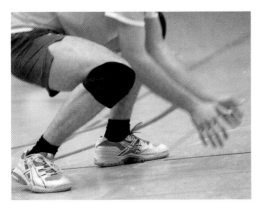

fine, too. The beach game is generally played barefoot, although you can wear socks or purchase specific booties if you prefer. Hats, visors, and sunglasses are common on the beach, but rules for indoor and outdoor games preclude wearing jewelry or clothes that might harm other players. Indoors, the gear is typically comfortable gym clothes and sneakers. There are specific volleyball sneakers for sale if you become a serious player. Second choice, if you have options, is a pair of crosstrainers, aerobic sneakers, or court shoes like those used in tennis or basketball. You can play in running sneakers or other types, but be careful not to roll an ankle since these shoes don't provide as much support for sideways motion as do court shoes.

Players should bring a bottle of water to games and, for outdoor play, wear sunscreen. Indoors, aggressive players often wear knee and elbow pads to prevent injury from contact with the ground when they dip or dive to get a shot.

YOUR FIRST TIME

Get an experienced player or coach to show you the main skills you'll need to play. The way you hit the ball back in high school is probably not the best technique, even if the shots seem the same. Novice volleyball players mainly use two types of hits: *bumping* or *digging*—when you put your hands together,

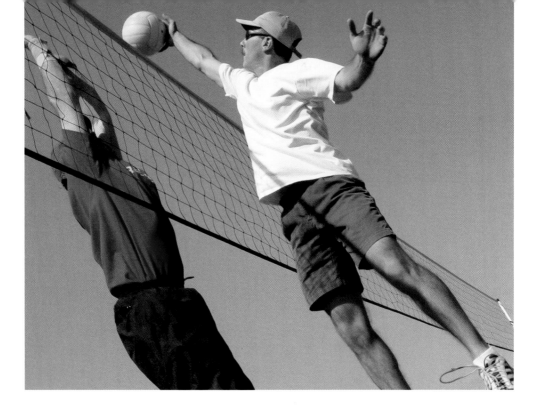

striking the ball with your wrists or forearms to pop it high in the air, setting it up for another teammate or directing it over the net; and *hitting* or *attacking*—when you strike the ball with one arm, often making a slight fist, to drive it over the net for a serve or during a rally. As your skills advance, you may learn to *spike* the ball by jumping up to drive it down onto the opposing court. Other advanced skills include diving to hit a low ball and blocking at the net.

You can practice volleyball hits alone by just hitting the ball into the air repeatedly or bouncing your shots against a wall at a handball court or the side of a house. Toss the ball high against the wall and as it comes down toward you, get into the proper position to bump it (hands and forearms together, elbows down, insides of forearms making a flat surface), and try to target an exact spot on the wall. Give the ball plenty of loft so you have time to get into position, and strive for accuracy over speed or power. Practice until you miss, then shake out your arms and legs, hold the ball in both hands, and rotate from the hips as far as you can in each direction. Catch your breath and try again.

When you find a friend to practice with, strive for precision in placement as you perfect your form. And once you can manage a few decent shots, look for a pickup game. It's also not unusual to simply sign up for a league and show up to play games.

When you arrive for a scheduled game, it's common to find people warming up on the court—if it's available—or stretching and warming up on the sidelines if another game is in progress. The coach or team captain will check the roster to make sure enough players are present for a game, and the team will forfeit if too few show up, so it's important to be on time.

Before the game begins, the referee will hold a coin toss. The winners can choose between picking their side of the court or serving first. After a warm-up, the ref checks the roster and the game begins. For games with six players or more, each team lines up in rows. When your team has the serve, the person in the back right corner serves the ball over the net to the other team. The receiving team has three shots to return it, and no player can hit the ball twice in a row. No matter who served the ball, a point is scored by the team that puts the ball over the net last before it hits the ground or goes out of bounds. (This *rally scoring* rule is fairly recent—a few years ago, only the serving team could score; and you may find the game still played that way in some venues.) The team that won the point gets to serve next. If they did not serve last, the players rotate position clockwise. A serve that fails to clear the net is a *fault*, and after one or two (depending on the rules for that game), the other team scores a point and gains control of the serve. Also, the server must be behind the rear boundary of the court until after striking the ball. And the server must wait until both teams are ready, then toss the ball and hit it with a hand or arm, not throw it, or use another part of the body to hit it.

While the serve must clear the net, hits during rallies can touch the net as long as they go over with no more than three hits from the team. You can hit the ball with any part of the body, but you aren't allowed to catch or throw it. And while you're not allowed to hoist up a teammate to reach the ball, you are permitted to grab him to keep him from committing an error such as touching the net.

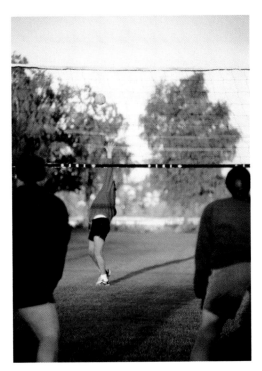

VOLLEYBALL

SECRETS TO SUCCESS

You can get out on the court using the skills you learned in grade school, but if you want to play well, have someone show you a few refinements. "You don't learn the proper mechanics in gym class," says Bill Maik, a trainer and volleyball instructor at the Sports Center at Chelsea Piers. For example, an experienced player or coach can show you how to make a solid platform with your arms to bump the ball and snap an overhand serve instead of punching it. "When you use your body correctly, it's fairly effortless to move the ball," says Maik, so anyone can be a solid player.

Because of the shifting surface, playing in sand requires more adjustment than games on hard courts. It's harder to run and jump when the ground is moving under your feet. And you'll usually have fewer players on a side, which means you need to cover more territory. After your first game, you'll feel sore in your ankles and calves from a workout that's unusual for your body. "It takes two to six weeks to get comfortable with the sand game," says Maik. To get accustomed to moving faster, you can run and jump in sand when you're off the court or play around on a wobble board to improve your

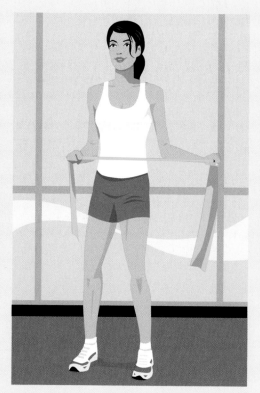

shoulder strengthener

Grasp a stretch band in both hands, shoulder-distance apart, with an overhand grip. Sit in an armless chair or stand in a stable posture. Press your shoulders down and back, away from your ears. Hold your elbows close to your sides. Lift your hands so your forearms are parallel to the ground. This is the start position. Don't move your entire right arm or your upper left arm as you pivot at the left elbow and swing your left hand away from the right, pulling it as far as you can with the wrist straight. Use the muscles in your left shoulder to assist the rotation but don't hunch or strain them. Release back to the start. Do 5 repetitions with the left arm, then repeat with the right. Next, rotate your fists so the palms face each other and repeat. Build slowly until you can do 3 sets of 12 reps.

balance and strengthen the stabilizing muscles in your feet and ankles.

For off-court practice for any style of volleyball, try a drill called *peppering*. You stand 12 to 20 feet away from another player and practice controlled bumps back and forth. Then, when you have learned the skills, you can add some spikes and digs.

If you want to get in shape to improve your game or prep for your first foray onto the court, try the moves below.

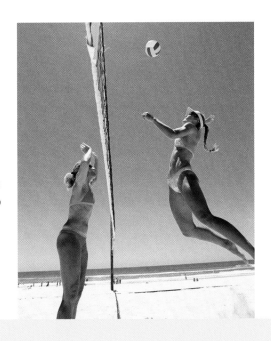

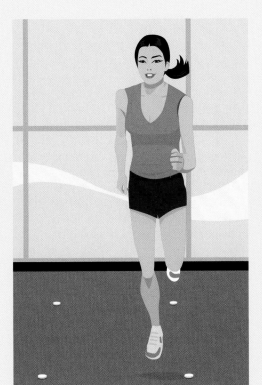

jump training

Use a marker such as chalk or 4 coins to set up this grid: Mark where you're standing (if you're using chalk, make a large box around your feet), then walk 2 comfortable paces to your right and make another mark, step 2 paces forward for the third mark and complete the square for the fourth mark. Walk back to your first mark and stand facing the fourth mark. Leap to the mark on the right, going as high as you can, landing softly on the balls of your feet with bent knees. Leap forward to the next mark. Leap left to the next mark, then leap back to the start. Reverse direction, leaping forward first, then right, back and left to complete 1 rep. Every time you leap, try to increase the height and soften the landing. Do 10 repetitions. Practice until you can do 3 sets of 10 reps, then move the markers farther apart and keep practicing.

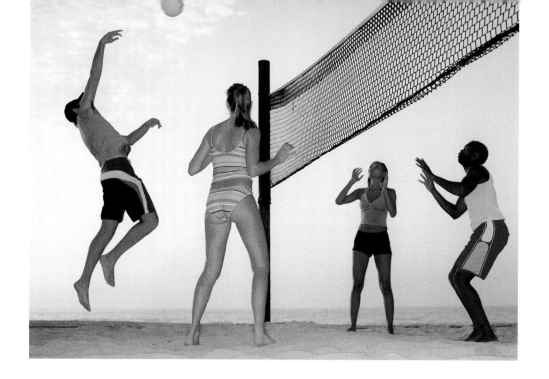

TACKLE THE TRUTH

You'll hurt your wrists and arms playing volleyball

Some of the most painful memories of those school volleyball games are of the red throbbing wrists and forearms you got after hitting the ball. Better quality volleyballs are softer than the ones you probably used in school. And your arms quickly get used to the impact. But when you hit hard, it can smart. If you'd prefer not to feel it, wear long sleeves or cut off tube socks and wear them over your arms for a little extra padding.

You have to dive in the sand to play beach volley-ball

Televised beach volleyball competitions are filled with tan hardbodies flying all over the court. That doesn't mean you have to do the same, although it can be great fun. The sand is a forgiving surface, which makes the game easier to play at an intense level without getting hurt. And even indoors, if you're properly conditioned and outfitted, it can be fun to dive for a heroic save. But nobody on the team will fault you if you prefer to stay on your feet as you're learning the game.

You have to be strong and powerful to play volleyball

Watch the pros and you see a lot of sky-high jumps, blocks at the net, power serves, and rocket-fast spiking of the ball into the opponent's court. But then, any sport at the elite level is played with a different intensity than you should expect in your early experiences in the game. It's wonderful when you learn an overhand serve and how to *spike*, but until then, focus on getting good at moving the ball where you want it to go, rather than driving it in any direction. Precision is more important than power. If you can learn how to bump the ball exactly where you want it to go, you'll be more valuable than someone who spikes it out of bounds.

GET MORE FROM YOUR SPORT

If you enjoy volleyball, consider taking up soccer and basketball; both are team sports that can be played with varying levels of intensity. Each of these games will help you hone your strategic skills, learning where your teammates are and how to coordinate passes and attempts to score. Tennis, racquetball, and handball are also helpful for learning how to place the ball accurately, anticipating the action, and working the court. And if you have access to a water-polo game, you can get a similar over-the-net team challenge with the added support and resistance of water. Consider taking up boxing, martial arts, fencing, or gymnastics to improve your foot speed, body awareness, and balance.

You'll have ample opportunity to play volleyball if you can find a net at your local park or beach. Suggest a game for family get-togethers or company outings. To find a weekly game, look for leagues at local recreation centers and parks. If you want to polish your skills in an intensive program, consider going to volleyball camp. There are a number of options. Two good choices: Bob Bertucci, the head women's coach at Temple University, offers a three-day program for adults (www.bobbertucci.com). Olympic gold medalist Pat Powers offers two-day camps held across the country (www.vbclinics.com). His camps combine juniors and adults (starting at age twelve) in one session. And if you want to get adventurous, keep an eye out for volleyball cruises featuring top pros and Olympians (www.volleyballcruise.com). Finally, if you're serious about playing beach volleyball, take a look at the South of the Border volleyball vacations in Mexico (www.sobvolleyballvacations.com).

RESOURCES

➡ **www.usavolleyball.org** is the site for the United States Volleyball Association, the governing body of both the sport and the national team. On this site, you can find links to local leagues plus the rules for indoor and outdoor games. There's also an archive of articles from *Coaching Volleyball* magazine, including a fascinating set of drills titled "Enhancing Visual Skills."

➡ **www.volleyball.com** is packed with useful information, including training tips and a camp finder, plus a great list of links to other resources.

➡ *Volleyball Skills and Drills* by the American Volleyball Coaches Association covers ninety skills as explained by ten top coaches from around the country.

VOLLEYBALL

Find it Near You

One key factor in the success of any fitness program is convenience. If you happen to live in or near New York City, or come to visit on vacation, you can head to Chelsea Piers for a chance to try dozens of activities. The complex offers 1.2 million square feet of fun for adults and kids—a huge playground along the Hudson River waterfront for all ages. But if you live elsewhere, the first challenge is locating safe and fun options for the sports you're interested in. Here's some guidance in locating a good match.

Word of mouth Start by asking other people about different sports venues. It's easy to get input if you know someone who plays the sport you want to try—and you'll almost always get an enthusiastic response to your inquiries. Don't skip this process just because you don't know anyone who participates in your chosen activity. The path to a personal recommendation is probably shorter than you'd expect. Try these leads to get going:
* a person who sells gear for the sport
* a coach at a school, college, or kids' program
* anyone athletic, such as a trainer at a local gym or someone who works at a park or at athletic destinations like ski resorts or ballparks
* anyone you see participating in the sport or a similar activity
* someone who runs a training program for coaches and instructors

Once you've found someone who actually plays the sport, ask him where he goes to play or where he went to first learn the skills needed. Also, ask for referrals to others he knows who play this sport, as well as additional resources for learning about it.

Most athletes are particularly fond of their own niche within their activity. For example, someone who fences with a foil may not recommend epée. And someone who rows in an eight may not suggest that you take up sculling in a single. Also, after years of experience, an athlete may have forgotten how hard it was to get started, or she may have developed her own preferences for a style of play that won't work for you—such as a round-robin tennis league if you're not competitive and just want to rally.

Keep these factors in mind as you sort through the information you're given. But also maintain an open mind, because a veteran's experience might save you a lot of trouble in your quest for the best coaches and venues.

Official organizations Every activity has an official association. Most sports actually have several—and therein lies the problem. Official organizations are rich sources of information and usually offer input on finding local options, but sometimes a professional-sounding group will represent a faction within a sport, or a single person promoting his training services, from which you can't expect to get an impartial referral. Try these ideas to determine if you've found a bona-fide organization:
* Start with the U.S. Olympic team's Web site, www.usolympicteams.com for information on your sport and look there for links to other groups. At the sport-specific pages you will often find information for beginners, plus help locating a local venue. Also, check the "links" section for connections to reputable associations for the sport.
* If your sport is an outdoor pursuit, try www.gorp.com, a Web site that has a plethora of information about a wide array of activities. From all the usual options—hiking, cycling, skiing—to caving and whale watching, you'll find tips on choosing destinations, gear, and gadgets, plus inspirational tales and photos.
* Type the name of your sport into a search engine such as Google. When evaluating the results, watch for words such as "American

Association of" and "National Federation" in the name of the group. These monikers are no guarantee of credibility, but they are often used by major reputable organizations.

* Look in sports magazines for references to groups. For example, many articles in *Golf Digest* mention the PGA or LPGA, which is a good sign that these organizations are well respected.
* At the library or bookstore, find books written by famous athletes or prominent coaches. Many of these books include a listing of organizations (usually located in the back). And check the author's bio for mentions of an association he belongs to.
* Look in the *Get More from Your Sport* section in each chapter of this book for references to Web sites for that sport.

Local resources To track down local groups, try these tips:

* Contact your town's chamber of commerce for referrals to organizations that coordinate events, leagues, or lessons in your area.
* Contact your local department of parks and recreation to inquire where the sport is played locally. Ask for the names of organizations that conduct local events and training.
* Post a sign on the bulletin board at the library, coffee shop, or grocery store to find neighbors who participate in the sport.

A good find Once you've found local contacts in your activity, evaluate them for quality. On Web sites, look for a link with a name like "About us" (it may not appear on the top or side of the page but only in the links on the bottom). Read the description of the group to see what affiliations it has, how large it is, how long it has existed, and, if you're lucky, a description of the group's philosophy or sponsorship. If you can't find this information easily, click around the site to get an idea of the position the group takes and the scope of its work. Also, enter the name in a search engine to see what others say about the group.

When you're confident that you've found a reputable sports group, contact them for help finding quality instruction and play opportunities in your area. Request advice in evaluating a program, what its standard parameters in instruction are, and what its average fees are. Also, ask if there is official certification for instructors as a qualification that you can look for when choosing a coach.

Now that you've amassed the information, ask your local contacts for suggestions about instructors, teams, or leagues. If possible, go watch them in action. Next, request a conversation with the instructors. Ask how they structure lessons for beginners, including the schedule and costs, what the expected results are, and what the required gear is. If the information seems like a good fit for your temperament and time frame, ask for more details about the logistics, such as a makeup schedule for missed classes and the length of the commitment for courses. Some suggested questions:

* Do you need to join a team for the whole season?
* Is there a minimum number of training sessions you can purchase?
* Are there discounts if you purchase multiple sessions or sign up with a friend?
* Are there refunds if events such as an illness prevent you from completing the term?

Try not to overcommit before you've tested the program. A ten-pack of sessions might represent a great savings, but not if you drop out after going five times. Almost every program will allow you a trial session for a small fee or no charge before you hand over your credit card. Also ask for referrals to other students who have gone through the same program and whom you can interview to learn about the experience, for example, what they like and don't like about it, what they wish they could change, and whether or not they recommend the teaching and motivation methods for beginners. Try to find out where the group goes out to after practice and go talk to them there, when they are relaxed and away from the coaches (plus, you might want to check out the post-play scene to see if you like it).

After all that work, you should know exactly what you're getting yourself into. Sign up, show up, and have fun!

Acknowledgments

This book draws inspiration and information from many years of athletics and journalism, including mentors and coaches too numerous to name. A few who stand out and deserve special mention: My mom, who set a great example as an active woman from my first recollections of fast-paced tennis matches to her 60-something pursuits: in-line skating, kayaking, 30-mile bike rides, toddler chasing, and more. Peg Moline, now the editor-in-chief of *Fit Pregnancy*, who taught me everything I know about fitness writing and editing. Many magazine editors along the way, especially Peggy Northrop, Lucy Danziger, Myrna Blyth, Beth Weinhouse, Ila Stanger, Dana Points, Lauren Purcell, Susan Crandell, Pam O'Brien, Stephanie Young, Carla Levy, Curt Pesmen, Nancy Smith, Alexandra Penney, Anne Alexander, Joanne Chen, and Donna Laurie. My coach Ed Hewitt and teammates from the women's rowing team at Columbia University, for my first real taste of "being an athlete"— the teamwork, the competition, the hard work, and the fun.

From starting gate to finish line, much thanks goes to: Ellie McGrath for making the connection. My editors, Becky Koh at Black Dog & Leventhal, and Annalyn Swan and Peter Bernstein at ASAP Media, for their coaching and cheerleading through the entire endurance event. The inspirational team at Chelsea Piers—Roland Betts, Tom Bernstein, David Tewksbury, Dana Thayer, and Erica Schietinger (this book wouldn't exist without you!) plus all the trainers, experts, and staffers who shared their stories, enthusiasm, and skills. The pinch hitters—Deborah Mead, Lorie Parch, Norma Strothenke, Stephanie Young, Elizabeth McGoldrick, Jo Ziegler, Caroline Afonso, Cris Louzada, and many other friends, relatives, and neighbors. And, of course, my home team and number-one fans, Bruce Strothenke and his little buddy Calvin.

Dedicated to the memory of strength, storytelling, and love
Dr. Robert J. Strothenke
1921-2006

All illustrations by Greg Paprocki

Photography Credits

Index